Dr. Hughes,
Thanks ;
work of interest in this
subject — I think!
— Barb

Elixir:
The American Tragedy
of a Deadly Drug

Barbara J. Martin, MD

3/24/14

ISBN-10: 0615898173
ISBN-13: 978-0615898179
Barkerry Press, Lancaster, PA, USA

DEDICATION

To those for whom death casts a long shadow

CONTENTS

CONTENTS

PREFACE AND ACKNOWLEDGMENTS

Each year, hundreds of thousands of US physicians prescribe antibiotics to about four million children with sore throats. These prescriptions are routinely filled and dutifully administered by mothers and fathers with the full intention of curing strep pharyngitis, an infection of the throat caused by a type of streptococcal bacterium. In the overwhelming majority of cases, the goals of recommending these commercially produced drugs are achieved: suffering is alleviated, no harm is done,[1] and parents successfully navigate another routine job of parenthood. Without much thought, Americans rely on the safety of prescription medications, because experience dictates that *they are generally safe.* Our reassuring history of prescription drug use in this country is largely due to the fact that the US government has established measures to ensure that pharmaceuticals are much more likely to help than to injure before they enter the marketplace.

Seventy-six years ago, Congress passed and President Franklin D. Roosevelt signed the Federal Food, Drug, and Cosmetic Act, which—for the first time in the history of the United States—required drug manufacturers to prove the safety of their products before they are sold. This historic act and important follow-up legislation have protected the American public from an unknowable number of pharmaceutical hazards, some of which would have otherwise been most assuredly fatal. We know this to be true, because we know what prompted passage of the drug law in 1938: the entirely preventable deaths of more than 100 Americans—many of whom were children—by a poisonous antibiotic solution, Elixir Sulfanilamide.

Elixir is the first comprehensive narrative of the deaths caused by Elixir Sulfanilamide and the myriad reactions to the fatal poisonings—from consumers, relatives of the victims, the drug manufacturer and his chief chemist, prescribing physicians, the wider medical community, the Food and Drug Administration (FDA), Congress, the White House, attorneys, and the media. My chief reasons for writing *Elixir*, the research for which began more than 10 years ago, were to understand how this event could have happened, how it unfolded, people's reactions to inadvertently doing harm, and efforts to prevent similar episodes. Another motive for writing *Elixir* was to understand, if possible, how similar drug-related poisonings have continued to occur throughout the world, specifically in developing countries where legislative safeguards against dangerous pharmaceuticals are limited or nonexistent.

My interest in Elixir Sulfanilamide began, logically enough, with my first knowledge of the product. In 2001, 15 years after I obtained my medical degree, I learned of the scores of deaths in the United States caused by this antibiotic solution, which was manufactured by The S. E. Massengill Company of Bristol, Tennessee, in 1937. I was informed of the event while taking a class in pharmaceutical regulation at the Kellogg School of Management at Northwestern University in Evanston, Illinois. The professor, Dr. Edward F. X. Hughes, mentioned the incident in a discussion of the history of drug regulation in the United States, and he revealed that the tragedy prompted the passage of the landmark law. As a physician, I was vaguely aware of the Food, Drug, and Cosmetic Act before taking the class, but I had not heard of the inciting disaster. I was immediately hooked by the story of deaths due to what should have been a lifesaving, innovative antibiotic. I soon found, however, that there were few reliable details in accessible sources. Thus began an enduring and meandering quest, spanning more than a decade, to discover what I could about Elixir Sulfanilamide, how it was created, how it was distributed, its effects on consumers, and its aftermath. Consequently it can be said, without exaggeration, that Dr. Hughes—unbeknownst to him until recently—is responsible for the origins of this book.

For reasons that I have trouble explaining to any rational degree, I thereafter began collecting, in fits and starts, numerous records pertaining to Elixir Sulfanilamide. My collection began mostly with government records. Crucial among these primary sources were those cited by medical historian James Harvey Young in his descriptive essay of the event, "Sulfanilamide and Diethylene Glycol," which was published in 1983.[2] This article was and remains, in my mind, the definitive synopsis of the tragedy. Young, best known for his book-length examinations of American medical quackery, cited in his essay various letters and other correspondence of the FDA, which were housed at the National Archives and Records Administration (NARA). These citations ultimately prompted me to visit the NARA facilities in College Park, Maryland, to view the voluminous files. Later I sought additional, supportive documents directly from the historical files (AF1258) of the FDA in Rockville, Maryland. For anyone interested in researching the Elixir Sulfanilamide tragedy of 1937, these sources represent an indispensable beginning. Although I provide a warning: The government records concerning Elixir Sulfanilamide are loosely organized and, despite their scope, hardly offer a cohesive story. To begin to craft the tale of Elixir Sulfanilamide into something resembling a linear narrative, it became necessary to collate and organize these vast official documents into some kind of sensible order. On more than one occasion, I swore that the job was impossible, if not futile. Nevertheless the government records on the Elixir Sulfanilamide tragedy are the foundation of any accurate account of the event.

My first goal was to identify the victims of Elixir Sulfanilamide, people who remained largely nameless in secondary accounts of the tragedy (including Young's article). Publicly accessible NARA and FDA records—which offer the victims' names, ages, race, locations, prescribing doctors, and relevant medical histories—enabled the construction of a detailed tally of the dead. Biographical information about these individuals was reliably supplemented and cross-checked with other primary sources, like census records and death certificates (the latter, when available by state regulations). In addition, contemporaneous news accounts of the deaths, either in the form of investigative reports or obituaries in local newspapers, complemented my research. In some cases, primary and secondary sources allowed for the identification of several living relatives of the victims, who were then contacted by phone or email for any additional information that might have been handed down within the family.

Similar investigations were used to obtain biographical information about other major actors in the Elixir Sulfanilamide story—including notable FDA staff, physicians who prescribed or investigated the deadly concoction, and key personnel of the Massengill company, the elixir's manufacturer. Likewise genealogical and web-based sleuthing allowed for the identification of living relatives of these individuals in several cases, and many of these people offered important biographical details. Colorful profiles of FDA agents and their involvement with Elixir Sulfanilamide were also occasionally found in the FDA's Oral History Transcripts (available at http://www.fda.gov/AboutFDA/WhatWeDo/History/OralHistories/SelectedOralHistoryTranscripts/default.htm), the agency's compilation of lengthy interviews with its retired personnel, which began in the 1960s. Descriptions of FDA field staff and their investigations were likewise supplemented by agents' reminiscences in periodicals such as the *Food, Drug, Cosmetic Law Quarterly* and the *Food, Drug, Cosmetic Law Journal*. Although the dating of these recollections, acquired some 20 to 30 years after the event, undercuts their complete accuracy—especially when compared with primary, contemporaneous government sources.

The foundation for essential information about the Massengill company; its president, Dr. Samuel Evans Massengill; the firm's general counsel, Frank W. DeFriece, Sr.; and chemist Harold Cole Watkins was the company's own comprehensive publication of its history, *Masengil Brothers and The S. E. Massengill Company, 1897-1971* (Knoxville, TN: Tennessee Valley Publishing; 1996).[3] Products offered by the Massengill company in the 1930s were found in the firm's catalogs. Further background about chemist Watkins was located by the Bethel Historical Society in Maine and also offered by Watkins's grand-nephew, Professor David C. Larsen (whom I was able to identify and locate through genealogical records and a circuitous web search). Of note, Dr. Larsen graciously met with me and shared rare photographs of the man who was responsible for creating Elixir Sulfanilamide. On request, the librarian of the Waterville Senior High School in Waterville, Maine, Julie Letourneau Ayers, dug up a senior portrait of Watkins with exceptional alacrity.

Over the years, various staff of local historical societies—notably the Tulsa Historical Society and the Mississippi Historical Society—located regional news coverage of the tragedy. The Tulsa County Medical Society provided the all-important minutes of the organization's contemporaneous investigation of the herald deaths due to Elixir Sulfanilamide in the city. The NARA records on Elixir Sulfanilamide contain files of many newspaper clippings related to the poisonings, and these were supplemented with other articles acquired through online sources, such as NewspaperARCHIVE.com, Google News Archives (now defunct, sadly), and ProQuest—the last of which was accessed online through membership to my excellent local library, the Evanston Public Library. Notably Evanston librarian Kathleen Lanigan cheerily retrieved numerous paper and electronic articles from dated and sometimes obsolete periodicals (including drug-trade periodicals) in response to my many, many interlibrary-loan requests. Throughout my life, particularly my academic life, I have met my share of librarians, some of whom were reasonably helpful and some of whom were downright obstructive. On my list of the best, Ms. Lanigan sits at the top.

Medical articles, specifically those contained in the *Journal of the American Medical Association* (*JAMA*), were acquired either at the University of Chicago's John Crerar Library or the Library of the Health Sciences at the University of Illinois at Chicago. Both of these libraries house expansive and important collections of historical medical journals, and they continue to allow crucial public access to them, in contradistinction to other academic libraries within the Chicago area. Very notably, the archives staff at the American Medical Association (AMA) responded that the organization did not have historical records pertaining to Elixir Sulfanilamide, outside of what was published in *JAMA*; although the Chicago-based medical group, and specifically the journal's editor-in-chief at the time, Morris Fishbein, were instrumental in the timely investigation of the poisonous compound. A clue to the fate of any internal AMA records on the Elixir Sulfanilamide tragedy is found in the FDA's Oral History Transcript of an interview with Dr. Fishbein. When questioned in 1968 about the event, Fishbein responded, "You should really go to the AMA to chase that up in the files. I think unfortunately they've destroyed a lot of files. I tried to look up something the other day, and they said, 'That's all gone. We don't have that anymore.'"[1] Contemporaneous information on Elixir Sulfanilamide was also surprisingly absent from the *New England Journal of Medicine* (save for a dedicated editorial and several, later passing mentions of the product). Perhaps in 1937 the journal had not yet established itself as a national, authoritative clinical periodical, which it is today. Alternatively the editorial staff may have maintained geographically narrow views of American medical practice and related news items, the coverage of which was confined at the time to the medical mecca of Boston specifically and the Northeast generally. An important reference for the development of sulfanilamide, the world's first widely distributed antibiotic, was John E. Lesch's comprehensive *The First Miracle Drugs: How the Sulfa Drugs Transformed Medicine* (New York, NY: Oxford University Press; 2007).

Essential history of landmark US drug laws in the early 20th century was largely derived from Charles O. Jackson's definitive *Food and Drug Legislation in the New Deal* (Princeton, NJ: Princeton University Press; 1970). The discussion of drug regulation in *Elixir*, while supplemented by sources other than Jackson's book (including news coverage of congressional activities), is admittedly derivative of this work. Jackson's book is generally considered required reading for all scholars of drug regulation in the United States. Legal records pertaining to Elixir Sulfanilamide were obtained through the Atlanta archives division of NARA, and thanks are given to Mary A. Martin for reading and interpreting selected court documents and providing general legal guidance. Important counsel, particularly on issues of privacy and copyright in the United States, was also provided by Pete Sahu. Useful information regarding copyright law in the United States, the definition of public domain, and interpretations of fair use were derived from several online sources, including the very user-friendly general-information website Public Domain Sherpa (www.publicdomainsherpa.com). Links available through the "US Catalog of Copyright Entries (Renewals)," at www.ibiblio.org/ccer/, and "The Online Books Page," at digital.library.upenn.edu/books/cce/, were indispensable for investigating the copyright status of specific books, periodicals, newspapers, and images.

The research for *Elixir*, the organization of sources, and the writing came sporadically, and I shelved the project more than once. The unanticipated result of my procrastination was an increasing access to any number of online sources, thanks to an explosion of digitized public records, government documents, newspapers, periodicals, and books within the last decade. Google Books and Internet Archive, in particular, have provided an unprecedented and growing access to any number of newly searchable public-domain works, which otherwise would have remained secreted in musty back corners of libraries. The phenomenon of digitization has allowed for the discovery of innumerable bits and pieces of the *Elixir* story. Separately these details might appear trivial, but together they add depth and color to the narrative and its main actors. I can only expect that continued access to even more digitized sources (including government documents), long after *Elixir* is published, will disclose further facts of the story, providing a wider picture of the tragedy. It is likely that these details will subtly change our understanding of the event, but some may dramatically alter or even upend my attempted historical record. As with any writer's attempt to document a historical event, any errors of omission, misconception, or misinterpretation are mine.

The beginnings of *Elixir* began with a detailed cataloging of the victims at my blog Pathophilia (see http://bmartinmd.com/elixir-sulfanilamide-deaths.html). The effort was and is intended to be a memorial to those who died as a result of the catastrophe and an homage to those who attempted to avert further disaster—like the scores of FDA men who confiscated the elixir in an age when mass communication was limited. The online identification of the victims was also meant to encourage living family members to come forward and provide personal stories of the event. In a few cases, the website enabled contact with victims' relatives, and their stories revealed tremendous family heartbreak.[5]

In 2008, I was motivated to begin writing *Elixir* in earnest, after news of a mass poisoning in Nigeria, which was due to a similar contamination of a liquid medication. Repeated incidents of injury and death as a result of tainted medicinal products, extending well into the 21st century, highlight the importance of revisiting this dark episode of American history. The *Elixir* narrative itself is admittedly wide in scope and shallow in depth, the necessary consequence of attempting to construct a story that involved hundreds of individuals across the United States. Opportunities remain for others to dive deeper into the personal stories of, specifically, the victims of Elixir Sulfanilamide.

My enduring thanks go to my immediate family for reading and providing essential criticism on *Elixir*: Maria Finitzo and Dr. Kerry T. Givens also provided much-needed encouragement. In addition to his feedback on the structure of the narrative, Dr. Givens provided his all-important perspective on medical terminology and facts. The necessary steps of publication, a potentially daunting process for any author (especially the author of a nonfiction work), could not have been negotiated without the sage advice of publishing expert Holly Brady.

The story of Elixir Sulfanilamide is one of hapless victims, government heroes, and exceedingly flawed men—the most prominent of which have been condemned by their neglect, ignorance, and denial—not their malice. *Elixir* is not meant to embarrass, chastise, or otherwise discomfit the descendants of those who were directly responsible for the deadly product. Specifically it is not my goal, to paraphrase Ezekiel (18:20), that the progeny bear any punishment for their forebears' transgressions. *Elixir* is not an accusation, but a morality tale: Our responses to inadvertently doing harm expose our moral core and dictate how we will be remembered.

—Barbara J. Martin, MD

1
AT LEAST SIX DEATHS IN TULSA

Saturday, October 9, 1937: A group of worried physicians telegraphed the editor-in-chief of a premier medical journal.

> ATTENTION IS CALLED TO AT LEAST SIX DEATHS IN TULSA
> FOLLOWING ADMINISTRATION OF ELIXIR OF SULFANILAMIDE
> SYMPTOMS OF ANURIA AND TOXIC DEGENERATION OF LIVER AND
> KIDNEYS[1]

The weekend dispatch stressed the urgency. The required brevity minimized the tragedy. In a span of 10 days, six young children had died in the Oklahoma oil town, and its leading physicians wanted answers and guidance from Dr. Morris Fishbein, editor-in-chief of *JAMA* and arguably the most influential physician in America. But instead of a sage reply from the revered and in-demand Fishbein, the doctors received prompt word from Dr. Paul Nicholas Leech.[2] As secretary of the AMA's Council on Pharmacy and Chemistry, Leech immediately wired back,

> YOUR TELEGRAM WILL BE BROUGHT TO DR FISHBEINS ATTENTION
> ON HIS RETURN THURSDAY STOP IN MEANTIME WOULD
> APPRECIATE RECEIVING FULL DETAILS CONCERNING DEATHS IF
> THIS OFFICE CAN AID YOU FURTHER PLEASE ADVISE

Telegraphy was the most rational way in 1937 to send an urgent message long distance. For 75 years, Americans had transmitted countless mundane, newsworthy, or even historic notes from coast to coast at relatively economy, especially when compared with the high cost of new long-distance telephone services. Telegrams had clarified business deals, announced personal successes ("DEAR MOTHER AND DAD GRADUATED OK"), and declared scientific conquests ("SUCCESS FOUR FLIGHTS THURSDAY MORNING–OREVELLE [sic] WRIGHT"). But wiring "full details" of the Oklahoma deaths to the AMA in Chicago, typically via Western Union, was problematic if not hazardous. Because telegram charges were based on letter counts, affordable dispatches had to be distilled to their essence and written in intuitively read sentences, without the use of costly punctuation. The rule accounted for the quaint use of "STOP" and "COMMA." Condensing the elements of six fatalities, complete with the appropriate medical jargon, was sufficiently challenging for the alerting physicians; but it was also risky given the series of unknowns. What if a cohesive or enlightening fact was omitted in the transmission for help? Here were the details, as they were known locally.

The first death was that of two-year-old Robert "Bobbie" Sumner, who succumbed at his aunt's home on Thursday, September 30th.[3] He had received less than three tablespoons of a bright-red liquid antibiotic, sulfanilamide, as treatment for a sore throat. Five days after beginning the medication, Bobbie stopped producing urine, a condition known medically as anuria. A kidney specialist was summoned. The boy was vomiting and feverish. His face was swollen, his abdomen was distended, and what little urine he passed was bloody. The veteran doctor was stumped. The child's apparent nephritis, or kidney inflammation, was different than any he had ever seen. He certainly knew that acute nephritis was an occasional consequence of scarlet fever, a system-wide disease caused by a type of *Streptococcus* bacterium, the same bug that causes "strep throat." However, scarlet fever produced a distinctive rash, and the nephritis, when it occurred, typically arose two or three weeks after the seminal infection, not in a matter of days.[4] The boy's fatal illness had lasted less than a week.

The day after Bobbie Sumner died, an 11-month-old girl and an eight-year-old boy expired, both at St. John's Hospital, one of two major inpatient facilities in Tulsa. Six days earlier, on September 25th, Mary Earline Watters, the infant girl, was diagnosed with strep throat by her physician, David Underwood. As he had done for Bobbie Sumner, Dr. Underwood prescribed a liquid preparation of sulfanilamide for the child's infection. Her condition deteriorated quickly. Two days after starting the treatment, she repeatedly vomited the medicine and struggled to breathe. Four days after starting the treatment, she stopped producing urine. Her parents rushed her to the hospital, where she was placed in an oxygen tent and given unspecified injections. A heroic, but futile, effort was made to transfuse her blood. (Dialysis, an artificial method of filtering the blood in cases of kidney failure, would not be performed in the United States until

1948.)[5] On the girl's death certificate, Dr. Underwood wrote the cause of death: "streptococcus nephritis." It was presumed that the antibiotic had been ineffective against Mary Earline's infection.[6]

Eight-year-old John "Jack" King, Jr., was glad to see his parents drive by as he walked home from school on Thursday, September 23rd. The boy felt so sick, he told his mother, that he wasn't sure how he was going to make it back to the house by himself. Once at home, Jack's parents quickly telephoned their pediatrician, Dr. Killis Reese, who prescribed a sulfanilamide elixir. During the course of a week, the boy drank about half of the medicine, roughly three tablespoons.[7] On October 1st, Dr. Reese recorded Jack's official causes of death as influenza and acute hemorrhagic nephritis.

And then there were three more dead children in Tulsa to describe to the AMA. Five-year-old Millard "Sonny" Wakeford and his younger sister had contracted sore throats. On Sunday, September 26th, Dr. Underwood wrote a prescription for the Wakeford children: "El Sulfanilamide," he scrawled. It was the third prescription for the liquid antibiotic he had written in two days. Sonny and his sister were each to take a teaspoonful five times a day. During the next few days, both children developed anuria and were hospitalized at St. John's. Sonny died on Monday, October 4th, exactly six weeks before his sixth birthday and eight days after beginning the treatment. Like in the case of the Watters girl, Dr. Underwood ascribed Sonny's death to streptococcal nephritis. Sonny's younger sister, however, slowly recovered.[8]

Another Tulsa physician, Dr. Logan Spann, also prescribed the liquid sulfanilamide on September 26th. His patient, six-year-old Joan Marlar, like the other children, was suspected to have strep throat. The otherwise hearty girl drank a total of about three tablespoons of the elixir. Joan's mother and older sister witnessed her progressive torment. During the course of nine days, Joan, anuric and semi-conscious, writhed with abdominal and flank pain.[9] She finally died at Tulsa's Morningside Hospital on Tuesday, October 5th. Her death was officially attributed to streptococcal nephritis.

And then Jack King's pediatrician, Dr. Reese, wrote another prescription for "Elixir Sulfanilamide," this time on Monday, September 27th. The patient was six-year-old Michael Sheehan, who also had a sore throat. Michael, an only child and a "strong, healthy boy," took all but one teaspoon of the four-ounce treatment and developed anuria. He expired on October 6th, nine days after beginning the therapy. He became the fourth child to die at St. John's Hospital under troubling circumstances.

In responding to the AMA, Dr. James Stevenson, president of the Tulsa County Medical Society, volleyed back only the most salient information about the children's deaths. On Sunday, October 10th, his follow-up wire highlighted the branded treatment and the most overt, deadly symptoms.

ELIXIR SULFANILAMIDE MASSENGILL THERAPY MANY CASES COMPLETE ANURIA WITH UREMIA TULSA COUNTY MEDICAL SOCIETY MEETS MONDAY NIGHT DESIRE ALL POSSIBLE INFORMATION AT ONCE WIRE OR PHONE ME MY EXPENSE

Stevenson did not write his response unilaterally. He had essential input from his physician colleagues and perhaps inadvertent assistance from a couple of motivated bystanders. As early as Thursday morning, October 7th, the day after the Sheehan boy died, rumors of the pediatric fatalities began spreading throughout Tulsa's medical community. By the end of the day, the gossip was heard from "every physician's lips" in the city.[10] Eager for more information, two representatives from New York drug firms, specifically one from E. R. Squibb and Sons and one from Winthrop Chemical Company, colluded to "get to the real truth of the matter." Dividing the hospitals between them, the two men learned that, in each case, the treating doctor had prescribed Elixir Sulfanilamide made by The S. E. Massengill Company. The Squibb rep went so far as to ship a sample of the product, which he had purchased directly from a local drug store, to his company's New York headquarters for analysis.[11]

The deaths were also keenly noticed by St. John's pathologist, 43-year-old Ivo Nelson. Nelson, a close friend of the elixir-prescribing Dr. Reese, suspected that the fatalities were not the result of streptococcal disease, as the pediatrician had officially recorded. Instead Nelson sensed that they were cases of poisoning. He first entertained the possibility of mercury toxicity. The element continued to exist in some medicinal preparations in the 1930s, particularly those intended for the treatment of syphilis. Acute, fatal kidney failure caused by mercury bichloride was well documented, and other clinical features of the Tulsa cases, like repeated vomiting, were consistent with the diagnosis.[12] But Nelson needed more information to confirm his suspicions.

Teaming up with a St. John's internist, Homer Ruprecht, Nelson catalyzed the systematic medical investigation of the six deaths in Tulsa. The two doctors, at least from a superficial perspective, were an unlikely pair.[13] Nelson, despite being of Swedish heritage, had dark features: olive skin, black hair, and dark-brown eyes. Five feet, six inches in height, Nelson was diminutive in physical stature only. He was often opinionated and brash, traits accented by a perpetually cocked head and an ever-present pipe in his mouth. The 37-year-old Ruprecht, on the other hand, was tall, affable, and quietly confident. And Ruprecht, unlike the typical pathologist, enjoyed interacting with living patients. Yet both men were intensely curious, pragmatic, and eager to argue their points on any number of medical topics, primarily because they made sure they knew their facts.

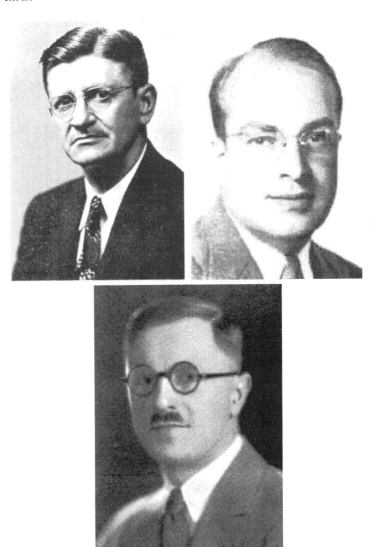

Top left, Ivo Nelson, MD, c1946; Top right, Homer Ruprecht, MD, c1944; Bottom, James Stevenson, MD, c1936 (All courtesy of the Tulsa County Medical Society)

Drs. Nelson and Ruprecht began to gather evidence to support their hypothesis that poison, not streptococcal disease, had caused the deaths of the Tulsa children. Nelson prepared to examine the bodies of the deceased, specifically those of 11-month-old Mary Earline Watters and six-year-old Michael Sheehan, both of whom had died at St. John's. Ruprecht interviewed the victims' parents, and the antibiotic elixir was found to be at least one consistent thread, confirming the drug reps' hasty probe. It was also learned that more prescriptions for the possibly poisonous medication had been written. Dr. Reese admitted that he had recommended the elixir to eight-year-old John "Jack" Voorhees on September 27th, and Dr. Underwood had prescribed the drug as recently as October 4th, the day that Sonny Wakeford died, to four-year-old Charlene Canady. If the medication was the deadly culprit, the children's lives were potentially in danger. It appeared that the Voorhees boy was already desperately ill.[14]

Certainly developing circumstances suggested that more subjects for Nelson's postmortem examination were possible. Three other Tulsa physicians had also prescribed the elixir, it was learned, each for a single patient. On the day that the Watters girl and Jack King died, October 1st, eight-year-old Kathleen Hobson began taking the liquid antibiotic for a cold and sore throat. According to family history, the girl hated the taste of the medicine so much that her mother and older sister had to hold her down to deliver the therapy.[15] The family struggle continued for three days as Kathleen's condition deteriorated. Like six-year-old Joan Marlar, Kathleen was admitted to Morningside Hospital with anuria. She died on Saturday, October 9th, the day that Tulsa physicians first wired the AMA. It was also the day that another suspect death occurred in the city: that of 20-year-old Glen Entler. Entler was one of two young men in Tulsa who had received the antibiotic solution for an entirely different indication: gonorrhea.

* * * * * *

The fact that the Tulsa physicians contacted the AMA and specifically Morris Fishbein in the immediate wake of the deaths underscores the historical importance of the medical association and that of *JAMA*'s editor-in-chief as premier guides for clinical practice and legitimate drug use in the United States—especially in contradistinction to the FDA or any other government agency in existence at the time.[16] Although he wasn't president of the AMA, the 48-year-old Fishbein was the de facto mouthpiece for the organization. Revered nationally for more than a decade, Fishbein had provided chief editorial services for *JAMA* since 1924, as well as for several other medical journals.[17] As such, he became the spokesperson for the nation's physicians and a popular go-to source for medical guidance. A graduate of the University of Chicago and Rush Medical College (also in Chicago), Fishbein was known for his militant quackbusting and his paternal relationship with the American public. He frequently wrote articles on sensible foods and common infectious diseases (like typhoid, diphtheria, and polio) for *The Saturday Evening Post, Good Housekeeping,* and *Reader's Digest,* and his regular, syndicated newspaper columns featured reassuring and friendly titles like "The Truth About Diet," "Your Baby's Health," and "The Family Doctor." Just four months earlier, Fishbein's status as a national medical authority had been sanctioned by *Time* magazine in a cover feature of the doctor. The article, which discussed the prospect of nationalized medicine, described the personification of the AMA:

[I]t is the worldly, alert Dr. Morris Fishbein who writes 15,000 words a week, makes 130 speeches a year, edits the A. M. A. *Journal* and *Hygeia,* manages nine A. M. A. special journals, is publishing a book *Syphilis* next month, is finishing *Diet & Health* and *Curiosities of Medicine* for publication this autumn. He syndicates a health column to 700 newspapers.[18]

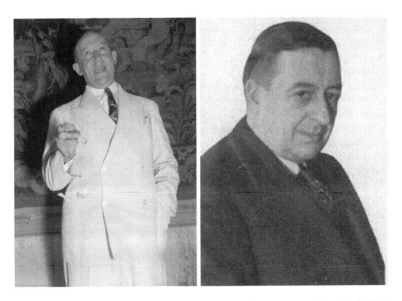

Left, Morris Fishbein, MD, c1938 (Library of Congress, Harris & Ewing Collection); Right, Paul Nicholas Leech, PhD, date unknown (*Chemical Bulletin.* 1941;28[3]:68)

To add to its national credibility, independent of Fishbein, the AMA provided important medical oversight to the nation's physicians through its Council on Pharmacy and Chemistry. An AMA subdivision, the Council was created in 1905 to examine the composition of industry-submitted pharmaceutical products for sale in the United States.[19] The Council was intended to supplement or supplant information from the decades-old US Pharmacopeia, a voluntary nongovernmental organization that produced standards for pharmaceuticals and published a national formulary roughly once every 10 years. From 1820 to 1905, the US Pharmacopeia had revised its formulary only eight times and was evidently ill-equipped to keep up with the exploding list of nostrums and more legitimate remedies that were being churned out at the beginning of the 20th century.[20] The AMA Council's raison d'être was to "list the new preparations, describe their actions and uses, denounce those that are clearly bogus, and place reliable information about them in the hands of every practitioner."[21] Assessments were regularly published in issues of *JAMA* and compiled in serial book form (*New and Non-Official Remedies*). The Council was "inclined to take the position that the approximate value of a new drug should be determined exhaustively, on patients as well as animals, before it is advertised to the profession." In the absence of federal legislation that required proof of the safety or efficacy of pharmaceutical products, the Council became the leading authority to review and endorse (or reject) commercially available medicines that were voluntarily submitted for inclusion in its widely read drug compendium. Consequently Leech, who was appointed secretary of the Council in 1932, was naturally and appropriately interested in the Tulsa dispatches. He responded, again immediately, to Dr. Stevenson's follow-up wire. The Council, Leech reported, had not examined any such antibiotic elixir.

NO PRODUCT MASSENGILL COMPANY ACCEPTED BY COUNCIL ON PHARMACY AND CHEMISTRY STOP SULFANILAMIDE IN ELIXIRS NOT RECOMMENDED STOP PHYSICIANS WOULD DO WELL TO USE ONLY ACCEPTED BRANDS AND DOSAGE FORMS STOP SEE EDITORIAL IN JOURNAL OCTOBER SECOND COMMA TEN ARTICLES IN JOURNAL SEPTEMBER TWENTY FIFTH AND COUNCIL REPORTS IN JOURNAL MAY TWENTY NINTH AND JULY THIRTY FIRST

Leech's wire referred the Tulsa physicians to a *JAMA* editorial that had been published just eight days earlier. Although the editorial acknowledged that the antibiotic sulfanilamide was "truly remarkable," indiscriminate use was discouraged. Drug-related toxicities—namely dermatitis (skin inflammation), photosensitization (skin sensitivity to light), agranulocytosis (a deficiency of white blood cells due to bone-marrow suppression), and sulfmethemoglobinemia (a cyanosis-producing blood disorder)—had been observed. Some cases of self-medication without a doctor's prescription—a potentially dangerous, but legal, practice in 1937— had necessitated hospitalization. The editorial admonished, "Responsibility lies considerably with pharmacists who are willing to sell dangerous drugs to anybody over the counter."[22] Warnings were also applied to use of the antibiotic with other drugs "until definite information is available as to toxic effects." Although the concurrent administration of sodium bicarbonate with sulfanilamide was apparently harmless, mixing the antibiotic with other sulfur-containing drugs, like magnesium sulfate (ie, Epsom salts), was ill-advised.

Leech also directed the doctors to a lengthy series of reports describing sulfanilamide's adverse effects in the September 25th issue of *JAMA*.[23] Likewise the Council had submitted its review of the antibiotic, related compounds, and proprietary US formulations in the May and July issues of the medical journal.[24] The reviewed drugs included sulfanilamide preparations from the major American pharmaceutical firms of Eli Lilly, Merck, Parke Davis, E. R. Squibb and Sons, and Winthrop Chemical (the latter two firms being the companies that employed the inquisitive drug reps in Tulsa). The preparations were in powder or tablet forms; no orally administered solution existed. The Council advised that the drug had "the apparent disadvantage of being relatively insoluble" and a tendency to crystallize out of solution.

2
THE BEST THING EVER DISCOVERED FOR GONORRHEA

Sulfanilamide, the first widely available antibiotic, was the revolutionary product of a revolutionary method for finding therapeutic drugs.[1] Its discovery in the 1930s, albeit in a circuitous route, validated the resolute commitment of the German chemical industry to systematically create, test, and sell drugs for human disease. It was the decades-long culmination of several, converging factors at the turn of the century in Western Europe, the most pressing of which was the need for product diversification in a market flooded with synthetic dyes. This mammoth industry, a prototype of the Industrial Revolution, was based on the production of stains from chemicals found in the abundant waste of coal tar, and the market for manmade pigments in the late 19th century was bloated and stagnant.[2] Sulfanilamide was also the indirect byproduct of a radical scientific breakthrough: the newly adopted germ theory, the idea that microscopic organisms can cause disease. To entrepreneurial dye chemists, and specifically those employed by the German dye conglomerate I. G. Farben,[3] the logical offspring of this theory was that dye-related chemicals—some of which had been found to adhere to and stain bacteria—might kill disease-causing germs without harming their human host.

The commercial strategy of I. G. Farben and specifically that of its subsidiary, Farbenfabriken Bayer (literally Dye Factory Bayer), the forerunner of Bayer Pharmaceuticals, was to repurpose its chemical assets through an "industrialized system of invention." This phrase, as it has been used by medical historian John Lesch, describes a systematic method for discovering and marketing products—specifically in the case of Bayer, therapeutic substances.[4] It was a fresh business model for dye and chemical companies, and it remains, more or less, the foundation of the pharmaceutical industry more than a century later. In the 1880s, Bayer executives made a conscious decision to expand and reapply their product base by investing the necessary capital and embracing the scientific methods of rational drug discovery. Bayer leaders Carl Duisberg and, later, Heinrich Hörlein, both of whom were academically trained bench-chemists, promoted the wide expansion of Bayer's laboratory and research facilities; the aggressive recruitment of university-trained chemists and physicians; the maintenance and cultivation of ties to independent academic centers; and the acceptance of experimental pharmacology—that is, the systematic testing of chemicals in animals and humans. The use of animal models of disease, and specifically animal models of infection, was embraced and considered essential to the scientific method. Experimental results in animals could support not only the efficacy, but the safety, of a therapeutic compound before its entry into the marketplace. These sizable acts, undertaken and fine-tuned over the course of roughly 50 years, were predicated on the hope that Bayer's vast supply of dye chemicals and any of their derivatives might yield safe drugs that had meaningful clinical benefits.

However, to imply that Bayer's transformation from a dye and chemical company to a pharmaceutical firm was based solely on economic desperation and a merely hypothetical ideal of medical treatment is misleading. There were concrete examples of chemicals, including those derived from coal tar and coal-tar dyes, that were found to be medically useful in the second half of the 19th century. Moreover some were commercial hits. In the 1860s, famed British surgeon Joseph Lister began using carbolic acid (phenol), a basic organic compound derived from coal tar, as a highly effective antiseptic for traumatic wounds.[5] Twenty years later, German chemists exploited the compound aniline, a component of coal tar and the basis for a series of commercially successful dyes. The general motive was to synthesize an artificial form of quinine, a natural and expensive extraction from the Peruvian cinchona bark and the most effective treatment for malarial fever at the time.[6] In 1883, German chemist Ludwig Knorr patented Antipyrine, which he synthesized from an aniline derivative. Although the compound had little activity against malarial parasites, it was successfully marketed by the dye company Meister Lucius and Brüning AG (the forerunner of Höchst)[7] as an effective antipyretic, or fever-reducing, medication.[8] In 1886, acetanilide, a compound also created from aniline, was likewise shown to reduce fever, and its relative safety was shown in rabbits and dogs.[9] The substance was then sold as an antipyretic by a competing dye firm, Kalle and Company, under the trade name Antifebrin. Sales of the brand-name compound (over the generic and less-easily pronounced acetanilide) were largely responsible for the company's dazzling growth. The success of Antifebrin prompted Bayer's Duisberg, newly promoted in the 1880s to supervise the company's research and patenting division, to enter the antipyretic market with a novel compound. He challenged Bayer's chemists to produce a similar fever-busting drug from the company's accumulated barrels of coal-tar waste. Two short years later, Duisberg had overseen the creation, testing, and marketing of Bayer's first synthetic trade-name drug, Phenacetin (generic name, acetophenetidin), and the company was able to exploit Europe's influenza epidemic of 1889-1892 by selling the product—which was more expensive, but better tolerated, than Antifebrin. By 1900, standard operating procedure at Bayer dictated routine analysis of all chemicals, dye or otherwise, for pharmaceutical properties.[10]

These early dye-related compounds were proofs of concept—sort of. Although medically useful for reducing the fever of infectious diseases and highly profitable as branded drugs, they did not eradicate disease. It was not until 1891, when preliminary, but tangible, results suggested that microbe-staining synthetic dyes had direct germicidal effects and might cure infections. German chemist Paul Ehrlich was the most visible champion of a "magic bullet" chemical therapy (or "chemotherapy") against infectious disease, and he demonstrated modest success with the coal-tar dye methylene blue in two patients with malaria.[11] Ehrlich's promising case studies, in which methylene blue exerted little toxic effect against his human subjects (despite coloring the urine green), motivated the government scientist to test a multitude of synthetic dyes, as well as non-dye chemicals, in animal models of several infections.

Ehrlich ultimately turned his attention to syphilis, after the cause of the venereal scourge, *Treponema pallidum*, was confirmed in 1905. He tested a number of arsenic-based compounds in animals injected with the causative spirochete. After several years of collaborative work, he realized a historic triumph with the synthetic compound arsphenamine in a rabbit model of syphilis. Once the drug's efficacy and modest safety were established in animals, arsphenamine was shown to eradicate the disease—albeit at the significant cost of arsenic-related side effects—in infected patients. Arsphenamine's relative success in humans triggered an unprecedented demand for the compound, and it was profitably marketed by Höchst under the trade name Salvarsan ("the arsenic that saves"). Thus, although the first chemically synthesized antimicrobial drug was not a dye derivative, arsphenamine was the first drug to fulfill the promise of rational drug discovery in infectious disease: from chemical creation to serial testing in animals to human use. The wild success of Salvarsan and that of a better-tolerated follow-up drug, Neosalvarsan, fueled the commercial search for other antimicrobial agents.

While straddling the dye and drug industries in the early 1900s, Bayer developed azo dyes—coal-tar derivatives into which a new chemical group, a sulfur-containing amide, was incorporated.[12] This chemical attachment made the azo dye more lightfast, because it conferred a stronger affinity for fabric proteins. Emulating Ehrlich, Bayer scientists reasoned that azo dyes would also readily fix to bacterial proteins and thereby halt bacterial growth and possibly cure infections. In the late 1920s, Bayer's Hörlein and a newly hired physician-scientist, Gerhard Domagk, were motivated by data showing that these azo dyes had some antibacterial properties, at least in the laboratory. Domagk was charged with investigating numerous variations of Bayer's sulfur-containing azo dyes in experimental models of infectious disease.

For his bacterial target, Domagk ambitiously chose *Streptococcus pyogenes*, a ubiquitous, spherical bacterium (or coccus) that causes pyogenic (pus-producing) wound infections and a host of other highly communicable diseases, like septic sore throat. In Domagk's time, streptococcal infections were a relentless public-health threat; control was limited to preventive antisepsis and quarantine. To Domagk, a World War I veteran, the torment of streptococcal infection was not an academic abstraction. He had specifically witnessed the gruesome aftermath of festering injuries in a war without antibiosis. First identified in wound pus and named *Streptococcus* in 1868,[13] the bacterium was cultured in pure form 15 years later from patients with erysipelas—a flame-red, infectious swelling of the skin and underlying tissues. In 1884, bacterial isolates from wound infections were labeled *Streptococcus pyogenes*, and by the early 1930s, the bacterial species was confirmed to be the cause of not only erysipelas and wound infections but serious systemic illnesses like scarlet fever and puerperal (childbed) fever.[14] In addition, streptococcal infection was linked to the delayed effects of rheumatic fever and nephritis.

With the incentive to test a number of Bayer's azo dyes,[15] Domagk found a substance in 1932 that showed no antibacterial activity in dish cultures of streptococcus but that exerted dramatic curative powers in streptococcal-laden mice.[16] This compound, which appeared to be safe when given in large doses to mice (and later to rabbits and cats), was a deep-red azo dye branded "Prontosil." Domagk showed that, without Prontosil treatment, his infected mice died within a day or two, their bodily fluids teeming with streptococcus. However, every mouse treated with Prontosil not only survived; they appeared cured of infection.

But before Domagk's remarkable animal data could be published, the interests of Bayer and those of its parent company, I. G. Farben, took precedence. Prontosil, being a corporate product with tremendous therapeutic and therefore commercial potential, required patent protection. On December 25, 1932, the German Patent Office issued its Christmas gifts to Bayer's inventive chemists: patents on Prontosil and several other azo dyes. Yet for unclear reasons the patents were not published until two years later, in January of 1935. One month after that, Domagk's article describing his animal experiments with Prontosil was published. "Ein Beitrag zur Chemotherapie der bakteriellen Infektionen" (A Contribution on the Chemotherapy of Bacterial Infections) appeared in the prominent German medical periodical *Deutsche Medizinische Wochenschrift*, with an unequivocal credit to Domagk's company above the title: "Aus den Forschungslaboratorien der I. G. Farbenindustrie" (from the research laboratories of I. G. Farben).[17] In the article, Domagk offered little to explain Prontosil's mechanism of antibacterial action. He simply observed, "It acts like a real chemotherapy only in living organisms."[18]

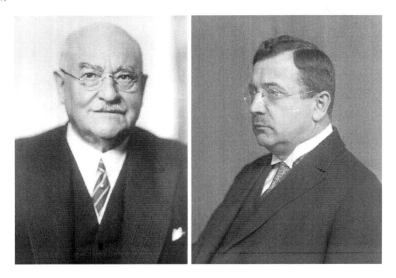

Left, Carl Duisberg, c1931; Right, Heinrich Hörlein, c1928
(Bayer AG/Corporate History and Archives, Leverkusen, Germany)

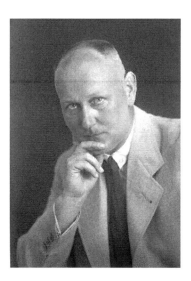

Gerhard Domagk, c1939
(Bayer AG/Corporate History and Archives, Leverkusen, Germany)

The first human test case of Prontosil remains uncertain but
unquestionably occurred before publication of Domagk's landmark article
in 1935. Two years earlier, a Düsseldorf physician publicly presented an
infant's dramatic recovery from a near-fatal case of sepsis after being
treated with Prontosil.[19] Domagk recorded the convalescence of his own
daughter, who developed a raging streptococcal infection after a needle
injury in her hand, with experimental Prontosil therapy.[20] Beyond
individual case reports, German clinicians were able to attest to the drug's
benefits in a range of human streptococcal infections—namely erysipelas,
septic sore throat, and scarlet fever. Promising results were also observed
in infectious complications of childbirth and miscarriage. These varied
case studies, published in the same February 1935 issue as Domagk's
report, described a two-year experience with the drug.[21] Clearly Prontosil
had been given to some German physicians for human trials shortly after
the conferred patent.

Yet Europe's wider medical community did not appear to be fully
aware of the revolutionary compound until Domagk's 1935 publication, at
which time French scientists promptly requested samples of the drug for
testing. When these were not readily forthcoming from Bayer/I. G.
Farben, investigators at the Pasteur Institute in Paris synthesized the dye-
drug themselves, despite French patents that had already been given to
Farben for Prontosil and a number of its chemical derivatives.[22] (The
Pasteur scientists circumvented French patent law, because medicinal
products in France were exempted from patent protection.) Shortly after

creating several Prontosil analogs, the French investigators attempted to replicate Domagk's work and assess the antibacterial properties of their own derivative compounds in infected mice. On an apparent whim, the Pasteur scientists decided to test the effects of a chemical component of Prontosil, the moiety sulfanilamide. To their surprise, they found that when sulfanilamide was given to infected mice, the animals survived just as if they had been given Prontosil.[23] Moreover the investigators were able to show that sulfanilamide, unlike Prontosil, was active against streptococcus in dish cultures. It became quickly apparent that sulfanilamide, a byproduct of Prontosil, was the lifesaving substance. The French scientists rightly deduced that once Prontosil was consumed, it was cleaved in two by the body to produce the active compound sulfanilamide. This phenomenon explained why Prontosil was ineffective against colonies of streptococcus in the laboratory, when the drug (or prodrug) remained intact. The Pasteur Institute's experimental results were published just nine months after Domagk's seminal article on Prontosil.[24] By revealing that the active portion of Prontosil was in fact sulfanilamide, the French undermined Farben's monopoly on the world's first distributable, branded antibiotic.[25] In 1908, almost 25 years before Bayer's chemists created Prontosil, an Austrian chemist published his synthesis of sulfanilamide and related compounds.[26] Owing to the remote dating of this work, the patent on sulfanilamide had long expired. By 1932, the product was in the public domain for general production and use.[27]

2D chemical diagrams of Prontosil (top) and sulfanilamide (bottom). Once ingested, the N=N azo bond of Prontosil is cleaved to produce sulfanilamide, the active compound.

Other European physicians were also intrigued by Prontosil. In London, Dr. Leonard Colebrook was especially interested in reports of the drug's activity against puerperal sepsis, or childbed fever. Colebrook finally acquired samples of Prontosil and its French equivalent in the latter part of 1935. After successfully treating infected animals with Prontosil in a series of experiments, he studied Prontosil's efficacy in 38 women with puerperal fever, a frequently deadly infection. In February of 1936, he reported in *The Lancet* how Prontosil treatment cut the historical death rate of puerperal fever by two thirds (from an average of 22% to 8%).[28] In the same issue, researchers at England's Wellcome Laboratories described the lifesaving benefits of sulfanilamide in infected mice—replicating the French investigators' findings.[29] Five months later, Colebrook supported his clinical data with another 26 cases of Prontosil-treated puerperal fever; in this case series, there were no deaths.[30] Moreover in a follow-up article, Colebrook and his associates showed that the blood from humans treated with sulfanilamide or Prontosil similarly stunted the growth of streptococcus in culture.[31] Ongoing investigations by UK physicians would eventually demonstrate the comparable clinical efficacy of Prontosil and sulfanilamide in puerperal fever.[32] However, they would also note that the two drugs differed in an important way, beyond their patent status. In addition to being in the public domain, sulfanilamide, unlike the dye-drug Prontosil, "had the further advantage of not turning the patient as red as a boiled lobster."[33]

In America, systematic investigations of Prontosil and sulfanilamide were delayed, at least in part, by insufficient importation of the drugs until 1936. Paramount US investigations of Prontosil and sulfanilamide were conducted at The John Hopkins University Hospital by Perrin Long and Eleanor Bliss, who replicated Colebrook's in vitro and animal experiments and confirmed sulfanilamide's efficacy in several cases of human streptococcal infections.[34] Notably Long and Bliss postulated a mostly bacteriostatic, rather than bactericidal, property for the drug. In other words, sulfanilamide stunted streptococcal growth—instead of killing the bacteria outright—and thereby allowed the body's natural immune defenses to eliminate the pathogen.[35]

But the real enthusiasm for sulfanilamide was generated by a high-profile case study. A few short weeks after the initial Hopkins work was publicly presented (in November of 1936), news reports were buzzing with the recuperation of the American President's son, Franklin D. Roosevelt, Jr., from a grave sinus infection. While hospitalized at Boston's prestigious Massachusetts General Hospital in December, the junior Roosevelt was treated with sulfanilamide tablets in a last-ditch effort. The dramatic recovery of the President's son after receiving the antibiotic was chronicled faithfully by the Associated Press and popular newspapers, including the *New York Times*.[36] "Young Roosevelt Saved by New Drug," the paper declared. On the heels of FDR, Jr.'s recovery, *Time* magazine reported that "some responsible doctors" were calling sulfanilamide "the medical discovery of the decade."[37]

Glowing anecdotes and scientific endorsement fueled widespread zeal for sulfanilamide among the American public and physicians alike. And zeal gave way to mania when studies described the antibiotic's efficacy in gonorrhea.[38] A venereal plague of humankind, like syphilis, gonorrheal infection most commonly manifest as urethritis in men (with painful urination and penile discharge) and as vaginitis and pelvic inflammation in women. The bacterial infection (from "impure sexual intercourse," admonished Sir William Osler's *The Principles and Practice of Medicine*) had been historically and notably resistant to all sorts of superficially promising or frankly desperate therapies during the last century. These included an orally consumed form of Indonesian pepper (*Cubebae fructus*), various antitoxin vaccines, locally applied Mercurochrome, and—specifically for infected men—electrically applied heat to the prostate (diathermy) and penile irrigations with any number of ostensibly antiseptic solutions (like potassium permanganate, silver nitrate, or mercury oxycyanide).[39] While general medical advice in the early 20th century was to "actively" treat gonorrheal urethritis with trials of antibacterial serum, this measure often failed. "Drugs," Osler's textbook cautioned, "are of little value."[40]

Consequently reception was high for any compound that offered plausible relief from gonorrheal symptoms. This perpetually unmet need was seemingly answered in May of 1937, when urologists at Hopkins reported their remarkable series of 19 infected men treated with sulfanilamide.[41] Symptoms of urethral discharge and burning vanished, in some cases, within two days of treatment. In most patients, the offending bacteria disappeared from the urine by four days. Lay reports, perhaps overstating the medical findings, startled readers by broadcasting that the drug was "the best thing ever discovered for gonorrhea"[42] and cured the disease within 48 hours. One American drug maker, Winthrop Chemical, advertised, "[I]t would seem that a revolutionary change is impending in the treatment of another plague of humanity."[43]

As a result, the US market became flooded with competitive brands of the antibiotic, including the patented prodrug, Prontosil (the original Bayer/I. G. Farben compound, in injectable form) and the unpatented sulfanilamide, the active metabolite of Prontosil, in powder and tablet forms.[44] The latter group included many identical formulations with distinctive brand names, an example of which was Winthrop Chemical's

Prontylin tablets, the drug specifically credited in press reports with saving the life of the President's son. In May of 1937, the AMA's Council on Pharmacy and Chemistry attempted to avert confusion by adopting "sulfanilamide" as the preferred nonproprietary term for the drug and stated, "It is regretted that certain firms in America are using proprietary names [for sulfanilamide]."[45]

3
SOMETHING IS WRONG WITH THE ELIXIR

To complement Dr. Stevenson's wired reply to the AMA on Sunday, October 10th, Dr. Ruprecht and Glen Entler's physician, Dr. Darwin Childs, drafted letters to the AMA, providing more complete information about Tulsa's suspected cases of poisoning.[1] Essential contributions from Ruprecht: There were now 10 known patients in Tulsa who had consumed the sulfanilamide elixir. Two of the four still-living patients were close to death. Two of the 10 individuals were young men with gonorrhea, and one of these patients "had received tablets of sulfanilamide over the period of two weeks without any bad effects." This person had visited a second doctor, who "put him on the elixir of sulfanilamide and the typical train of symptoms followed shortly afterwards." Ruprecht's letter tended to exonerate sulfanilamide in its standard tablet form and implicated the elixir preparation as the cause of illness. Dr. Childs, perhaps most important, rushed a sample of the liquid drug to Chicago for chemical analysis. He added in a parallel letter,

> My patient, a 20 year old adult, who had an acute gonorrhea, took a total of 220 grains, as represented by 55 teaspoonfuls of the elixir of sulfanilamide. Twenty-four hours after the ingestion of this amount, he began to have symptoms of an acute nephritis, and forty-eight hours later he was totally anuric. He died [Saturday, October 9th] four days after receiving the last dose. The clinical picture and autopsy reports of this case closely resemble each of the other cases.

> It is my opinion, and the opinion of the other physicians here who have had such cases, that something is wrong with the elixir of

sulfanilamide and that probably your chemistry department will be able to give us some light on this matter.

On Monday, October 11th, Secretary Leech of the AMA wired the headquarters of The S. E. Massengill Company, the maker of the questionable elixir, in Bristol, Tennessee.

KINDLY TELEGRAPH COLLECT COMPLETE STATEMENT OF COMPOSITION ELIXIR SULFANILAMIDE MASSENGILL

While Leech waited for a response, members of the Tulsa County Medical Society officially reviewed the local deaths. By Monday evening, pathologist Ivo Nelson had performed autopsies on four of Tulsa's victims: 11-month-old Mary Earline Watters, six-year-old Sonny Wakeford, six-year-old Michael Sheehan, and Dr. Childs's patient, Glen Entler. The common factor, the elixir, was undeniable. Aided by Dr. Ruprecht, Nelson presented his findings to his "horrified associates" in attendance at the society meeting, including Dr. Underwood who had prescribed the drug on four occasions.[2] Nelson's postmortem findings were consistent with a toxic reaction: necrosis of the kidneys and degeneration of the liver.

For Nelson, implicating the elixir as the cause of the pathologic findings was perhaps easiest in the case of the youngest victim, Mary Earline Watters. She was an infant, so there was little chance that organ damage was due to other causes, Nelson argued. Also she had been bottle fed, which reduced the possibility that she had ingested a toxin through her limited diet. Nevertheless "the doctors were not easy to convince," according to the era's melodramatic press coverage. The *Kansas City Journal-Post* reported the society members' reactions.

> They could not at first believe they had prescribed a poisonous medicine, imperiling the lives they cherished. But Dr. Nelson was prepared. He had mustered his facts thoroughly as only a scientist can. Terrified, the doctors listened while he mowed down every alternative explanation advanced by their trained minds. Bewildered and aghast, they were forced to accept his conclusions.

By contrast, the society's official minutes of the meeting sterilized the drama. Discussion among the member physicians that Monday evening, whether heated or cool, elicited the following conclusions: that sulfanilamide is a "new" drug, requiring "further study and very careful use under the supervision of a licensed physician"; that the deaths are associated with the elixir version of the antibiotic and not tablet preparations; and that evidence against the elixir is "adequate to [indict] but insufficient to convict."

In his presentation to the medical society, Nelson demonstrated a high level of nitrogen in the form of urea in the victims' blood. The condition, known medically as uremia, was an accepted marker of renal failure.[3] Autopsies showed inflammation of the body cavities (polyserositis); degeneration of the central portion of the liver; and profound abnormalities in the cells lining one part (the proximal portion) of the kidney's microscopic filtering tubes. Notably the renal abnormalities observed by Nelson were different from those caused by streptococcal nephritis. The latter condition was known at the time to show abnormalities of the glomeruli, the parts of the kidney where the blood is initially filtered.[4] In Nelson's autopsy cases, the glomeruli were "intact." Mercury poisoning was also an unlikely cause of death. In addition to the fact that there was no overt history of ingesting the element (although the exact composition of the liquid antibiotic was not yet established), Nelson did not report lesions in the gastrointestinal tract, a hallmark of poisoning with mercury bichloride. Motions were carried by the society members to prohibit the sale of any sulfanilamide preparation that had not been accepted by the AMA's Council and to ensure that sulfanilamide was used only under the direction of a physician. At the instigation of the society, the local professional organization of pharmacists, the Tulsa Retail Druggists, urged its members to comply.[5]

The next day, Tuesday, October 12th, The S. E. Massengill Company wired its response to the AMA, collect. In addition to providing the ingredients of the liquid drug (while requesting that secrecy be preserved), the company implied that its product had been market tested and was safe. The claim was made despite the fact that physicians from Tulsa had already lodged a direct complaint with the company. Since early September, the firm had distributed gallons of the product nationwide; therefore, the company reasoned, more deaths would have occurred if the elixir was, in fact, lethal.

ACCEPT CONFIDENTIALLY ELIXIR SULFANILAMIDE CONTAINS SULFANILAMIDE FORTY GRAINS TO EACH FLUIDOUNCE DISSOLVED IN A MIXTURE OF TWENTY FIVE PERCENT WATER AND SEVENTY FIVE PERCENT DIETHYLENE GLYCOL WITH MINUTE QUANTITIES OF FLAVOR AND COLOR STOP WAS GIVEN CLINICAL TESTS AND WIDELY USED IN PRACTICE WITHOUT UNTOWARD RESULTS EXCEPT YESTERDAY SPRINGER CLINIC TULSA OKLAHOMA MADE COMPLAINT STOP WILL APPRECIATE ALL INFORMATION YOU MAY HAVE OR ACCUMULATE STOP

Reading beyond the company's defense and disregarding its plea for confidentiality, a shocked Secretary Leech immediately telegraphed Dr. Ruprecht in Tulsa.

[...] PRODUCT CONTAINS MUCH DIETHYLENE GLYCOL AS SOLVENT THIS IS TOXIC AND REPORTED TO CAUSE NEPHROSIS POSSIBLY MAY BE OXIDIZED TO OXALIC ACID SEE JOURNAL PHARMACOLOGY AND EXPERIMENTAL THERAPEUTICS VOLUME FORTY TWO PAGE THREE FIVE FIVE COMMA NINETEEN THIRTY ONE STOP SUGGEST PATHOLOGISTS DETERMINE IF OXALATE POISONING IS INDICATED STOP WILL MAKE CHEMICAL EXAMINATION OF YOUR PRODUCT WHEN RECEIVED

Leech was now directing Ruprecht to a scientific article with the unwieldy title, "The pharmacology of ethylene glycol and some of its derivatives in relation to their chemical constitution and physical chemical properties."[6] In 1931, pharmacologists from Western Reserve University in Cleveland, Ohio, Ruprecht's alma mater, reported their analysis of the toxicity of ethylene glycol and that of its chemical cousins, including diethylene glycol. These substances had well-known industrial uses, specifically in the manufacture of varnishes and thinners, and ethylene glycol was the essential component of Prestone, a branded antifreeze for car radiators made by the Union Carbide and Carbon Corporation. A few investigators in the 1910s and 1920s had advocated the use of ethylene glycol as a substitute for the solvent glycerin in liquid medications. However, four cases of severe poisoning from drinking radiator fluid, two of which were fatal, were reported in 1930.[7] Consequently the safe use of ethylene glycol and its derivatives, in a therapeutic context, was highly dubious. After injecting various glycols into laboratory rodents, the Western Reserve scientists determined that diethylene glycol, while not as toxic as ethylene glycol, damaged the kidneys and could be fatal. In his wire to the Tulsa physicians, Leech raised the possibility of oxalate poisoning. Oxalic acid was a known metabolite of ethylene glycol, and the presence of oxalic acid in the urine (specifically in the form of calcium oxalate crystals) was a known sign of ethylene-glycol poisoning.

Three days later, on Friday, October 15th, Drs. Ruprecht and Nelson wired their most complete autopsy findings of the Tulsa patients to *JAMA*.[8] The deceased victims now included Charlene Canady, who died on October 12th. She was the fifth child to die at St. John's Hospital. Another young man, 25-year-old Earl Beard, was in grave condition. But there were survivors—namely the Wakeford girl and Jack Voorhees, who was slowly recovering from symptoms of poisoning.[9] Ruprecht and Nelson discovered that, among those affected by the liquid antibiotic, urine production typically stopped within two days after taking as little as one-half ounce. They also observed that death, if it occurred, happened between two and seven days after the onset of anuria. Their postmortem findings were similar to what they had presented to the Tulsa County Medical Society four days earlier, with an important addition: There was no evidence of oxalate crystals, the characteristic finding of ethylene-glycol poisoning. The authors, instead, likened their pathologic findings to those of dioxane poisoning.

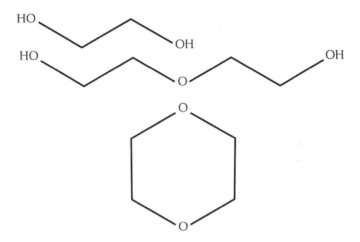

2D chemical diagrams of ethylene glycol (top),
diethylene glycol (middle) and dioxane (bottom)

Information on the toxicity of dioxane, another industrial solvent and chemical cousin of ethylene glycol, was published in 1935.[10] In laboratory animals, the solvent initially increased urine production and then produced anuria and death. Postmortem findings in animals were limited to the liver and kidney, with the latter organ showing abnormalities that were very similar to Nelson's autopsy findings. The initial increase in urine production with dioxane was attributed to "early damage which diminishes the concentrating power" of the kidney.

Ruprecht and Nelson concluded their wired case reports to *JAMA*: "Federal inspectors arrived today."

4
RETURN OUR EXPENSE

News of the Oklahoma deaths finally arrived at the FDA on Thursday, October 14th, five days after doctors in Tulsa first wired Morris Fishbein at the AMA. A New York physician "associated with a large drug manufacturing concern" telephoned the federal agency and repeated the rumors, "presumably through professional or trade contacts, that fatalities had occurred at Tulsa."[1] Perrin Long, the Johns Hopkins physician who had reported the impressive anti-infective powers of sulfanilamide, also notified the FDA, on October 15th. Long had received firsthand information of the Tulsa deaths from a "friend" at E. R. Squibb and Sons. He had also learned the makeup of Massengill's elixir through rapidly leaked information from the AMA's telegraph volley with the manufacturer. As one of the world's experts on sulfanilamide, Long defended the antibiotic to the FDA in a quickly penned letter.

> In my own experience and that of many others, there has been no reason to believe that sulfanilamide injures the kidneys. It is my opinion that something must have happened in the preparation of the elixir or that something happened either to the products in the elixir or to the sulfanilamide as it was prepared. I think it highly important that this be looked into because it is not only a very sad accident but it is also very necessary that none of the Massengill elixir be sold until the whole matter is cleared up. Otherwise an epidemic of death may occur over the country at large.[2]

Scientists at the AMA's Chemical Laboratory also wanted to determine if "something" had "happened in the preparation of the elixir."

Although diethylene glycol was strongly suspected to be the fatal ingredient in Massengill's Elixir Sulfanilamide, it was unknown if the solvent had affected the possible toxicity of the antibiotic or vice versa. It was also unknown if there had been any errors in the company's manufacturing process. "Indeed the possibilities are unlimited," warned Dr. Fishbein on Monday, October 18th. Fishbein, who by this time had returned to his *JAMA* office in Chicago and was evidently fully updated on the Tulsa deaths, continued the public alert: "[W]e are here concerned with a preparation not standardized by any reliable agency, semisecret in composition, and apparently hastily rushed into the market to meet an overenthusiastic reception of a new remedy."[3] But unlike Dr. Long, Fishbein hedged in his endorsement of sulfanilamide. He called the drug "very valuable" but also cautioned that it could be "exceedingly dangerous" if used at high doses or without a doctor's prescription. Fishbein's hesitation may have been due to the fact that he had been burned at least once by his hasty support for another novel drug, dinitrophenol, a weight-loss compound.[4] Widespread and indiscriminate use of dinitrophenol in the 1930s showed that it could produce cataracts and agranulocytosis (like sulfanilamide), among other problems. Fishbein now feared that the unguarded use of sulfanilamide could lead to similar deleterious effects in a high percentage of consumers, particularly those engaged in self-treatment. He admitted to the press that he knew of no law precluding over-the-counter sales of the antibiotic, including those of the new liquid version. In fact, the AMA was aware that there had been "widespread purchases [of sulfanilamide] by youths attempting to treat themselves for venereal disease."[5]

For its chemical analysis, the AMA laboratory used one gallon of Massengill's product, which it had received, by request, directly from the company. In addition, AMA chemists obtained samples of the drug on the open market and (finally) received the small elixir bottle from Tulsa physician Darwin Childs, which he had secured from a city pharmacy.[6] The chemists noted the contents of the doctor's bottle: It held "approximately 50 cc [50 cubic centimeters, a little more than 3 tablespoons] of a reddish, somewhat viscous liquid, having an aromatic odor resembling raspberry and anise, a sweet taste, and resembling glycerin in general physical character." Quick distillation experiments confirmed the product to be a solution of approximately 40 grains (2.6 grams) of sulfanilamide per fluid ounce of "menstruum." The menstruum, or solvent, was 72% diethylene glycol and about 16% water. The chemists then assessed the solid residue of Massengill's antibiotic elixir and found sulfanilamide to be intact—meaning that diethylene glycol had not chemically altered the antibiotic. Further assays did not reveal other potentially toxic substances like lead, arsenic, or significantly, mercury. These initial laboratory data supported the contention that diethylene glycol in Massengill's preparation was the lethal ingredient and had not affected the chemical integrity of the antibiotic. Conversely sulfanilamide had not chemically altered the already toxic diethylene glycol. To complement the AMA's chemical analysis, scientists at the University of Chicago began conducting toxicity experiments on laboratory animals.

* * * * * *

Immediately after the FDA learned of the Tulsa deaths, the agency dispatched its Kansas City station chief, career veteran William Hartigan, along with Junior Inspector Walter Donaldson to Tulsa. Racing 250 miles by "motor car," the men arrived in Tulsa on the morning of Friday, October 15th, and wired their findings to the FDA's Central District chief in Chicago, James "Jimmie" Clarke.[7] (This was the same date that Drs. Ruprecht and Nelson telegraphed their case reports to the *JAMA* office in Chicago.) Simultaneous events were happening quickly, according to the FDA correspondence. Clarke, in turn, updated his bosses at FDA headquarters in Washington, DC, on Saturday, October 16th.[8] In addition to confirming the current death tally in Tulsa (now eight children and one young adult), Clarke reported that Hartigan had rushed three elixir samples by air express to an FDA laboratory in Baltimore, Maryland, and had embargoed all wholesale and retail lots of Massengill's product in the area. Clarke's wire also relayed a disturbing piece of new information: "STLOUIS NOTIFIED VIA WESTERNUNION RUMOR HERE SIMILAR CIRCUMSTANCES."

With the assistance of the newly arrived FDA agents, the Tulsa County Medical Society continued its investigation of the city's deceased children who "had a peculiar kidney ailment, following sore throats," reported the local press.[9] Despite rumors of similar cases in the St. Louis area, per Clarke's dispatch, confusion remained as to why "the particular treatment would affect children in Tulsa and not [...] children or patients in other places where [sulfanilamide] has been used to much greater extent." To that end, cases of unexplained death in Tulsa would be reexamined, and local tests of the elixir on guinea pigs were initiated, independent of the animal experiments in Chicago.[10] Station Chief Hartigan indicated to reporters that the government's investigation in Tulsa would be cautious and possibly protracted. Hartigan cited his agency experience with numerous cases of paralysis in Oklahoma City in 1930. That investigation, consuming months, had led to the discovery of adulterated Jamaica ginger, or "jake," which had been tainted with an organophosphate, a known neurotoxin. The jake, sold legally throughout the country as a medicinal compound, had been consumed enthusiastically during the era of Prohibition because of its high alcohol content. The FDA had been instrumental in seizing contaminated lots of jake in several states, and government chemists had identified the offending agent only after an extended series of laboratory analyses.[11]

However, Dr. Fishbein—despite his guarded view of sulfanilamide— believed that an extended analysis of Massengill's elixir was largely pro forma. In a *JAMA* editorial that was prereleased to newspapers and radio stations on October 18th, the editor fingered the death-causing ingredient to the nation, without much question: "It would appear to be clear that the diethylene glycol rather than the sulfanilamide was responsible (for the Tulsa deaths)."[12] Fishbein's certainty may well have been informed by preliminary and as-yet unpublished data from ongoing animal experiments at the University of Chicago. Scientists collaborating with the AMA observed that, within a matter of days, treated rats, rabbits, and dogs showed effects that were remarkably similar to the signs and symptoms of the Tulsa victims: Death, always preceded by anuria, occurred in animals that received variable, divided doses of diethylene glycol, Massengill's elixir, or a synthetic version of the product (which had been mixed up by the AMA for the experiments).[13] Conversely sulfanilamide alone did not produce the same renal symptoms or death. Fishbein concluded his broadcasted editorial, "This tragic experience should be a final warning to physicians relative to the prescribing and administration of semi-secret, unstandardized preparations."[14]

Despite the understandable speed with which Fishbein acted to warn a vulnerable public, the finality of the AMA editorial (and probably its chastising tone toward physicians who had innocently prescribed the elixir) was resented by the Tulsa doctors. On Tuesday, October 19th, they were still waiting for an official word from the AMA on the analysis of Dr. Childs's elixir sample, and, perhaps taking a cue from Station Chief Hartigan, they believed that a more complete investigation was necessary before final judgment could be pronounced.[15] An anonymous Tulsa physician involved with the local animal tests told the *Tulsa Daily World*, "The guinea pigs which have been given the drug [...] look like they might die any time, but we still do not feel ready to release a formal statement because it really is a very serious situation." He added, "It seems the physicians here who have observed the conditions thoroughly should be in a better position to make a thorough analysis."

FDA Chief Walter Campbell was also more circumspect than Fishbein about the cause of the Tulsa deaths, at least publicly. "We do not know as yet the explanation of the fatalities," he told the Associated Press on Tuesday, October 19th.[16] "It has been reported that the solvent, diethylene glycol, is probably the responsible agent. We know that there is something radically wrong," he admitted. Campbell had already launched a government investigation of all liquid sulfanilamide preparations on the US market, by air-mailing letters to his three district chiefs in New York, Chicago, and San Francisco on October 18th.[17] He advised:

> The tragic results at Tulsa, Oklahoma, following the administration of sulfanilamide elixir made with diethylene glycol, indicate the necessity of immediate investigation of preparations of sulfanilamide already placed on the market by numerous pharmaceutical houses and coming into existence in new form almost daily.

> For the present, it is suggested that this investigation be restricted to liquid preparations since these are more likely to undergo change than are the tablet and other solid preparations.

Regardless of whether similar liquid versions of sulfanilamide, if they existed, posed the same risk as Massengill's product, an urgent and complete withdrawal of the proprietary elixir seemed imperative.[18] Campbell advised the press that the FDA was seizing all shipments of the "poisonous drug."

For his part, Dr. Samuel Evans Massengill, president of The S. E. Massengill Company, conducted shrouded damage control. On the day that FDA agents Hartigan and Donaldson arrived in Tulsa (Friday, October 15th), the company sent out hundreds of telegrams nationwide, recalling the elixir without explanation.[19] To its customers, the firm advised: "DO NOT USE ELIXIR SULFANILAMIDE SHIPPED. RETURN OUR EXPENSE." To Massengill's salesmen: "ELIXIR SULFANILAMIDE DISCONTINUED. PICK UP AS RAPIDLY AS POSSIBLE ALL SOLD IN YOUR TERRITORY." To jobbers, druggists, and doctors: "HAVE WITHDRAWN PRODUCT ELIXIR SULFANILAMIDE. PLEASE RETURN UNUSED STOCKS IMMEDIATELY." The attempted recall coincided with an expected visit from the FDA's Chief Medical Officer and a veteran inspector at Massengill's headquarters in Bristol, Tennessee.

5

MUCH PREJUDICE AGAINST TABLETS

The S. E. Massengill Company of Bristol, Tennessee, began in 1899 as a fraternal venture between East Tennesseans Samuel Evans Massengill and his older brother, Norman, both of whom were natives of the quaintly named Appalachian village, Piney Flats.[1] Sons of a country physician, the two brothers began selling common fluid extracts and tinctures out of a rented storeroom in Bristol, a modest city about 15 miles northeast of their hometown. The hilly community of Bristol, with a population of about 10,000, was largely unremarkable; although it was a mild geographic oddity, owing to the fact that it straddled the border between northeastern Tennessee and southwestern Virginia. More important, however, for the Massengill brothers was the fact that Bristol was commercially strategic. It allowed for the easy rail distribution of medical supplies to the generally disregarded physicians of Appalachia, a market that the Massengill brothers hoped to dominate.

Samuel Massengill's interest in a pharmaceutical career, by his own account, arose after observing a drug-sales call made to his father in the spring of 1897. The junior Massengill, who was looking for a way to pay for his own ongoing medical education (which consisted of a disconnected series of lectures), was evidently impressed by the drug rep's "various colored pills."[2] Presumably cash-strapped and motivated by the prospect of commission work, Massengill made several inquiries into pharmaceutical sales positions and ultimately landed a job with a wholesale drug company based in Boston, Massachusetts. Years later, Massengill rallied his own sales force with homey tales of his early experiences in the mountainous South as a detail man for the New England firm.

When I began my work as a salesman there were no good roads anywhere I worked. It was before the automobile was invented, and my transportation was mostly by buggy or horseback. Most of the good prospects were widely scattered in the country districts. It was impracticable to reach hotels for lodging, but the people were hospitable. A familiar response to a request to stay overnight was, "If you can put up with our fare, light and come in." At the time most of the practice was done with tinctures, fluidextracts, powders and cathartic pills. The doctor with his long-blade pocketknife, called a physician's knife, mixed his powders from his saddle bags which he placed across his knees. I have often speculated about the great amount of confidence and faith this act must have inspired in the patient.[3]

Massengill lamented that, because the mixed powders "lasted too long," they undermined repeated, frequent drug sales. He continued his reminiscence, describing his early troubles when attempting to sell new-fangled, compressed tablet drugs, the shelf lives of which were comparatively short.

There was much prejudice against tablets, and it was well founded, for they were all hard, insoluble and generally bad [...] Doctors claimed their patients could not swallow them. I directed over and over again that the patient should be instructed to place a tablet in his mouth, take a mouthful of water, forget about the tablet and swallow the water.[4]

When Massengill finished his last round of medical lectures at the University of Nashville in 1899 (the final year that the school bestowed medical doctorates after a mere three sessions of lectures), he abandoned a career in clinical medicine.[5] Instead Massengill, with his older brother, established a full-scale distribution center in Bristol for the Boston drug company. The local outfit was christened "Masengill Bros.," and the fledgling company began producing its own competitive versions of unpatented drugs. With the help of a teenage neighbor, Rhea Harkrader, Massengill began cranking out his own versions of time-sensitive, revenue-generating pills with a new $25 hand-operated tablet press. Harkrader later wrote of his summer employment with "Dr. Sam," as his boss was called (or liked to be called), in the tiny enterprise.

[...] Dr. Sam mixed the drugs which were packaged in bottles or small paper boxes sealed, then labeled to identify contents. Another part of my job was to bottle and label castor oil, spirits of ammonia, etc.

which were received in large casks for bottles. Too, I remember operating the first tablet machine. It was a clumsy affair, requiring a complete turn of the crank to make and eject a single tablet. The powder which was mixed and kept to the proper consistency by Dr. Sam fed down from a small V-shaped bin, and the faster I turned the handle, the faster the tablet popped out. It was a continuous operation.[6]

Such a homespun, unchecked process, repeated by drug entrepreneurs nationwide, provided little-to-no assurance that tablets contained a consistent amount of an active ingredient, were reasonably safe, or even dissolved in the body once consumed. This freewheeling nature of drug manufacturing in the United States, the unhappy norm at the start of the 20th century, also invited outright fraud. American firms could sell proprietary nostrums that included little of what was advertised, largely inert substances, or even potentially dangerous ones. Moreover medicinal products could be promoted to treat all sorts of conditions, without any scientific basis whatsoever. In a widely read and influential series of articles in *Collier's Weekly*, muckraker Samuel Hopkins Adams outed a number of the more egregious offenders in 1905.[7] The purported antiseptic Liquozone, a "liquid oxygen" produced by the Liquozone Company of Chicago, was nearly 99% water. The witch hazel in Pond's Extract, made by the Pond's Extract Company of New York, was promoted to treat "all diseased conditions of the mucous membranes," and its maker attempted to bolster sales by shamelessly exploiting a meningitis epidemic in New York City. Many products, like Lydia Pinkham's Compound for "women's troubles," Paine's Celery Compound for depression and fatigue, and Peruna for catarrh and tuberculosis, merely contained high levels of alcohol. Other heavily promoted treatments were sources of cocaine for the discerning "fiend."

These rogue companies, many of which existed solely for the purpose of selling a single dubious product, were distinct from the more legitimate US firms that would become the foundation of the modern pharmaceutical industry. Companies like Charles Pfizer and Company[8] and Merck (as the US subsidiary of the German family partnership) were established in the 1800s as suppliers of fine chemicals, many of which were imported into the United States and some of which were found, mostly by accident, to have medicinal uses. By the turn of the century, it was the generally prevailing, haphazard business model of America's chemical industry, which had not yet adopted the systematic search for and development of therapeutic compounds—a model forged and embraced by Bayer/I. G. Farben to emerging success. But there were a few exceptions: Eli Lilly and Company of Indianapolis, Indiana, was founded in 1876 for the explicit purpose of discovering and creating new drugs; E. R. Squibb and Sons of Brooklyn, New York, was known for the purity of its chloroform and ether, two widely used anesthetics; and the Abbott Alkaloidal Company of Ravenswood, Illinois, produced "dosimetric granules" of its plant-alkaloid drugs to enable the fine-tuning of drug dosages.[9]

These comparatively ethical and well-intentioned companies aside, criticism of dubious nostrums at the turn of the century paralleled the exploding US market for them. In addition to Adams's articles, growing demand for legislative reform was fueled by other exposés in popular magazines, such as the *Ladies' Home Journal.* There was also a heated backlash against deceptive drug ads in venerable medical journals, including *JAMA*, and the righteous influence of government officials, like the outspoken Harvey Wiley, Chief Chemist of the Department of Agriculture.[10] The groundswell for government intervention gave Congress the necessary political nerve to pass the Food and Drugs Act of 1906, the first US law that enabled the federal regulation of drug manufacturing.[11] The law addressed the production and interstate sale of drugs, prohibiting adulterated or misbranded products. To its credit, the law defined adulteration in the broadest sense, addressing any deviation of the labeled strength, quality, or purity of a drug. Among the law's definitions of misbranding were infractions related to the nondisclosure of potentially harmful ingredients. Specified among these were alcohol, morphine, cocaine, heroin, and cannabis. However, the law did not mandate that drug manufacturers list their products' inactive ingredients—simply that, if they did so, they must be truthful. In addition, the law did not prevent unsafe drugs from entering the market, for there was no provision that a manufacturer had to conduct tests to demonstrate a product's safety. The 1906 law was also relatively toothless: Infractions were defined only as misdemeanors, with each infraction necessitating a small, predetermined fine (eg, "not exceeding two hundred dollars for the first offense") or limited jail time.

Massengill advertised his company's prompt compliance with the 1906 law, claiming, "[W]e were among the first to file our guaranty with the government and were assigned Serial Number 1871 under which all our products are guaranteed."[12] The law was also viewed by Massengill as a dictum to employ professionals who could "assay and control not only raw materials but also the finished drug products." He began hiring pharmacists and boasted in his company catalogs:

We have an analytical laboratory equipped for testing and assaying of all standardized products which is under the direction of a chemist who has had a long experience and is especially proficient in this class of work.

We test all chemicals and drugs entering into our pharmaceuticals and standardize all of our finished products directed to be standardized by the [US] Pharmacopoeia and apply the same system to all others where there has been a reliable standard found.[13]

By 1910, Samuel Massengill, president of his company, had 18 employees in Bristol, including his older brother. The firm, which declared that it would "discontinue jobbing the medical products of other houses,"[14] offered more than 1,600 items to area physicians. Products ranged from absorbent cotton and antitoxins to medicinal wines and saddlebags. The overwhelming majority of these goods were repackaged from commercial suppliers, but Massengill also ramped up his on-site production of tablets. This was accomplished not only with the original rotary press but with two single-punch tablet machines, a rotating tablet-coating pan, and a rotating tablet-polishing drum. To produce ointments, a rotating pot mill and grinder were purchased. And to give the appearance of product exclusivity, Massengill branded many of his refurbished drugs with the -gill suffix of the family name. For example, a boric-acid powder for wounds was sold as Aseptogill; gastric "sedative" tablets containing various bismuth compounds were labeled Bismogill; and any number of powders, ointments, inhalants, or lotions containing menthol were called Menthagill.[15] Thus Massengill's business model was largely one of reselling and, to a lesser extent, manufacturing and compounding nonproprietary pharmaceuticals that were then branded to appear exclusive. He was not in the business of drug innovation, and his own general manager later conceded that "especially during the early years Dr. Massengill looked toward several large companies and the products they announced for guidance in developing products for the Massengill Company."[16]

Despite the lack of innovation or, at the very least, a regular commitment to it, Massengill's company grew steadily from a small, one-room warehouse to a multi-acred plant in Bristol. The firm's growth was probably aided by a lack of regional competition for manufactured drugs. And having conquered the local drug market, Massengill expanded nationally by creating a plant and distribution center at Kansas City, Missouri, in 1922. Warehouses were subsequently purchased in New York City in 1926 and San Francisco, California, in 1934. Sales offices were established in the US territories of Hawaii and Puerto Rico. By 1937, the company (now called The S. E. Massengill Company) had more than

500 employees, a "well equipped laboratory, with five chemists and four pharmacists [and] a bunch of guinea pigs and equipment for tests."[17] Massengill himself boasted that his company was "the largest pharmaceutical manufacturer for the entire South."[18]

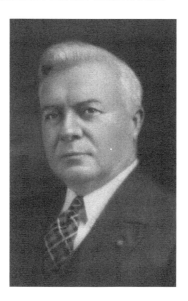

Samuel Evans Massengill, MD, date unknown
(Courtesy of the Bristol Rotary Club)

The firm's 1936 catalog, which offered hundreds of tablets, capsules, elixirs, or ointments, read like a drug compendium on the cusp of modern medicine. Products like antimony wine, mercurial ointment, and rhubarb elixir shared index space with aspirin, novocaine, and phenobarbital. The catalog promised, "Every step in the manufacture of our general line of pharmaceuticals is under the supervision of skilled workmen and strict chemical control, and the physician may rely upon our products for prompt and full therapeutic effect."[19] The company's net annual sales for the year, while modest on a national scale, totaled more than $1.6 million and represented approximately 40,000 accounts with doctors, hospitals, and wholesale or retail druggists throughout the United States.[20] By the late 1930s, Massengill's personal wealth was estimated at $11 million.[21]

Despite the friendly moniker of Dr. Sam, Massengill's corporate mind-set grew, along with his wealth, into one of formality, if not rigidity, and his oversight was reflected in the mood of his official portrait: stern and imperious. A six-day, 48-hour work week was strictly enforced. Written rules for on-site employees prohibited conscious *or unconscious* humming, whistling, or other distracting noises, like "boisterous" laughing or talking. A fan of the mute employee, Massengill posted "Silence" signs throughout the company's headquarters, after admiring similar admonitions at the renowned Mayo Clinic. Ever mindful of appearances, Massengill also drafted a list of 20 "Don'ts" for his national sales force (approximately 200 strong in 1937). These rules specified, among other things, when to wear or remove caps and hats and scolded, "Don't get the idea that you (or ourselves) have any principles, either religious, political or racial that you must defend or propagate while drawing a salary and expenses from The S. E. Massengill Company."[22]

Massengill's commercial success and social prominence in Bristol were reflected in a customized home. In 1910, he built a stately Victorian mansion for his wife, the daughter of a prominent landowner in nearby Johnson City, Tennessee, and his two children. The foundation was composed of stone blocks weighing two tons each.[23] Massengill employed a live-in driver, according to the year's census, at a time when less than 1% of Americans owned a car. (The necessity of a driver for Massengill is unclear; his home was approximately one mile from his office.) A self-proclaimed "avid but mediocre golfer," he constructed a miniature golf course on the front lawn of his corporate campus, which featured a small lunchroom, a raised goldfish pond, a screened aviary, and "numerous painted plaster of paris gnomes and dwarfs."[24] Employees were allowed to use the lunchroom and golf course during their strictly clocked lunch breaks.

Massengill's community status also drew on the fact that his ancestors were among the first white settlers of the area, information that he was pleased to highlight.[25] Similar knowledge of others' relations informed his hiring decisions. "[Massengill] would closely interrogate applicants from families whose reputation labeled them lazy. On the other hand, applicants from industrious families were often 'hired on' for the initial trial period to confirm that the incumbent possessed the 'families'" commitment to work."[26] Accordingly Massengill was a fan of nepotism. Among several hired relatives: his son-in-law, Frank W. DeFriece, who became the company's chief legal counsel in 1932. Educated at Columbia University School of Law, DeFriece was a Democrat but by no means a fan of President Franklin D. Roosevelt and his New Deal economic programs of the 1930s. DeFriece was a vocal critic of FDR's controversial National Recovery Act, which fostered the organization of unions. He believed that the act "greatly complicated the management of employees," and he felt "strongly that many of these new laws were not only ill-advised and bordering on socialism, but were downright illegal."[27]

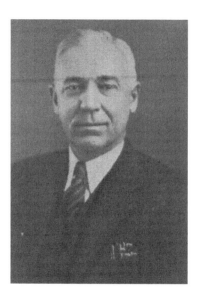

Frank W. DeFriece, Sr., date unknown
(*National Cyclopaedia of American Biography*, 1952)

In the summer of 1937, Massengill, a seasoned businessman at the age of 66, recounted a brief history of the US pharmaceutical industry for his sales representatives.[28] It was a disparaging and often gossipy account of the competition, which perhaps revealed more about Massengill's insecurities than it did about his competitors' shortcomings. Among his list of aspersions: George S. Davis of Parke Davis and Company "was said to have gambled heavily [...] and caused the financial ruin of his company"; Dr. Upjohn's pills were comically "friable"; Squibb's ether was overrated; Abbott's shipping department was surprisingly small; and the Searles of G. D. Searle and Company "exaggerated [their] importance in the pharmaceutical industry." Massengill was also quick to cite others' violations of the Food and Drugs Act, including fines against Sharp and Dohme, John Wyeth and Brother, and William R. Warner and Company. Of Wyeth and Warner, he scorned,

> Both of these companies are just shadows of the former substance. Both firms have been frequently and recently fined under the Food & Drug[s] Act, as might be expected, for when a firm in our line gets too low financially to stand the expense of proper supervision or falls into the hands of exploiters, a lowering of standards will follow.[29]

In fact, the FDA had brought charges, albeit relatively minor, against The S. E. Massengill Company on three occasions during the 1930s.[30] In one case, the company's Fluidextract of Colchicum, a gout treatment, was found to be overstrength. In another, Massengill's Tincture of Aconite was determined to be below its stated concentration. Fines of $150 and $250, respectively, were paid; although the company claimed that the overstrength colchicum product was "probably better on this account" (despite the greater risk of drug-induced toxicities, including bone-marrow suppression), and the understrength aconite product was attributed to the compound's naturally limited shelf life.[31] The government's third case, the seizure of Massengill's "Special" Elixir Terpin Hydrate and Codeine, a steadfast cough suppressant, was based on one charge of adulteration and two charges of misbranding. The case was successfully prosecuted in a New York federal court on the misbranding counts, and the product was forfeited and destroyed. Massengill's chief counsel later argued that the outcome was a "rather unusual victory" for his boss, because he was acquitted of the adulteration charge, "[t]he only one of the counts which was considered of any importance."[32]

6
AT LEAST 2 SHEETS IN THE WIND

In 1937, The S. E. Massengill Company, like so many drug companies before it, launched its own tablet versions of the unpatented sulfanilamide.[1] However, by mid-year the company's salesmen reported a demand for a liquid version of the antibiotic.[2] It appeared that a general bias against tablets still existed, particularly in the South.[3] Moreover a liquid drug would be much easier to administer to children. There were also rumors that liquid preparations for oral consumption were already on the market.[4] This information reached its way from Massengill's sales force to the company's chief chemist, Harold Cole Watkins. Whether Massengill personally urged or ordered Watkins to produce a liquid version of sulfanilamide is unknown; although it is not unreasonable to entertain the possibility—especially given Massengill's enthusiasm for drug marketing and his penchant for micromanagement.

After returning from a vacation in July of 1937, Watkins began testing liquid vehicles for the relatively insoluble powder of sulfanilamide. He turned his attention to the glycols, a group of chemically related alcohols, on the basis of their similarity to glycerin, a common solvent in liquid pharmaceuticals.[5] After several weeks of work, Watkins discovered that he could dissolve up to 75 grains (nearly 5 grams) of sulfanilamide in one fluid ounce of a clear, odorless, sweetish glycol known as diethylene glycol. However, at this strength the antibiotic powder tended to come out of solution when cooled. So Watkins reduced the concentration to 40 grains of sulfanilamide per fluid ounce and settled on the following mass-quantity recipe[6]:

Sulfanilamide, 58½ pounds
Elixir flavor, 1 gallon
Raspberry extract, 1 pint
Saccharine soluble, 1 pound
Amaranth[7] solution 1/16, 1½ pints
Caramel, 2 fluid ounces
Diethylene glycol, 60 gallons
Water, quantity sufficient to make 80 gallons

Watkins was evidently unaware that the FDA had advised against the use of glycols in foods, on the basis of limited safety data, and that Union Carbide, a chief maker of diethylene glycol, discouraged use of the solvent in any consumed product. Watkins was also evidently ignorant of relevant scientific reports, specifically the Western Reserve study of 1931 and an article published only months earlier, which also described the lethality of diethylene glycol in laboratory animals.[8]

Watkins proceeded to mix an initial, 40-gallon "trial batch" of Elixir Sulfanilamide at Massengill's headquarters in Bristol, probably sometime in late August, and he personally transported this supply to the company's shipping room.[9] Two more batches of the elixir, 80 gallons each, were produced at Bristol, and the formula was sent to Massengill's Kansas City branch, where the ingredients for another 40 gallons were combined in a large "stone jar."[10] Supplied instructions to the compounders were remarkably simple: "Dissolve sulfanilamide in diethylene glycol, add the other ingredients and mix." For raw materials, the company obtained sulfanilamide powder from Gane and Ingram, a chemical manufacturer in New York. Diethylene glycol was purchased, at 23 cents per gallon, from the Carbide and Carbon Chemicals Corporation, a division of Union Carbide, in West Virginia.[11] In total, 240 gallons of Elixir Sulfanilamide were produced.

Commercial lots of the elixir were bottled in one-gallon and one-pint volumes. The cork stopper of each filled bottle was covered with a company sticker, reading "Quality Pharmaceuticals." In addition, hundreds of elixir samples were produced in one- and two-ounce aliquots; these were to be freely and liberally distributed to physicians by company salesmen. Shipments of the product from Massengill's headquarters in Bristol to his warehouses in San Francisco and New York began on September 4th. A total of 30 gallons were sent to California, and New York received more than eight gallons.[12] Beginning at least as early as September 8th, commercial lots were shipped from Massengill's warehouses directly to retail pharmacies, doctors' offices, and hospitals throughout the nation. The product's label failed to list the ingredients, other than sulfanilamide, and instructed consumers to continue the treatment "until recovery." Pint bottles were sold to retail outlets for $1.65; gallon bottles went for an economical $12.00.[13] Invoices to retail customers stipulated, "All articles herein mentioned within the scope of the food and drug act, June 30, 1906, as amended, are guaranteed to conform to said Act. The S. E. Massengill Co." In conjunction with the mass distribution of the product, a promotional brochure announced, "Our research department has just released an Elixir Sulfanilamide [...] It is ideal for your patients who can take liquids—but little else. Also, it is not unpleasant to take, so is suitable for children."[14] Commercial shipments of Elixir Sulfanilamide continued through October 15th, the same date that Drs. Ruprecht and Nelson telegraphed their autopsy findings to *JAMA* and the same date that Massengill sent out his first recall telegrams.

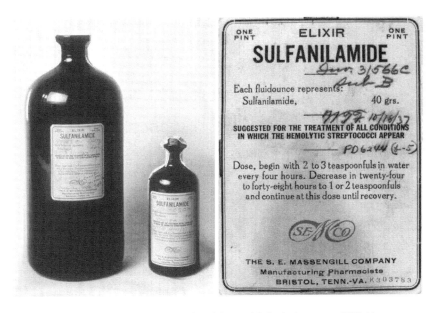

Bottles of Elixir Sulfanilamide and label close-up (FDA)

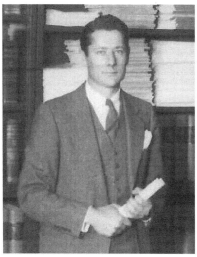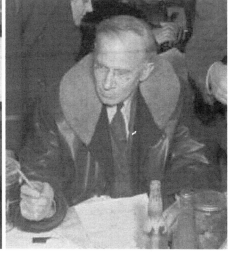

Left, Chief Medical Officer Theodore Klumpp, MD, c1940 (FDA);
Right, Chief Inspector William T. Ford, c1937 (FDA)

When the FDA received word of the Tulsa deaths, the agency's
Chief Medical Officer, Dr. Theodore "Ted" Klumpp, and Chief
Inspector William "Billy" T. Ford left immediately for Massengill's
headquarters.[15] There in Bristol, on Monday, October 18th, they found a
distressed company president, who offered his "full cooperation" to the
agents. But in his defense, Massengill claimed that he had done "all that
was humanly possible" to retrieve the at-large bottles of his sulfanilamide
elixir. He cited his recall telegrams of Friday, claiming that he had sent out
a total of 1,100 wires from the company's headquarters or its branch
offices.[16] He admitted to Klumpp and Ford that no toxicity tests, and
specifically no animal tests, were performed before the 240 gallons of
elixir were bottled for distribution. The product was merely referred to the
company's control laboratory, where it was assessed for its looks, aroma,
and palatability. Yet Massengill resisted the mounting evidence that
diethylene glycol was responsible for the Tulsa fatalities. Instead he
suggested that overuse of the antibiotic was to blame. "The drug
sulfanilamid[e] had been so exploited by physicians and the press that
everyone in the country was going wild with it and using it for everything
and now the disastrous effects of it were coming out," he pleaded.
Massengill also proposed that the adverse effects of his product were
caused by other drugs taken with it.

When they interviewed Watkins, Klumpp and Ford found
Massengill's chief chemist shockingly glib and cocksure. He blithely
described his previous compounding of a colloidal sulfur solution for

Massengill, which had caused "the sudden death of a number of people" until the sulfur content was halved.[17] The Harvard-educated Klumpp, typically a paragon of equanimity, was shocked: "Mr. Watkins told about this event as if it were an ordinary incident in the business of making and marketing pharmaceuticals," he wrote. Watkins also claimed that the company was importing and distributing a cinchophen-based analgesic, despite well-established evidence that the substance was toxic to the liver.[18] In response, an exasperated Klumpp lamented in his official report of the interview,

> It would seem that a great many drugs are being compounded and placed upon the American market without adequate testing. The expressed or implied attitude of certain drug manufacturers seems to be that drugs can be tested on the American public. If they fail to kill, or injure in such a way that the injury can be detected and traced to its source, the products have then met their trials successfully. The conclusion is inescapable that such drug manufacturers are perfectly willing to wait for reports of death or injury for information concerning the toxicity of their drugs.[19]

In a more succinct and graphic commentary to Hopkins physician Perrin Long, Klumpp later charged,

> [T]he only criteria of [Elixir Sulfanilamide's] safety and value as a medicine were that the ingredients were mixed, did not immediately explode, and the color, taste and smell of the product were satisfactory to their so-called control department.[20]

Watkins affirmed to Klumpp and Ford that no meaningful laboratory or animal tests were conducted on Elixir Sulfanilamide before its distribution. But the chemist hastened to add that "a few guinea pigs" were injected with the drug after reports of the Tulsa fatalities.[21] All of these animals were "perfectly well," Watkins declared to a suspect Klumpp. The chemist also boasted that, in the last few days, he had drunk a half-cup of diethylene glycol and "teaspoon doses" of the elixir itself. Instead of experiencing anuria after the self-experiment, Watkins claimed that, on the contrary, his urine production had actually increased. While Klumpp seriously doubted that Watkins had taken the poison in any form, he also suspected that, if the chemist's urine production had actually increased, it was probably the result of early diethylene-glycol poisoning (like the published effects of early dioxane poisoning). In his official report of the visit, Klumpp concluded that Watkins's act, regardless of its plausibility, was merely a token gesture. "Instead of properly testing the article prior to its distribution," Klumpp wrote, "the chemist attempts to attone [sic] for it by a display of heroics."

To his credit or obliviousness, Watkins claimed direct responsibility for "the origination of new products, the suitability of the formulas, and the control of methods of manufacture of both old and new products" at the Massengill company. He admitted that the formula for Elixir Sulfanilamide was his creation and asserted "scientific responsibility" for it (although other Massengill employees had mixed up most of the product for distribution). Details of the man who called himself accountable for Elixir Sulfanilamide are patchy and incomplete. During their interview with Watkins, Klumpp and Ford learned that the 57-year-old chemist obtained an undergraduate degree in pharmacy in 1901 from the University of Michigan.[22] While a student, Watkins received a research fellowship and shared the Ebert Prize of the American Pharmacists Association in 1902 and 1906 with a University of Michigan pharmacy professor for their chemical study of plants in the poppy family.[23]

Information from Klumpp's FDA report, Watkins's family history, public records, and alumni registries reveal that Watkins led a highly itinerant life after leaving college. Residences or employment are documented in Omaha, Nebraska (1903-1906), Portland, Maine (1906), New York City (1907-1908), Anacortes, Washington (1908-1910), Spokane, Washington (1910-1911), Vancouver, Washington (1911-1912), Portland, Oregon (1912), Ogden, Utah (1912-1913), Sacramento, California (1913-1917), and Brooklyn, New York (1917-1920). Watkins reportedly worked for one year (c1907) in the analytical department at Merck in New York City and for three years as an assistant chief chemist for the drug importer and wholesaler McKesson and Robbins in Brooklyn. Between that time, Watkins was "employed by various wholesale drug and pharmaceutical houses as a chemist," wrote Klumpp. Public records reveal that, in 1914 Watkins, at the age of 34, married a 23-year-old Norwegian immigrant in Oakland, California. Their first son was born the following year in Sacramento.

Apparently unknown to Klumpp and Ford was the fact that Watkins had been convicted of petty embezzlement in 1917. While working for a wholesale drug firm in Sacramento, Watkins pleaded guilty to stealing a platinum evaporating dish from his employer.[24] The stolen dish was sold by Watkins in November of 1916 to a local metal assayer for $85. (The assayer, in turn, sold the dish to a San Francisco outfit for nearly $200.) Watkins, while managing the firm's laboratory and analytical chemistry department, had become financially overextended due to his "very poor business ability," concluded the magistrate who presided over the criminal case. The chemist threw himself on the mercy of the court, presenting—

according to the case record—"quite a sad spectacle" as a "weak looking fellow" with his pregnant wife and "little baby boy" at his side. After pleading guilty, Watkins was committed to the custody of the county sheriff until the $3,000 bail was delivered. Through a letter-writing campaign to the probation officer, Watkins avoided jail time. Previous employers in Nebraska, Oregon, Washington, and Utah, who were surprised by Watkins's "troubles," uniformly praised the chemist's trustworthiness and previous work. They particularly noted his avoidance of alcohol and gambling. One employer exulted, "I regarded him as one of the cleanest, brightest chemists I ever knew, and predicted for him a very bright future, and cannot help but think that if given a chance he certainly would make good, even yet." Watkins was subsequently granted a five-year probation, which he may have promptly violated by moving to Brooklyn and finessing his way into McKesson and Robbins.[25]

In 1922, Watkins was living with his young family in Scranton, Pennsylvania, where his second son was born.[26] In Scranton, Watkins was employed by the Scranton Distributing Company, a supplier of patent and proprietary medicines.[27] Klumpp wrote that the company went defunct "following certain difficulties with the Federal Alcohol Administration" and that Watkins was involved in the troubles in some unspecified manner. According to a contemporaneous news report, the Internal Revenue Service shut down the company on March 16, 1921, charging that the firm was putting an excessive amount of alcohol into its health tonics.[28] Scranton city directories of 1924 and 1925 indicate that Watkins established his own business, the Watkins Products Company. He is absent from the 1926, 1927, and 1928 Scranton directories and then reappears in 1929, as president of Nature's Products, Inc. His listed residence was Fleetville, a country-road intersection about 15 miles north of Scranton. Around this time Watkins, as Watkins Laboratories, was caught peddling a weight-loss product to produce a "perfect slenderness" and a "trim, youthful athletic look." To avoid charges of mail fraud from the Solicitor of the Post Office, he agreed to stop selling the compound.[29]

Although the product was not identified in FDA reports, the dubious item was probably "Takoff," Watkins's name for a mail-order compound he advertised (as Nature's Products of Scranton) in the trade journal *American Druggist* in 1928.[30] The submitted announcement boasted,

Takoff is a new obesity treatment manufactured by Nature's Products, Inc., Scranton, Pa. It is said to have been thoroughly tested in a two year period on the Pacific Coast where it met with considerable success. It is the result of eight years of research by a leading Denver physician and contains no glands or other harmful products. A further novelty appeal is lent by its directions which require a user to eat three square meals a day. It is packaged in an attractive metal box lithoed in color and will be backed by national magazine and newspaper advertising as well as a policy of no free goods, no private agreements or price cutting. It will retail at $2 and $5, trade prices to be $16 and $40. Samples and particulars on request.[31]

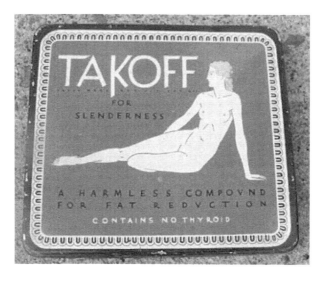

Photograph of a tin for "Takoff" from Nature's Products of Scranton, PA (Courtesy of Barb Lesniewski, Country Lady Antiques)

In February of 1929, Watkins placed advertisements for a weight-loss formula in newspapers, presumably at his own cost. The ads touted, "EAT WHAT YOU LIKE," with the following caveat:

This would be fine and has been recommended but many when they follow this advice get headaches, pains or gas, heartburn, sour stomach, or a tired feeling which shows that their stomach is not acting as it should and needs help. If you have any of these troubles write Harold C. Watkins, Box 298, Scranton, Pa., for information about a formula worked out by a chemist and used for 17 years with amazing success in such cases.[32]

Another advertisement from Nature's Products, in the March 1929 issue of *Motion Picture* magazine, promoted Takoff by barking the headline, "Reduce Without Risk, Without Diet, Without Exercise."[33]

Moreover $10,000 "in cash" was offered to "anyone proving that Takoff contains thyroid or any other harmful substance." The "magical formula" was purportedly a "harmless vegetable compound" created by a Hollywood physician. A five-to-eight-pound weight loss was promised with a $2, nine-day, mail-order treatment.

According to the 1930 US census, Watkins was living with his wife and two sons in the tiny rural township of Benton, Pennsylvania, in Lackawanna County, about 16 miles north of Scranton. In the public record, his occupation appears to have been originally recorded as "chemist" and then overwritten with "farmer." Watkins's sources of income during the early 1930s are unclear. In the Scranton city directory of 1930, he is listed as a chemist with the Smo-Ko Company, a maker of tobaccoless cigarettes. The cigarettes were hawked by the firm as a remedy for colds and other respiratory ailments. University of Michigan alumni directories and registrar files indicate that Watkins moved his family at least two more times before landing in Bristol, Tennessee. In 1932, he provided an address in Rahway, New Jersey; the following year, he submitted two different addresses in Seymour, Indiana (about 60 miles south of Indianapolis). According to Klumpp, Watkins was "idle part of the time" during the early 1930s, although he held "a number of small jobs."[34]

In 1935, after 32 years in at least 13 different locations at an unknown number of jobs across the country, Watkins relocated to Bristol, where he began his employment with The S. E. Massengill Company. Per the firm's policy, Dr. Massengill would have personally interviewed Watkins before he could be hired; although it is extremely unlikely that Massengill ever knew of Watkins's criminal record in Sacramento or his run-in with the federal government in Scranton. The chemist probably traded in on his respectable education and a few, select recommendations to gain employment. Watkins's responsibilities as chief chemist with the Massengill company were "to examine labels, criticize formulas, and search out, test and recommend new formulas."[35] Within the company, he was regarded as "a reputable pharmacist." Consequently it was "the natural inclination [...] to rely upon such a man," Chief Counsel DeFriece later offered. Watkins's position within the Massengill firm was one he appeared to be proud of, as evidenced by his somewhat curious offer of a business card to Klumpp at the October 18th interview.

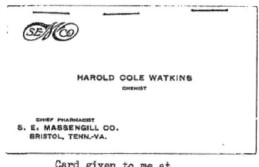

Card given to me at
interview by Mr. H. C. Watkins
in the office of Dr. S. E.
Massengill - Bristol, Tenn.
Oct. 18, 1937

 An examination of the early, Dickensian life of Harold Cole Watkins may explain his character and specifically his gypsy-like existence as an adult. Born January 25, 1880, in the bucolic and progressive village of Paris, Maine, Watkins was the first child of George Watkins, the "tireless" publisher of the county newspaper, the *Oxford Democrat*, and Annah Cole Watkins, the youngest daughter of a local judge.[36] The union of George and Annah produced two more children in quick succession: Mabel Russell was born in 1881; Edith May, in 1882. However, the young family was short lived. Annah died of consumption in 1883, when Harold was three years of age. The following year, his toddler sister Mabel died, also of tuberculosis.

 In February of 1885, George, at the age of 31, married the daughter of a local merchant. It was the same year that he sold the *Oxford Democrat* and moved with his second wife and two children to Portland, Maine, about 50 miles south-southeast of Paris. George became a partner in a printing and publishing firm in the coastal city, and his wife reportedly tried to make a pleasant new home for her young stepchildren. However, the woman was sickly, possibly suffering from tuberculosis as well, and she died in childbirth (along with her infant) 21 months after her wedding. Harold was six years old.

 After the death of Harold's stepmother, four-year-old Edith, who was frail by family accounts (possibly also due to tuberculosis), was sent to live with the family of her father's cousin, Dr. Alden Bessey, in the town of Sidney, Maine. It was believed that the physician's medical expertise and the rural air would sustain the girl's health to greater advantage than the Portland climate. For a short time, Harold remained with his father in Portland, where both boarded with a local family. But by the end of 1887, Harold, too, was sent to live in Sidney, about 70 miles northeast of

Portland, with the family of a farmer whom he had never met. How this particular arrangement came about is unclear.[37] While living in Sidney, Harold and Edith were able to see each other periodically, and their father wrote to them regularly, according to family history. On the occasions that George visited his children, he would travel 55 miles by train from Portland to Augusta, Maine; from there, he would hire a buggy to cover the remaining 15 miles or so to Sidney.

Four years after the death of his second wife, George prepared to marry again, this time to the oldest daughter of a Scottish sea captain. But in a jarring turn of events, George, who had been "troubled for some time past with a cough," was found dead in a Portland hotel bed on the evening of his scheduled wedding date, March 6, 1890. Death was apparently spontaneous and due to a massive pulmonary or gastric hemorrhage. Local reports of the event suggest that 10-year-old Harold and seven-year-old Edith were with their paternal grandparents in Paris, Maine, at the time; although family history implies they were in Portland for their father's third wedding. Regardless it was in Paris, according to the *Oxford Democrat* obituary for George, where the children viewed their father's corpse on its arrival for burial.[38]

Consequently in the first 10 years of his life, Harold Cole Watkins endured the deaths of his mother, a sister, his stepmother, a newborn half-sibling, and his father. Probate and other records indicate that, after their father's death, Harold and his sister were taken in by their cousin, Dr. Bessey. County records also reveal that Harold and Edith inherited a little more than $3,200 from their parent's estates, about half of which was consumed by property taxes and previously expended support for the children. The remainder of the inheritance was placed in the hands of their permanent guardian, Dr. Bessey. He was by reputation a highly devout Christian who, by all appearances, proceeded to use the funds reliably for Harold's and Edith's upbringing. With his newly blended family—consisting of a second wife, two sons by a first marriage, a daughter by a second marriage, and Harold and Edith—Dr. Bessey moved to Waterville, Maine. About 10 miles northeast of Sidney on the Kennebec River, Waterville was a busy, pleasant mill town and, to its credit, a growing educational center. For his secondary schooling, Harold attended Waterville High School, graduating at the age of 17.[39] Dr. Bessey, either by example or actively, probably encouraged Harold to pursue a medically related career. Harold may have also been influenced by Dr. Bessey's two sons, both of whom became physicians. After graduating from high school, Harold worked for two years as a clerk for H. H. Hay & Sons, a drugstore in Portland. At 19, Harold traveled 900 miles west to attend the University of Michigan School of Pharmacy in Ann Arbor.

A diligent search of school records and newspaper articles reveals a single photograph of Harold Cole Watkins, at the approximate age of 17. According to his World War I registration card, Watkins at 38 was "tall" and "slender" and had light brown hair and blue eyes. Family photographs from the late 1910s or early 1920s (shared with the author) reveal a man of medium-to-slight build who appeared to be well below six feet in height. (According to family history, Harold's father was a "small, slight man.") Watkins, in his late 30s or early 40s, had a full crown of dark, straight hair, parted rakishly on the side and combed forward. He routinely wore pince-nez glasses and sported a full mustache. Family photographs also suggest that Watkins was a proud and doting father.

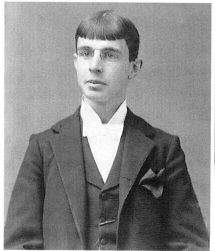 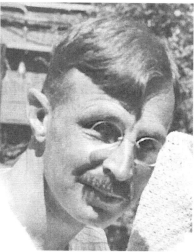

Left, Senior high school portrait of Harold Cole Watkins, c1897 (Courtesy of the Waterville High School library); Right, Harold Cole Watkins, c1920 (© 2014 David C. Larsen. All rights reserved)

To complement the photographs of Watkins, a character portrait was provided by his sister, Edith, in 1917. In a letter to Watkins's probation officer in Sacramento, she pleaded her brother's unfortunate history as an orphan and the fact that he was "dumped into a big family," where he did not receive the care and attention he needed as an adolescent. Edith described her brother as a "sensitive boy," who "took things in a harder way than the reprimands were intended." Consequently her brother "got a habit of retreating into himself and became selfish," she wrote. Edith entreated,

[F]or really I can't believe he is criminally bad, [although] I do think he is impulsively inclined and needs oversight just now until he has learned better self-control, and you could easily guide him for I suppose [...] he is a "weak man."

* * * * * *

When Klumpp and Ford finished interviewing Massengill and Watkins, Ford stayed behind "indefinitely" in Bristol to oversee the recall of Elixir Sulfanilamide.[10] The veteran FDA agent thought it would be necessary to personally account for all seizures, so that he could "refrain from bringing pressure on the manufacturer to hasten return of such lots." The FDA's district chiefs were instructed to advise Ford of all nationwide seizures and "informal" disposals of Massengill's elixir (like flushing it down the toilet). To expedite the recall, Ford first had to coax Massengill to send out more explicit telegrams, conveying the lethal nature of Elixir Sulfanilamide. Follow-up wires sent on October 19th to the company's branches and commercial clients now included the phrase, "PRODUCT MAY BE DANGEROUS TO LIFE."[11] A particularly vexing issue, however, was accounting for the hundreds of salesmen's and physicians' samples in circulation. In a telegram to District Chief Jimmie Clarke, Ford expressed several days' frustration in his attempt to get at least a partial list of salesmen and a nod from "the old boy" Massengill to send follow-up wires to them. The job apparently required Ford, not a young man himself at the age of 63, to hotfoot it around Bristol, checking out the town's various watering holes. He finally wired his success, albeit in an overtly peeved state:

Dear Mr. Clarke:

Here is your list of salesmen out of Bristol + copy of [the follow-up recall] wire.

Had some job finding the old boy around town, & a worse one inducing him to send wires—guess he was trying to drown his troubles—& at least 2 sheets in the wind.

He was in no condition to supervise the sending of 61 telegrams. So yours truly did it for him, getting him to O.K. the charge to W[estern] U[nion].

Hostily

W. T. F[ord]

As told you over the phone, will see Monday [October 25th], when heads of that Dpt. get back to town, if they really know what they did with the 1 oz. physician samples. Each salesman (including all branches) got a 2 oz. case sample.[12]

An added headache for Ford was the revelation, after direct questioning, that several other Massengill products contained glycols, including ethylene glycol.[13] These products were indicated for a range of conditions but were apparently not *primarily* intended for oral consumption. Nevertheless Ford was appropriately concerned about their shipment and use. When Ford confronted Massengill, he encountered hesitant cooperation. "Massengill did not exactly refuse to list shipments," Ford relayed, "but said he would prefer not to, 'because your inspectors will run all around to our customers, frighten them, and hurt our business.'" Ford was also skeptical that a complete list of glycol-containing drugs had been provided, despite assurances from Watkins. The wary inspector, also a pharmacist by training, advised, "I have been biding my time and attempting to trip him on it, and may before I finish or get the facts some other way." Ford's chief priority was, however, to obtain the names and locations of elixir consignees by negotiating the voluntary cooperation of Massengill's clerical force. Federal law did not obligate the company president to share his shipping records with the FDA.[14]

7
A TECHNICAL AND TRIVIAL CHARGE OF MISBRANDING

Although The S. E. Massengill Company attempted to recall Elixir Sulfanilamide through its less-than-candid telegrams and then FDA-fortified wires, the government did not rely solely on these efforts. Chief Campbell jumpstarted the agency's seizure of the liquid sulfanilamide—a process that nevertheless required considerable cooperation from Massengill, given what little government agents could do under existing law. It was sufficiently tricky to merely justify a legal confiscation. On October 19th, Campbell informed the Associated Press that, because of the "present inadequate Federal law," seizure of the product would have to be based in part on "a technical and trivial charge of misbranding."[1] By Campbell's understanding and inference, an elixir should contain alcohol; on the basis of information from the Massengill company and the AMA's laboratory analysis, Elixir Sulfanilamide did not.

On Wednesday, October 20th, the US attorney for the Northern District of Oklahoma filed a libel "praying seizure and condemnation of 1 gallon of elixir sulfanilamide at Tulsa."[2] The libel was a required step in the government's confiscation of a dangerous drug. Interstate shipping of Elixir Sulfanilamide from Massengill's Kansas City branch to Oklahoma constituted a violation of the Food and Drugs Act, the government alleged, because the product was adulterated and misbranded. The US attorney's rationale for the official seizure was slightly different from that of Campbell (specifically Campbell's interpretation of misbranding, as reported by the press). The product was *adulterated* (not misbranded), the US attorney argued, because "its purity fell below the professed standard under which it was sold [...] since it was not an elixir of sulfanilamide but was a solution of sulfanilamide in a mixture of diethylene glycol and water." On the other hand, the product was *misbranded* because the "'Quality Pharmaceuticals' sticker was false and misleading when applied to an article consisting of a solution of sulfanilamide in diluted diethylene glycol." Furthermore, the attorney loosely argued, the "label gave the firm address as Bristol, Tenn.-Va.; whereas it had been manufactured at Kansas City, Mo."

But the government's rationale for seizing Massengill's product on the basis of the definition of "elixir" was highly debatable, and Massengill would later contest this point. The Food and Drugs Act, remarkable for its brevity, did not spell out such granular information. Contemporaneous professional sources defined an elixir as an aromatically flavored syrup containing about 25% alcohol[3]; however, other sources merely described "elixir" as a liquid medication. In addition, there were "non-alcoholic" elixirs that substituted glycerin for alcohol.[4] The latest version of the *National Formulary* provided recipes for 54 elixirs, 52 of which contained alcohol (from 3% to 78% by volume).[5] The exceptions: an aqueous elixir containing glycerin, and an elixir of chloral hydrate and potassium bromide made with distilled water.

Evidently drawing on this uncertainty, the AMA publicly undermined the government's rationale for seizing Massengill's Elixir Sulfanilamide. An anonymous editorialist in *JAMA*, presumably Dr. Fishbein, acknowledged the ambiguity of the term "elixir," writing that the definition "has undergone some changes in the practice of pharmacy," with the use of solvents like glycerin instead of alcohol.[6] Furthermore, the editorialist claimed, there was no legal definition of the term and urged the US Pharmacopeia or "some group with legal power" to define the word in practice. One can imagine Campbell's irritation at the medical journal and, by extension, the ever-intrusive Fishbein, particularly on this point. Regardless of the FDA's legal footing, however, the agency chief pressed on with the confiscation. Campbell wanted a tally of every last ounce of Massengill's poisonous Elixir Sulfanilamide.

A "pugnacious Kentucky lawyer," as *Time* magazine described him, Campbell began his lengthy civil service career in 1906 at the age of 29.[7] He was personally selected by the Bureau of Chemistry's controversial chief and media hound, Dr. Harvey Wiley, to organize and manage the men who were newly hired to enforce the Food and Drugs Act of 1906. Despite Wiley's preoccupation with administrative politics and his own publicity, he perceived Campbell's intuitive leadership skills, which overrode the fact that Campbell had not performed as well as others on the required two-day civil-service examination. Campbell, or "Wat," as he was known to his friends, also had brief experience enforcing the comparatively rigorous food and drug law of his native state.[8]

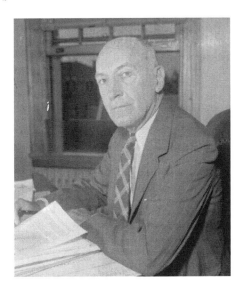

FDA Chief Walter G. Campbell, c1939
(Library of Congress, Harris & Ewing Collection)

Early accounts of the Bureau of Chemistry, the forerunner of the FDA, indicate that Campbell was a fan of results over bureaucracy. He organized a highly flexible team of food and drug inspectors and fostered investigative tactics that, at times, required ingenuity, if not outright trickery. (Other than requiring a court-ordered libel of condemnation, the Food and Drugs Act of 1906 was actually mum on exactly how food and drug inspectors could enter a commercial establishment to seize its goods and exactly how merchants were obliged to cooperate.) Likewise Campbell did not advocate strict rules about an inspector's appearance, but the "very well dressed" lawyer promoted, by example, sartorial neatness. It was a mimicked quality that likely increased the odds that an FDA agent could access company property in an official capacity. At the very least, smart attire gave the appearance of government authority, if the agency did not have it in crystalline law.

Initially the Bureau of Chemistry concentrated its investigative efforts on tainted or substandard food, while comparatively little attention was paid to drugs. The Bureau's partiality to food enforcement has largely been attributed to Chief Wiley's preferences, but a Supreme Court decision in 1911 also undermined the government's power to enforce the 1906 law, or at least the spirit of it, with respect to drug marketing. In

1910, the Department of Agriculture, in *US v Johnson*, brought misbranding charges against the Dr. Johnson Remedy Company of Kansas City, Missouri.[9] The company promoted a combination of sugar pills, alcoholic solutions, and petroleum ointments as "Dr. Johnson's Mild Combination Treatment for Cancer." In addition, the products' labels read, "Complies With the Food and Drug[s] Act, June 30th, 1906," a stinging claim that likely forced the government's hand to pursue legal action. The company vigorously defended itself through appeal, however, and the high court essentially agreed with the company. The Food and Drugs Act was not violated, the ultimate court ruled in a divided decision, because the law applied only to false claims about a drug's ingredients, not to false therapeutic claims. In other words, a drug manufacturer could write on the product's label that the active ingredients cured any number of ailments, even cancer, so long as the ingredients were accurately printed. Follow-up legislation, specifically the Sherley Amendment of 1912, attempted to shore up the breach[10]; however, this amendment required that the government prove fraudulent intent on the part of the drug manufacturer—a difficult, if not impossible, standard. Also the Bureau could not pursue therapeutic claims made outside of a product's label. Drug advertising was the purview of the Federal Trade Commission (FTC), not the Bureau of Chemistry. And the FTC was severely restricted in its ability to prove fraudulent marketing, according to a 1931 Supreme Court decision. In the case of *FTC v Raladam Company*, the high court ruled that the government had to demonstrate injuries to competing firms on the basis of an unfair marketplace.[11]

Exceptionally well-liked and respected, Campbell rapidly ascended the Bureau ladder, but he accepted his promotions modestly and often reluctantly. Campbell was ever mindful of the fact that he was not a scientist, and he wanted to avoid resentment in the chemist-dominated organization. In 1914, he was appointed chief of the Bureau's Eastern District, and in 1917, he became assistant chief of the entire organization. Campbell refused to helm the agency in 1921. (Wiley had resigned from the Bureau under pressure in 1912, owing to administrative and political differences within the Department of Agriculture.)[12] Instead Campbell accepted the qualified title of acting chief, until a permanent replacement could be found.[13] But finally in 1927, he was persuaded to lead the Department of Agriculture's newly established Food, Drug, and Insecticide Administration, which became simply, in 1930, the Food and Drug Administration. Campbell's rise to the top of the regulatory group paralleled his ever-growing frustration with the 20-year-old Food and Drugs Act.

Campbell got his chance to complain publicly about the law's inadequacies in 1930. When called before Congress to answer allegations that the FDA had allowed the trade of substandard drugs, Campbell countered, "I am hopeful that the time will come when the regulation of the traffic in food and drug products will be by the terms of a license statute rather than by the terms of a law that has no more power and no more teeth than are to be found in the present food and drugs act."[14] To boot, enforcement of the anemic law was undermined by the FDA's limited manpower. While the agency had 234 "scientific employees" at the time, only 61 were designated as inspectors, and they were charged with surveying up to 50,000 drugs on the American market.

Campbell provided considerable input into a 1933 bill that was officially drafted by Rexford Tugwell, then-Assistant Secretary of Agriculture, and backed by physician Royal S. Copeland, a Senate Democrat from New York.[15] The bill, S. 1944 (also known as the Tugwell-Copeland bill), was designed to 1) remove the government's burden of proving a drugmaker's fraudulent intent; 2) widen the definition of misbranding to include therapeutic claims; and 3) loosen the definition of adulteration to include drugs that were dangerous (when used according to printed directions). Campbell, through the FDA, led a concerted publicity campaign to promote the bill, specifically through the agency's notorious "Chamber of Horrors" exhibit. The exhibit was a popular, traveling display of the most egregious drugs on the US market—like Crazy Water Crystals, a salt laxative advertised as a cure-all; Koremlu cream, a thallium-containing depilatory; Marmola, a weight-loss tablet with desiccated thyroid; and Radithor, a tonic of distilled water and radium isotopes.[16] However, the FDA campaign was ultimately quashed by charges that the agency was violating the Deficiency Appropriation Act of 1919. The law prevented government agencies from lobbying their causes to Congress. Consequently the FDA's campaign was silenced, and opposition to new drug legislation gained steam.

Follow-up bills made substantial concessions to industry and were particularly lenient about false advertising. Campbell found them distasteful, but the FDA chief was also a realist. Major compromises would have to be made, he conceded, if a new law were ever to become reality. One particular flash point was the control of drug advertising. The FDA and the FTC each justified exclusive control, and congressional views were informed by political ties to one agency or the other. A powder-keg disagreement on the issue killed yet another drug-reform bill in the summer of 1936, and a persistent dispute on the subject held a similar bill in limbo when Massengill's elixir hit the market.[17]

* * * * * *

The large, headache-inducing job of taking Elixir Sulfanilamide out of
the hands of consumers was forecasted by the FDA's quick inventory at
Massengill's distribution center in Kansas City, Missouri (which happened
to be Tulsa's elixir source). On October 18th, the acting chief of the
FDA's Kansas City branch, Leo Cramer, reported that a little more than
four gallons were on hand of the 40 produced there and another five-and-
a-half gallons that had been shipped from Bristol.[18] The bulk of the
remainder had been sent out as commercial packages from Massengill's
Kansas City warehouse to scores of wholesalers, retail druggists, or other
consignees in a total of 10 states: North Dakota, Minnesota, Wisconsin,
Iowa, Illinois, Missouri, Kansas, Oklahoma, Arkansas, and Texas. In
addition, hundreds of ounce-sized samples had been shipped directly
from Kansas City to Massengill's salesmen for their at-will disposal.[19]
Massengill's initial recall telegrams of October 15th, Cramer learned, had
prompted the return of 27 unopened pint bottles, 21 opened pint bottles
(some of which contained as little as four ounces), and a one-gallon bottle
that was about five-sixths full. In the best possible light, the hasty tally
meant that more than 36 gallons of Elixir Sulfanilamide were still at large,
not counting the salesmen's samples. After the distressing inventory,
Massengill's local production manager told Cramer that, if the elixir had
indeed caused harm, it was due to either "improper dispensing" or the
simultaneous use of other drugs.

The FDA's inventory at Massengill's San Francisco branch was
slightly less ominous. Of the 30 gallons (in pint, gallon, and sample bottles)
shipped from Bristol, more than four gallons had been distributed
regionally as commercial packages between September 23rd and October
13th. Shipments, most in pint-sized bottles, were scattered among two
physicians' offices, one hospital, and more than a dozen pharmacies.
Some of the shipments in California had gone to nearby Oakland, but
most were dispersed, in seemingly random fashion, among small towns in
the middle of the state. In addition, two pints each had been shipped to
Meeker, Colorado, and Eugene, Oregon. By the morning of October
19th, the FDA learned that only two, one-pint bottles had been returned
from drug stores.[20]

In New York, FDA inspectors first showed up to Massengill's
Greenwich Village warehouse in the late afternoon hours of October 18th.
The branch manager, Athel Price, was initially, if only superficially,
cooperative. He admitted knowledge of the elixir recall, but he claimed
that he did not know the reason. Before closing hours, the visiting agents
were allowed a cursory interview with Price, who professed that his entire
stock of Elixir Sulfanilamide "had already been returned to the home

office." However, when the agents followed up the next morning to check the branch's shipping records, Price resisted further inspection, and the FDA men had no explicit authority to examine the company's ledgers. Price's obstinacy could only be broken by a personal telegram from Dr. Massengill that morning ("GIVE GOVERNMENT AGENTS FULL INFORMATION DO NOT CONCEAL ANY FACT"), but not before city health inspectors—who, by this time, were also on the scene—had lost their patience. As payback for Price's stalling, the city officials confiscated not only the remaining elixir at Massengill's New York warehouse, but all of the company's sulfanilamide formulations, including its tablets. When Price asked an FDA inspector to intervene, the government man shrugged at the city's strong-arm tactics. He could only honor the independence of the two regulatory bodies, he offered—probably with some level of veiled satisfaction. The FDA men were then able to discover that, of the more than eight gallons of elixir that had been sent from Bristol to New York, 15 pints (in 10 shipments) had been distributed between September 19th and October 11th throughout New York State, Connecticut, and Pennsylvania.[21] In addition, six pint bottles had been sent from New York to a company distributor in Puerto Rico, and all of the 30 one-ounce samples had been given out to regional salesmen. The FDA's initial inventory therefore revealed that nearly 23 pints (almost three gallons) of Massengill's elixir remained available within New York's distribution area.

Yet most of Massengill's elixir had been sent out from the company's Bristol headquarters, where Inspector Ford discovered, with the ultimate help of Massengill's clerical force, that more than 400 shipments had been sent directly to consignees.[22] These commercial packages, representing more than 110 gallons, were dispersed among 15 states, from Michigan to Florida; but most of the shipments were concentrated in the Deep South, specifically Mississippi, Alabama, and Georgia. Bristol was also the direct source of hundreds of distributed samples, representing about two-and-a-half gallons.[23] Consequently the FDA's first pressured inventories revealed possibly, if not probably, that more than 150 gallons of Massengill's product remained available for public consumption within 31 states and Puerto Rico. About 26 ounces had killed 10 people in Tulsa including, now, Earl Beard. The 25-year-old had died in a local hospital on October 16th after consuming about five ounces of an eight-ounce prescription as treatment for gonorrhea. He had been ill for a week.[24] If the Tulsa experience was any indication, Massengill's at-large elixir had the potential to wipe out thousands.

* * * * * *

The critical job of retrieving Elixir Sulfanilamide was hindered by the limited forms of mass communication in 1937. At the time, there were two major outlets, radio and newspapers, and radio was certainly the more promising method for transmitting swift warnings to the American public. The vast majority of US families, 82%, owned at least one radio set in 1937,[25] and Dr. Fishbein attempted to exploit the medium on October 18th by prereleasing *JAMA*'s editorial warning over the airwaves. But radio ownership in the United States was geographically uneven and tied to income. In New England and the Pacific Coast states, more than 95% of families owned radios. In the US South, however, where a large percentage of Massengill's elixir was distributed, ownership rates were much lower. Less than 60% of families in some southern states owned radios. In Mississippi, only 42% of families had radios, and ownership was even lower among African Americans. Moreover the use of radios in rural America (unless families owned battery-operated radios) was limited by the meager electrification of farmlands in the 1930s.

For those citizens with access, newspapers represented an important, supporting medium for conveying the dangers of Elixir Sulfanilamide. Yet many newspaper editors, for unclear reasons, did not view the elixir story as front-page news, at least not initially. During the week of October 18th, news of the elixir-related deaths and the wide distribution of Massengill's poisonous drug were trumped by ongoing, international events—namely the Spanish Civil War, the escalating conflict between China and Japan, and the travels of the Duke and Duchess of Windsor to meet Hitler. Domestic reports focused on the crash of a passenger plane in Utah, yet another selling wave in the stock market, and the kidnapping of a greeting-card magnate in Chicago. When attention was given to the elixir story, publishers were apparently reluctant to provide or chase down important details, and they relied, in many cases almost completely, on wire services. On October 19th, papers like the *New York Times* and the *Washington Post* tucked wire stories on inside pages and gave readers only general descriptions of the product, like a "new preparation" from a "Tennessee firm."[26] Perhaps fearing libel charges, news editors were evidently loathe to name names or print photographs of Massengill's elixir bottles to aid identification of the product. Early news reports also incorrectly focused on the potential dangers of sulfanilamide or spoke in unhelpful generalities like, "Think Medicine Causes Deaths."[27] To add to the public's confusion, some papers chased the breaking wire copy of Fishbein's warning with an evasive and disingenuous rebuttal from Massengill: "We are not sure what there is about the compound that is deadly," the company president hedged, "[a]nd neither does the medical association know positively."[28]

In Massengill's hometown, newspapers were vague to the point of deceit. On October 19th, the *Bristol News Bulletin* merely warned against the indiscriminate use of sulfanilamide with the headline, "Strong Drug Is Recalled," and the subhead, "Sulfanilamide Valuable But Not To Be Used Without Prescription," which was followed by a three-paragraph, below-the-fold wire story of Fishbein's warning.[29] The paper failed to mention Massengill, his company, or the elixir by name. "Dr. Fishbein said the preparation in question was only recently placed on the market by one firm," couched the severely truncated write-up. A sister paper, the *Bristol Herald Courier*, did not begin covering the story until days later and also failed to identify the drug's manufacturer when reprinting curtailed wire dispatches. Both papers were owned and published by Charles Harkrader, who oversaw two other area newspapers.[30] The local publisher was the older brother of Rhea Harkrader, the Bristol teenager previously hired by Massengill to run his company's first tablet press. The historical and neighborly bond between Massengill and the Harkrader family likely informed the very tight-lipped coverage of the Elixir Sulfanilamide story in Massengill's backyard.

Consequently to ensure the removal of Massengill's elixir from the market, a massive and far-reaching footwork campaign by the FDA's Field Inspection Service was necessary. All of the elixir shipments from Bristol, Kansas City, San Francisco, and New York had to be traced to their several hundred consignees: wholesalers, retail druggists, physicians, and hospitals scattered among 31 states and Puerto Rico. To confound the FDA's physical seizure of Massengill's elixir, endpoints for many of these commercial shipments were tiny, otherwise-unheard-of settlements—like Wedowee, Alabama, and Doe Hill, Virginia. And all of these consignees, whether urban or rural, would have to be investigated for the dispensing of prescriptions or over-the-counter sales, which would then have to be traced to an unknown number of consumers. In addition, hundreds of distributed samples had to be located. Thus the successful confiscation of the entire volume of Elixir Sulfanilamide would require the voluntary and speedy cooperation of hundreds, if not thousands, of people. Not only did the government rely on the assistance of Massengill and his employees (including approximately 200 salesmen).[31] Numerous pharmacists, prescribing doctors, and treated patients would have to comply willingly and honestly, if only begrudgingly. Accounting for Elixir Sulfanilamide was no mean feat, and the doggedness of the FDA, under the direction of Campbell, to find and retrieve bottles and sample vials of Massengill's elixir cannot be overstated. To examine the federal effort is to appreciate the FDA's resolve to protect the American public. But the study is not confined to this point alone. It is also a revelation of 1930s medical care,

American poverty, and civil liberties (or popular notions thereof). As well, the study uncovers the timeless human traits of evasiveness and deceit. For the FDA agents who encountered such dissembling, their investigations would reveal more deaths.

* * * * * *

In Tulsa, Station Chief Hartigan and Junior Inspector Donaldson proceeded with their door-to-door confiscation of the elixir after learning that at least 33 residents had received prescriptions.[32] It was known, thanks to the FDA's coordinated work at Massengill's Kansas City branch, that a little more than four gallons had been distributed among eight city druggists, and Hartigan and Donaldson were then able to scrutinize pharmacists' files for potential victims, ostensibly on the basis of legal sanction from the local US attorney. The inspectors determined that half of these retail outfits had dispensed the elixir to consumers. One drug store had given out 24 prescriptions, including those for seven of the 10 deceased victims. Armed with the names of the elixir recipients, Hartigan and Donaldson spent a sleepless and "harrowing week" from October 15th to the 22nd, bearing "the grim tidings" as "they awoke families with their frantic knocks upon the doors."[33] During their home visits, the inspectors learned that most of the at-risk Tulsans had taken at least a portion of the elixir; in some cases, the entire prescription had been consumed. At least several of these consumers reported no ill effects whatsoever from the drug. And while a typical pattern was seen in the 10 known individuals who were terminally affected by Elixir Sulfanilamide, it was uncertain if the initial absence of symptoms in other patients precluded the chance of delayed effects. The plan in those cases, per 1930s medical care: observe and hope for the best.

When Hartigan and Donaldson interviewed the parents of the 10 deceased Tulsans, several families insisted on retaining the prescription bottles.[34] Jack King's mother bluntly stated to the FDA men that the elixir "killed my child." The remaining portion of the prescription, Mrs. King told Hartigan, was in the possession of her brother, a Tulsa attorney. When Hartigan interviewed the lawyer, he declared that "the circumstances could not be described as anything other than 'murder,'" and that he would hold the bottle "as evidence for a possible legal action."

Avoiding culpability, legal or otherwise, was apparently on the mind of Dr. Logan Spann. The 31-year-old was the treating physician of Joan Marlar, one of two children who had died at Tulsa's Morningside Hospital. Hartigan and Donaldson were initially perplexed in their investigation of this case. They could not find any record of a sulfanilamide prescription for the girl in their canvass of pharmacy files.

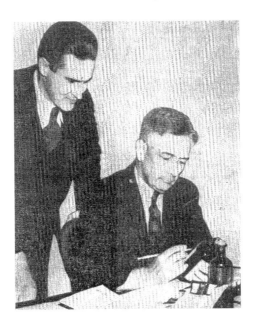

Junior Inspector Walter Donaldson (standing) and
Station Chief William Hartigan (seated)
(*Kansas City Journal-Post.* October 31, 1937)

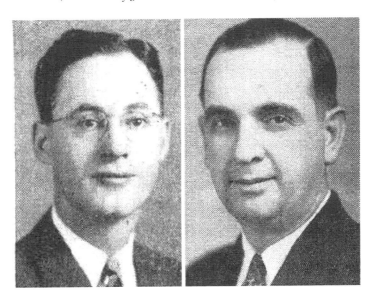

Left, Logan Spann, MD, c1953; Right, Pharmacist T. Roy Barnes, c1952
(Courtesy of the Tulsa County Medical Society)

Yet Joan's mother insisted to the agents that Dr. Spann had provided a prescription for Elixir Sulfanilamide for her daughter. Moreover she gave verifying details: The prescription had been dispensed on September 26th by the Getman Drug Store and cost one dollar. But Dr. Spann, when interrogated, flatly denied to Hartigan that he had written a prescription for Massengill's elixir.[35] The agents then revisited the Getman Drug Store to view the prescription files for September 26th. In the store's record book, the on-duty pharmacist and the proprietor, Roy Getman, were able to locate a prescription number, 121426, that, in fact, had been written by Dr. Spann; however, there was no copy of the actual prescription. Both men emphatically denied to the inspectors that they had removed the file. Hartigan recorded the ensuing events in his official report.

> Mr. Getman now with emotional alarm and consternation, drove us in his automobile to the home of T. Roy Barnes, another prescription pharmacist, employed at the Getman Drug Store. Mr. Getman in our presence questioned Mr. Barnes concerning the removal of prescription 121426 written by Dr. Spann from the prescription files. Mr. Barnes informed Mr. Getman that Dr. Spann had removed prescription 121426 from the prescription file.

> A hurried drive by Mr. Getman took us to the home of Dr. Spann. In the presence of Mr. Donaldson and Mr. Hartigan, Mr. Getman asked Dr. Spann if he removed prescription number 121426, dated September 26, 1937 for [Joan Marlar] from the file at the Getman Drug Store. Dr. Spann stated in reply, "He did not pull this prescription for Elixir Sulfanilamide out of file." Dr. Spann further states, "Mr. Barnes removed the prescription and gave it to me, and I threw it in the waste paper basket." Mr. Hartigan asked Dr. Spann if the prescription under investigation was for Elixir Sulfanilamide-Massengill. Dr. Spann said it was for Elixir Sulfanilamide in the amount of three ounces. Directions, One teaspoonful every four hours. The prescription was given over the telephone and was typewritten at the drug store.

> Mr. Hartigan forcefully inquired of Dr. Spann why he had lied, and lied, and conspired to obstruct the finding of facts by the inspectors in the investigation of deaths suspected of being caused by Elixir Sulfanilamide-Massengill. Dr. Spann walked away without making an answer.

Mr. Getman with the inspectors (Donaldson and Hartigan) made a second call at the home of Mr. Barnes. Mr. Getman recited to Mr. Barnes what Dr. Spann had stated.

Mr. Barnes, stated to Mr. Getman[:] Dr. Spann came into store, went to the prescription file, and asked Mr. Barnes for this prescription. Mr. Barnes was unable to recall the number from memory. Mr. Barnes admitted he pulled the prescription from the file and gave it to Dr. Spann. The last recollection he has is that Dr. Spann crumpled it up in his hand.

Mr. Hartigan told Mr. Barnes that although he had appeared to be an ethical pharmacist, and desirous of aiding the inspectors in the investigation of prescriptions written and dispensed for Elixir Sulfanilamide-Massengill, his actions as just disclosed, were detestable.

Hartigan did not record the date that Dr. Spann retrieved Joan Marlar's prescription record, but it can be deduced that the doctor attempted to alter the store's file sometime between Monday, October 11th, the date that Dr. Nelson presented his autopsy findings to the Tulsa County Medical Society, and October 22nd, the date that Spann was first interviewed by Hartigan.[36]

Mounting evidence in Tulsa further implicated Elixir Sulfanilamide as a poisonous product. On October 20th, autopsies performed by Drs. Nelson and Ruprecht on two of the medical society's experimental guinea pigs showed tell-tale findings. Pathologic changes in dysfunctional kidneys mirrored those of Tulsa's human victims.[37] Dr. Stevenson, the society president, nevertheless assured readers of the *Tulsa Tribune* that "there was no reason for further alarm"; sulfanilamide could only be distributed locally in tablet form, he promised.[38] In its in-depth coverage (in contradistinction to that of other newspapers), the city journal also highlighted the recovery of eight-year-old Jack Voorhees, whose convalescence from Elixir Sulfanilamide was attributed to aggressive oral hydration ("a gallon of water and two quarts of fruit juice" daily) and the fact that he never experienced complete anuria. The *Tribune* also confirmed rumors of deaths in the St. Louis area—information that was corroborated by Dr. Fishbein. "All the patients there were Negroes," the paper reported, "and were being treated by a Negro physician."

8
THE PRESCRIPTION WAS A LEGITIMATE ONE

Unaware of the Tulsa deaths, a young St. Louis pathologist sent his necropsy report to *JAMA* on October 19th. The doctor, Omer Hagebusch, "thought that this information should be in the hands of as many physicians as possible, and THE JOURNAL was the best means of accomplishing this end."[1] His dispatch:

> In the last several days I have seen four deaths in patients using a product called "Elixir of Sulfanilamide" and sold by Massengill & Company.

> These patients, all Negroes, were treated by a Dr. Weathers of East St. Louis, Ill. In all he has given the drug to about thirty people, but of the six people treated recently four are dead and have come to autopsy. One is expected to die at any time, and one may recover.

> All have had similar symptoms: vomiting and diarrhea, subnormal temperatures, slow respiration, anuria, edema of the face, hands and feet, a progressive anemia and then death.

> All four autopsies have shown the same findings [...]

Dr. Weathers's deceased patients were 26-year-old J. D. Kimbrough, a laborer; four-year-old Maurice Slaughter; five-year-old George Nixon; and 60-year-old Joseph Henry, a railroad switchman. The victims had died over the course of three days, from October 15th to the 18th, after each had drunk a few ounces of Elixir Sulfanilamide.[2] Weathers had prescribed

Massengill's product with the intention of curing a range of infections, and the elixir had been routinely compounded with other substances like phenolphthalein (a coal-tar laxative) and codeine.[3] Likewise Weathers had recommended the product in compounded solutions to 70-year-old Alexander Brooks and 38-year-old Gertrude Black, who—by the time of Hagebusch's autopsy report—showed signs of diethylene-glycol poisoning.

As information grew about Massengill's elixir and its consequences, it became evident that identifying vulnerable consumers was difficult, if not impossible. If Weathers's experience (as reported by Dr. Hagebusch) was any guide, about 20% of treated patients would experience fatal poisoning, given recommended dosages of the product.[4] Yet, despite the unpredictability of the elixir's effects, when symptoms of poisoning did emerge, they were consistent. Nausea and vomiting began either immediately or within a few days of consuming Massengill's drug. These symptoms were typically followed by backache and abdominal or flank pain. Often, but not invariably, urine output dropped; in all but a few cases, it ceased completely.

Like the prescribing doctors in Tulsa, the unsuspecting Weathers first attributed his patients' progressive conditions to unchecked infections. For instance, Weathers diagnosed J. D. Kimbrough with encephalitis, but the patient may have actually been suffering from uremic encephalopathy, a brain disorder due to uremia and the accumulation of unspecified toxins (which are otherwise cleared by functioning kidneys). An alternative explanation for Kimbrough's symptoms was the direct toxic effects of diethylene glycol on the nervous system, a phenomenon not well-recognized until the 21st century.[5] Belly pain was sufficiently prominent in a few elixir-consuming patients to suggest an "acute surgical abdomen"—a condition indicating internal crisis, like a ruptured appendix. According to Weathers, all of his terminal elixir-treated patients, including Alexander Brooks and Gertrude Black—who died on October 21st and 24th, respectively—"lapsed into a comatose condition and passed out quietly."[6] Their seemingly peaceful deaths contradicted, specifically, the torment of six-year-old Joan Marlar in Tulsa.

Thirty-four-year-old Henri Hudson Weathers, identified repeatedly in contemporaneous sources as a "Negro" or "colored" physician, maintained a busy medical practice in East St. Louis, where he served a largely African-American population.[7] The son of schoolteachers, Weathers was born in 1903 in Rolling Fork, Mississippi, the home of antebellum cotton fields along the Mississippi River flood plain. The time and place of Weathers's upbringing dictated that he become a sharecropper after completing a segregated primary-school education; however, Weathers's parents sent him 200 miles north to continue his secondary education in Memphis, Tennessee. From there, Weathers traveled to Nashville, where he enrolled in and graduated from Fisk University, a liberal arts college founded shortly after the Civil War for the higher education of freed slaves.

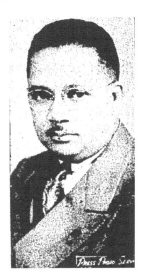

Henri H. Weathers, MD
(Press Photo Service; printed in the *Chicago Defender,* July 24, 1943)

For a young black American interested in medicine, there were two legitimate options in the 1920s: Howard University in Washington, DC, and Fisk's sister graduate school, Meharry Medical College. The very limited, accredited educational choices for aspiring doctors of color were a direct casualty of the reform of medical training in the early 20th century. Only decades earlier, the quality of US medical education varied widely. Nineteenth-century Americans who wished to practice medicine could obtain their training by apprenticeship; through a series of generally ad-hoc lectures at proprietary medical schools (in the style of Dr. Massengill's education); or at more rigorous, university-based medical colleges. The options produced a motley group of clinicians, ranging from the competent to the utterly dangerous. Although the AMA had attempted to standardize medical training for allopathic physicians a number of times during the second half of the 19th century, the movement did not gain public or political support until several scientific advances informed the practice of medicine. Chief among these were the newly recognized germ theory and the follow-up notion that the suppression of microorganisms, through hygiene and antisepsis, could prevent infectious diseases.

Encouraged by shifting public opinion, the AMA formed the Council on Medical Education in 1904 (the year before it created the Council on Pharmacy and Chemistry) and commissioned a survey of medical education in the United States from the Carnegie Foundation for the Advancement of Teaching. The results of the survey, contained in the historic Flexner Report of 1910, confirmed the highly variable quality of medical education and specifically condemned the training provided by proprietary schools.[8] The report's academic ideals were The Johns Hopkins School of Medicine and Harvard University, both of which stressed college-level premedical education and four years of scientifically based graduate training. Informed by a public duty to raise health standards, the Flexner Report motivated state licensing boards in the 1910s to implement uniform requirements for medical education. Obtaining a medical license became tied to the periodic grading of a graduate's medical school. In some states, a graduate was refused licensure if his school was graded lower than "A." The immediate result: a reduced, but comparatively elite, number of scientifically minded young doctors.

When Tulsa physicians Ivo Nelson and Homer Ruprecht, for instance, enrolled in their respective medical schools—the University of Oklahoma and Western Reserve University—in the early 1920s, admission specified premedical instruction at the college level.[9] Prospective matriculants had to take three semesters of chemistry (including the perennially dreaded organic chemistry), two semesters of physics, and two semesters of biology—requirements that have persisted, more or less, to this day. The reformed structure of medical curricula—two years of basic science classes, such as gross anatomy and microbiology, followed by two years of clinical instruction—has also endured. Nelson was one of 40 graduates in his medical class of 1926. Two years later, Ruprecht graduated with 58 classmates from Western Reserve.

To an even greater extent, the reform of medical education constrained the already very limited options for African Americans. Excepting Meharry and Howard, the Flexner Report all but damned the handful of black medical schools that existed at the time, and by extension, the survey didn't have much to say for black graduates. Nevertheless the report recognized the potential of Meharry and Howard and urged their development.[10] When Weathers enrolled in Meharry in the early 1920s, the financial stability of the school and its AMA grading were tenuous. However, fundraising efforts by Meharry's white president infused much-needed cash into the school's laboratory facilities and associated hospital,[11] and the school was able to advertise itself as a class "A" medical college with departments of medicine, dentistry, pharmacy, and nursing during Weathers's attendance. In further appeal to prospective students, the school boasted, "All departments recently organized," and stipulated that enrollees must have undergone at least two years of preparatory college-level work.[12]

After completing his medical education in 1927, Weathers had the option of applying for a postgraduate-training position at one of 12 "Negro Hospitals" approved by the AMA's Council on Medical Education and Hospitals to offer internships.[13] Among them was St. Louis No. 2, also known as the St. Louis City Negro Hospital, a 375-bed facility where Weathers elected to perform his internship and complete another three years of postgraduate work in surgery.[14] In 1931, Weathers then established a rapidly growing practice across the Mississippi River in East St. Louis, while maintaining clinical privileges at several black-only or segregated hospitals in the area. Along the way, he endured, like other African-American doctors, racially based exclusion from the AMA and its constituent state and county medical societies.[15]

In a two-column, page-three story, the *St. Louis Post-Dispatch* confirmed on October 19th that four elixir-related deaths had occurred in the area.[16] Weathers responded to the inquiring paper that he began prescribing Massengill's elixir eight days earlier (two days after Tulsa physicians first wired the AMA with their concerns). The doctor had already discussed his suspect cases with the FDA's St. Louis chief, Austin Lowe, the previous night.[17] Weathers told Lowe that he had visited all of his surviving elixir-consuming patients. Many had experienced "no bad effects whatever" from the elixir, and "in fact results in some cases were most gratifying," Weathers reported. The claim suggested that Massengill's antibiotic solution cured the infections of patients, when they were not adversely affected by diethylene glycol.

Lowe submitted the preliminary findings of his local investigation to Jimmie Clarke at the FDA's Central District office in Chicago.[18] Lowe discovered that, astonishingly, a representative of the city's medical association and officials at the Bureau of Vital Statistics were completely unaware of any deaths related to Massengill's elixir, despite the fact that Morris Fishbein had phoned the St. Louis Board of Health on the morning of October 18th to inquire about the rumored fatalities. Two agents from the health board specifically advised Lowe that "a careful review" of records dating back to October 1st showed "nothing that could possibly be of value." It was a highly unreliable claim, not only because of the known deaths of Dr. Weathers's patients, but because a sizable volume of Massengill's elixir had been distributed within the greater metropolitan area.

From Massengill's two local salesmen, Lowe learned that two-and-a-half gallons of elixir had been distributed among three physicians, three pharmacies, and one wholesaler in St. Louis.[19] More than seven gallons had been shipped to southern Illinois, with most lots distributed within East St. Louis. Massengill's reps were asked to retrieve what they could, but the detail men discovered that the St. Louis wholesaler, Meyers Brothers, had no bottles on hand. Although one pint had already been returned to Massengill's Kansas City branch, the remaining five pints had been sent out to local druggists. Officials at Meyers Brothers advised the reps that a search of their records to identify the recipients would be a "tremendous job." It would be easier to locate the bottles by surveying area drug stores, the company said. So while Massengill's two detail men searched for the outstanding product on foot, government agents began sifting through the company's 20,000 sales slips.[20]

These painstaking efforts led to the identification and early recovery of five pints of elixir from three pharmacies in East St. Louis and a pharmacy in Lovejoy, Illinois.[21] It was an important development, because it established another unequivocal chain of interstate commerce of Elixir Sulfanilamide: this time from Massengill's Kansas City branch to Meyers Brothers in St. Louis to drug stores in East St. Louis. Given evidence of elixir shipments from Missouri to Oklahoma and now to Illinois, where deaths had occurred as a direct result of drinking the antibiotic solution, the investigation was an undeniable federal matter. Station Chief Lowe officially documented the FDA's method for tracking down bottles of Massengill's elixir in southern Illinois. Phone warnings were coordinated with follow-up visits from field inspectors, as well as conscripted analysts and "laboratory helpers":

> All of our inspectors and analysts [...] were used for rapid coverage as possible. All station cars and personal cars of Messrs. McCarthy, Ahlmann, Field and Ahern were pressed into use. Laboratory helpers Allen and Meyers were used as drivers for analysts inexperienced in traffic. In addition I by phone reached most of the men in the Alton [Illinois] area and at other outlying points advising each to dispense no more of the product and to hold any lots on hand for our investigator who was enroute. We were thus able to cover practically all the primary consignees in our territory that day and early the next day.[22]

But Lowe and his FDA men also found that six druggists in East St. Louis had sold the elixir, in variable amounts, to eight additional retail pharmacies in Illinois. Nevertheless "[c]overage on these houses was also very rapid," the station chief assured his Chicago boss. Elixir found at the primary and secondary consignees was either destroyed or seized by the government. The FDA agents rapidly turned their attention to pharmacy records and discovered that at least 70 prescriptions for Massengill's elixir had been dispensed from 14 retail druggists and three doctors' offices in the greater metropolitan area.[23] Two East St. Louis pharmacies had dispensed the overwhelming bulk of these prescriptions (about 70%).

The difficulty of tracking down these prescriptions, most of which had been written by Dr. Weathers and another African-American doctor, was magnified by very limited pharmacy records. Dispensing data were casually recorded and woefully incomplete—revealing only a common name and maybe the patient's age. Time-pressured investigators were left to find "Willie Smith" or "Betty Jean 9 months old." In other cases, there was no identifying information whatsoever. Agents interrogated the prescribing doctors and dispensing pharmacists, often fruitlessly, for leads on vulnerable citizens and scoured post office records and relief rolls for clues. The FDA's determined efforts to locate consumers of Massengill's elixir and any remaining product are exemplified by the case of "Otis Jamieson," an otherwise unknown man who had received a four-ounce prescription for Elixir Sulfanilamide from an East St. Louis drug store. Without leads on Jamieson's location, FDA men identified and visited all local families with the same surname. Despite their cogent pursuit, the government agents could not find the elixir-consuming Otis Jamieson, and his fate was evidently never determined.

Yet the overwhelming majority of elixir recipients were located, and they "very gladly gave up these prescriptions," Lowe recorded. It was discovered that many of these patients had consumed some portion of the medicine without any adverse consequences, but that others had experienced recurrent nausea, which had led to the discontinuation of the product. This early side effect of diethylene-glycol poisoning may well have been a lifesaving one. The FDA also learned that some consumers had discarded the product at the instigation of their prescribing physician. But the agency was obliged to follow up to ensure the proper disposal of Massengill's elixir. In one case, a patient told a field agent that she had simply tossed a partially empty prescription bottle out of her window into a back alley. To mitigate any risk of harm to urban scavengers, the inspector was obliged to comb the backstreet, where he found the bottle intact, with a little more than one ounce of remaining liquid. Although a small amount, it was enough to kill in unpredictable fashion.

In St. Louis, the FDA found another errant ounce of Elixir Sulfanilamide in the hands of William Schroeder, a 50-year-old brewery employee. Schroeder's physician, Dr. Louis Murray, had dispensed six ounces of the product on October 14th as treatment for Schroeder's urethritis.[24] The prescribed treatment was from a one-gallon bottle that Murray had purchased directly from one of Massengill's local salesman on

October 13th (despite the fact that the Massengill company had already received a wired complaint from Tulsa about the product). Two days after starting the treatment, Schroeder was nauseated and in excruciating pain. Murray advised his patient to discontinue the product and proceed to the hospital, but Schroeder refused to go. The following day, October 17th, Murray received Massengill's first recall telegram. Two days later, a follow-up wire revealed the dangerous nature of the elixir. On October 21st, an FDA agent found Schroeder at home and attempted to confiscate the remaining ounce, but Schroeder also refused this request, stating that he wanted to keep the liquid drug for legal proceedings. Gravely ill with acute nephritis, Schroeder was finally taken on October 22nd to the city's Barnes Hospital, where he died two days later.

It is noteworthy that Massengill's two local salesmen willingly assisted the FDA's confiscation of outstanding bottles of Elixir Sulfanilamide within the metropolitan area, and Lowe recorded their essential help. The company's St. Louis rep, in particular, was "most cooperative" and "very reliable," wrote Lowe; however, the detail man also advised the FDA station chief that the deaths, if due to the company's product, resulted from "oxidation" of the substance on contact with the air. In an illogical attempt to bolster his argument, he added that the adverse effects only resulted when the drug was administered from one-gallon containers, and that "no illness has yet been traced to the pint bottles."[25] Whether the Massengill rep independently invented this explanation or was merely repeating one of many developing excuses for the elixir's effects from company headquarters is unknown. Regardless his argument was scientific nonsense and demonstrably false. While many of the deceased patients in Tulsa and the St. Louis area had had their elixir prescriptions filled from Massengill's one-gallon bottles, others had not. Dr. Weathers, an otherwise reserved man who did not court public attention, attempted to clarify where fault lay in no uncertain terms to the *Post-Dispatch* on October 21st. It was an exceptional, if not remarkable, act for a mainstream—that is, white—newspaper to quote the assertive claim of a resident black man in 1937, notwithstanding his professional status. Perhaps responding to Massengill's charge that the elixir's adverse effects were caused by the concurrent use of other drugs—for instance, in compounded formulations—Weathers declared:

> There has been an impression created that the error causing the East St. Louis deaths was made locally, either on my part or by the [...] East St. Louis drug stores filling the prescription, so I wish to point out that the prescription was a legitimate one and that the error, if any, was made by the [...] pharmaceutical company which prepared

the elixir. Sulfanilamide has been used extensively and successfully by physicians in other sections of the country.[26]

Nevertheless newspapers continued to misinform, and confusion about Elixir Sulfanilamide remained among the nation's physicians, despite published explanations from Weathers and, most important, Morris Fishbein. Drawing on unpublished data from ongoing animal studies at the University of Chicago, Fishbein told the Associated Press on October 19th, "[L]aboratory experiments made it quite evident that diethylene glycol, not sulfanilamide [...] was responsible for the deaths."[27] By contrast, Ohio's health director, perhaps attempting to explain the apparent absence of deaths in his state (to date), indicated that only certain lots of the product were accidentally tainted. "[I]t was entirely possible that physicians had been given contaminated shipments of the drug," he told a local paper, while citing the occasional "bad lots" of diphtheria and smallpox antitoxin.[28] Tennessee's state chemist, reporting from Nashville, wrongly informed the Associated Press on October 21st that the "manufacturer of this product inadvertently made a mistake in its preparation."[29]

But given that diethylene glycol was an intended and major ingredient in Massengill's product, an inquiry into recent, unexplained deaths in the St. Louis area was undertaken by local and FDA officials (despite assurances from the city health board that no suspect deaths had occurred that month). Among the FDA's identified victims was 23-year-old manicurist Hazel Fea, who had succumbed to a "mystifying" case of acute nephritis on October 10th at Barnes Hospital in St. Louis.[30] The coroner's initial presumption was that Fea had died after ingesting mercury bichloride. However, the FDA discovered that, about six days before her death, Fea began taking Massengill's elixir, which had been prescribed for an "abdominal ailment." Fea had received the liquid drug directly from her physician, Dr. Philip Dale of Granite City, Illinois, who had dispensed the product from one of Massengill's pint bottles. It was also discovered that Dr. Dale had given the elixir to three other patients, including his wife, all of whom had suffered "no ill effects."

News of more elixir-related fatalities trickled in from outside Lowe's territory, including Massengill's home state. On October 21st, the *St. Louis Post-Dispatch* printed a one-sentence notice of the death of C. W. Miller, a gas-station attendant in Memphis.[31] The local paper, the *Commercial Appeal*, provided more in-depth coverage of the married 25-year-old and how he had obtained the fatal drug without a doctor's prescription.

Mr. Miller, friends of his family said, took the elixir to cure a venereal disease which he believed he had contracted. He sent a negro to the drug store with a note telling the druggist of his suspected ailment. The drug clerk prescribed the elixir of sulfanilamide.[32]

In response to the direct sale of the elixir, the Memphis and county medical societies "planned war against 'over-the-counter' drug prescriptions," reported the Associated Press.[33] Concurrent news revealed the elixir-related death of a Mississippi pastor in Knoxville, Tennessee. The 65-year-old Reverend James Byrd, while away from home on clerical business, died in the early morning hours of October 21st at a city hospital. He had taken about 13 doses of Massengill's elixir, after receiving a prescription from his longtime friend and hometown physician, Dr. Archibald "Archie" Calhoun of Mt. Olive, Mississippi. Byrd's death, the source of which was traced to the southern town, signaled a wave of yet-to-be recognized deaths in the Deep South, where shipments of Massengill's elixir were concentrated.

9
NOBODY BUT ALMIGHTY GOD AND I

Mississippi native Archie Calhoun was a highly respected doctor in the tiny, devout community of Mt. Olive, a town exemplifying the Bible Belt of the US South. One of two physicians in Mt. Olive, Calhoun catered to a racially mixed, rural population out of a two-room, second-floor office, which was conveniently located above his brother's drug store. The 53-year-old doctor, who was also the county health officer, began prescribing Massengill's elixir in late September after receiving a sales call from a company rep. Calhoun's brother bought three pints of Elixir Sulfanilamide, directly from the firm's Bristol headquarters, on September 27th. He was also able to purchase one gallon of the product from the company on October 13th.

One of Calhoun's first elixir-treated patients was a visiting cousin, who took four ounces of the product and then another four-ounce treatment with apparently favorable results.[1] Possibly given this satisfactory outcome, the doctor prescribed Elixir Sulfanilamide to at least 13 other individuals, including his office nurse.[2] Some of these patients experienced "very gratifying" results, but others became gravely ill. An ensuing series of deaths among these patients began to trouble the doctor. One of the first surprising and perplexing fatalities among Calhoun's elixir-consuming patients was that of John Gibbons. However, the likelihood that Massengill's product killed the Mississippi farmer remains uncertain.

Implicating Elixir Sulfanilamide as the cause of Gibbons's death was and is confounded by the 71-year-old's symptoms of an enlarged prostate and probable cardiac disease.[3] The prostate is a walnut-sized gland between the bladder and the penis, and its enlargement, a common condition in older men, often causes voiding problems. Because the gland hugs the urethra, the tubal conduit for urine from the bladder, a growing prostate can squeeze the tube, much like a pinching clip on the neck of a water-filled balloon. A sufficiently enlarged prostate can trigger the retention of urine, with subsequent distension of the bladder and acute discomfort—which were the farmer's documented symptoms before Calhoun prescribed Massengill's elixir on October 4th.

Shortly after recommending the treatment to Gibbons for "prostate gland trouble," Calhoun referred his patient to a Jackson, Mississippi, doctor, who promptly admitted the man to the city hospital for "acute retention of urine" and a "malignant" prostate. Gibbons's inpatient therapy consisted of snaking a rubber catheter into his bladder, through the urethra, to enable voiding. Once the bladder was emptied, it was irrigated with a boric acid solution through the same catheter. The solution was a common remedy for bladder infections and intended to stop any bacteria in the urine from growing. It is notable that, during hospitalization, the farmer's urine output did not appear to be suppressed; but gauging urine production in this case would have been difficult, owing to the fact that Gibbons's bladder was regularly irrigated.

While waiting for surgery—specifically a prostatectomy, a partial resection of the prostate gland to eliminate pressure on the urethra— Gibbons experienced a devastating cardiac event. Likely a massive heart attack, the event occurred four days after his hospital admission. It was treated emergently, but futilely, with intravenous injections of Coramine (a branded nicotine-like stimulant), adrenalin, and Digafoline (a branded digitalis preparation). Sometime after Gibbons's death, it was determined that he had taken six or seven doses (about two ounces) of Massengill's elixir before going to the hospital, but the lack of obvious renal symptoms during Gibbons's hospitalization and particularly his precipitous demise make an elixir-related death uncertain. Nevertheless Calhoun was startled by his patient's abrupt death; although the doctor had no clear reason to question the prescribed elixir. The unfortunate event occurred on the same day that Tulsa physicians, 600 miles away, were preparing to wire the AMA with their first concerns about Massengill's product.

By contrast, the death of Leffie Easterling, a 25-year-old African-American farm laborer from nearby Collins, was typical of diethylene-glycol poisoning. Easterling began suffering severe abdominal pain, nausea, and vomiting on October 4th, four days after Calhoun prescribed Elixir Sulfanilamide as treatment for gonorrhea. The doctor went on to recommend another elixir to Easterling, this one containing morphine, for the patient's puzzling abdominal pain. By October 8th, the young man had stopped producing urine; the following day, Easterling, like farmer Gibbons, was dead.[1]

The next suspect death among Calhoun's elixir-treated patients occurred on October 14th. The doctor prescribed the drug to Katie Stuckey, also of Collins, for "renal colic" (possibly kidney stones) on October 9th (the date of Gibbons's and Easterling's deaths). Two days later, the farmer's wife and mother of eight "could retain nothing on her stomach," and her urine output plummeted. She was admitted to nearby Magee General Hospital, a modest one-story inpatient facility in an adjacent town, where she slipped into a coma and died, five days after her first dose of Massengill's elixir. Calhoun also provided elixir prescriptions to Mrs. Gussie Mae Grubbs, a 22-year-old "Negro" with cystitis; Edie Sullivan, a 49-year-old farmer with a "large carbuncle on the back of the neck"; and Otis Coulter, a 36-year-old farmer with gonorrhea. All became anuric, and all died in succession, within eight to 10 days of beginning their prescribed treatments.[5]

On the date that Otis Coulter died, Tuesday, October 19th, Calhoun's brother received a telegram from the Massengill company. It was the wire that Inspector Ford had urged Massengill to send, warning that the "product may be dangerous to life." Calhoun felt like the rug had been pulled out from under him. The unexpected deaths of his patients (with the possible exception of Gibbons) now made horrifying sense. Immediately the doctor tried to warn his remaining, vulnerable patients. That night, he drove to the home of every person to whom he could remember prescribing Massengill's elixir.[6] If possible, he wanted to obtain urine specimens to ensure that their kidneys still functioned. However, for Nola Penn, the wife of a prosperous county farmer, the doctor's visit was too late. She was already gravely ill at Magee General Hospital, where Katie Stuckey, Edie Sullivan, and Otis Coulter had died. Calhoun prescribed Elixir Sulfanilamide to Mrs. Penn on October 9th for the treatment of, ironically, a kidney infection. She entered the hospital after eight days of treatment, on October 17th, having consumed a total of five tablespoons. Her admitting symptoms were abdominal pain and poor urine output, and her condition deteriorated quickly. She died on the night of October 20th, the day after Dr. Calhoun began his frantic house calls and the day after her 62nd birthday.[7]

For Calhoun, these fatalities were agonizing, but he was especially distraught over Reverend Byrd's death. Calhoun treated his "closest personal friend" for cystitis, prescribing the liquid antibiotic on October 11th. Shortly thereafter, the Baptist leader left for Knoxville to conduct a series of clerical meetings. FDA records indicate that Byrd developed rapidly progressive symptoms consistent with diethylene-glycol poisoning. Vomiting, diarrhea, and anuria began within days of starting the treatment. Byrd was hospitalized in Knoxville on October 17th. Two days later, blood tests indicated acute and severe renal dysfunction. Byrd's blood level of urea nitrogen (BUN) exceeded 160 milligrams per deciliter (mg/dL), about eight times the normal value. His creatinine level, another critical marker of renal function, was 7.5 mg/dL, about six times the acceptable upper limit.[8] Byrd died in a Knoxville hospital on October 21st with his family at his bedside. It was the same date that Mississippi state health authorities publicly confirmed the elixir-related deaths of Byrd, Otis Coulter, and Nola Penn.[9] A staff physician at the Magee General Hospital told the Associated Press that an autopsy on Coulter's body showed "marked kidney destruction." Likewise a postmortem examination of Mrs. Penn revealed that her kidneys were "practically destroyed."

The following day, Dr. Calhoun publicly revealed that six of his elixir-treated patients had died of poisoning, but that his other treated patients showed no signs of illness.[10] Nevertheless, "they are like people facing a death sentence," he warned the Associated Press, "Nobody knows what tomorrow may bring." In a chaser to the wire coverage, Morris Fishbein provided a running tally of known elixir-related deaths across the nation: There were now 30 to 37 fatalities, he estimated. He also confirmed that there was no known antidote for the toxic product.

Fishbein's public statement echoed his private answer to the Massengill company, which audaciously asked the AMA to recommend a remedy for its poisonous drug on October 20th[11]:

> PLEASE WIRE COLLECT BY WESTERN UNION SUGGESTION FOR ANTIDOTE AND TREATMENT FOLLOWING ELIXIR SULFANILAMIDE

The AMA bluntly responded:

> ANTIDOTE FOR ELIXIR SULFANILAMIDE-MASSENGILL NOT KNOWN TREATMENT PRESUMABLY SYMPTOMATIC

In fact, the AMA had already solicited, by telegraph, treatment recommendations for diethylene-glycol poisoning from three experts on the toxicity of sulfanilamide and that of the various glycols.[12] The responses were merely supportive shots in the dark. One expert recommended gastric lavage (known commonly as "stomach pumping"), oral and intravenous calcium, and symptomatic treatment of kidney dysfunction. Another wired, "Cannot suggest any possible antidote or treatment," although he offered that a "[f]ifty per cent dextrose solution with or without sodium bicarbonate intravenously might be tried." The third expert concurred that a highly concentrated dextrose solution might relieve the edema (an abnormal accumulation of bodily fluid) caused by kidney failure.

Anguished by the deaths of his patients and facing an uncertain future with his still-living, but at-risk, patients, Calhoun expressed his torment in a lengthy, public letter to the *New Orleans States* on October 22nd.[13] He confessed:

Nobody but Almighty God and I can know what I have been through in these past few days. I have been familiar with death in the years since I received my M. D. from Tulane university school of medicine with the rest of my class of 1911. Covington County has been my home. I have practiced here for years. Any doctor who has practiced more than a quarter of a century has seen his share of death.

But to realize that six human beings,[14] all of them my patients, one of them my best friend, are dead because they took medicine that I prescribed for them innocently, and to realize that that medicine which I have used for years in such cases suddenly had become a deadly poison in its newest and most modern form, as recommended by a great and reputable pharmaceutical firm in Tennessee; well, that realization has given me such days and nights of mental and spiritual agony as I did not believe a human being could undergo and survive. I have spent hours on my knees, once I had done all any physician could do for his patients. I have known hours when death for me would be a welcome relief from this agony.

After expressing his pain, Calhoun marveled at the elixir-consuming survivors,[15] unable to explain their ability to tolerate the poison.

It seems like a miracle to me. I have spent hours driving to see every one of them, white and Negro. I have checked and rechecked their condition several times a day. Why they are not dead like the first six who died I do not understand. For some obscure physical reason, their bodies were able, apparently, to throw off the poisonous effects of the medicine.

It is miraculous to me. I do not understand it. But I am grateful to Almighty God. Those six deaths weigh heavily enough on my mind and heart. Six more! I shudder when I think of it as a possibility. To me those six yet living who took that elixir have been like six human beings standing under sentence of death ever since I got the warning from the pharmaceutical house that made and sold it, that it was poisonous in that form. I have lost track of how many miles I have driven, trying to counteract the results of the fatal mistake of the men who prepared that medicine.

Like Dr. Long of Johns Hopkins and Dr. Weathers of East St. Louis, Calhoun exonerated sulfanilamide in its tablet and powder forms. He then explained his reasons for turning to a liquid version of the product from the "great and reputable" Massengill company.

I want to make it clear to the lay world that there is nothing poisonous or unfamiliar in sulfanilamide as a medicine in itself. It is invaluable in cases involving the urinary tract. I have used it for years. Hitherto it has come in two forms, a powder taken in capsules, and in tablets. I could not ever tell without checking my records how many hundreds of times I have prescribed it. But in capsule and tablet form it is very distasteful to many patients.

Within the past few weeks a representative of this big Tennessee pharmaceutical firm came to me with a liquid preparation of this drug, called Elixir Sulfanilamide, that was easier for patients to take than sulfanilamide in capsule or tablet form. He induced me to get it and administer it to my patients. The high standing of the firm he represented was all the recommendation their products needed. So I got some.

I am informed now that diethylene glycol, a solvent in the elixir, is responsible for its poisonous effect, its toxicity.

Calhoun described his reaction to Massengill's recall wire of October 19th, which warned of the elixir's hazardous nature. His reaction likely echoed the sentiment of physicians and pharmacists who had dispensed the antibiotic solution with nothing but good intentions.

Imagine my feelings. My heart sank. I stood reading that telegram with cold sweat streaming down my forehead. Then I started out to warn all those 12 patients who had taken this elixir on my prescription, and to do all in my power to save their lives.

The doctor again marveled at his surviving patients, unable to explain how they escaped the effects of the elixir: "violent nausea," "acute abdominal cramps," and "complete cessation of the function of the kidneys." Without an explanation, he nevertheless gave a cautiously optimistic prognosis for their survival.

In lay language, they seem "out of the woods." I believe that they are going to live, now, though I do not know why. Any doctor after a quarter of a century of practice can tell you human beings who have refused obstinately to die; who have lived when as far as their physician could tell, they were condemned to death by causes beyond their physician's control. That is the case with these six who live yet. They seem on the road to recovery. They have been spared the death of agony that was the portion of the other six. I thank God on my knees for that.

But it seems to me that somebody should be responsible for the preparation of that elixir that brought an agonizing death to six innocent patients.

Newspapers and magazines spun further melodrama from the fact that Calhoun's office nurse, Evelyn Sharbrough, had taken Massengill's drug. She was yet another "elixirite," reported *The Delta Weekly* in a regrettable turn of phrase.[16] (The paper also waggishly dubbed the deadly product, "Styx Elixir.") Sharbrough was the last of Calhoun's patients to take the product, a wire report claimed on October 23rd, the date of the nurse's 29th birthday. "And if it works on her as it did on the six," the story ominously continued, "she'll be the last to die."[17] The write-up projected a stoic professionalism on the "young, brown-haired" woman, who "refused to stop working." Sharbrough had consumed four doses of the elixir (or one-half ounce per FDA records) before Calhoun received Massengill's warning telegram. "I feel fine and have had no ill effects yet," she told a United Press reporter, while making a home visit to another elixir recipient.[18] "We're visiting the other patients or hear from their relatives who are reporting constantly to us. The doctor thinks they are all out of danger." Indeed, on October 25th, the "courageously frank" Calhoun publicly confirmed that his other elixir-consuming patients were "safely out of the woods."[19]

People who casually survived Elixir Sulfanilamide were objects of curiosity, if not marvel. "Boy Thrives on Death Elixir," professed the *Times-Picayune* on October 24th.[20] The Louisiana paper featured the story of four-year-old Ecton Terrebonne, Jr., of Westwego, a suburb of New Orleans. The child had taken Massengill's elixir for about two weeks without experiencing any ill effects whatsoever, his mother told the newspaper. "[T]he doctor wanted to give him some pills," she explained, "but his throat was so sore that he couldn't swallow them. So he gave him this medicine in a bottle. It looked like when he gave him that he got better right away." When interviewed, the child remained "[b]lissfully unconscious" of the fatal nature of the drug and said that it "didn't taste so bad." His mother attributed her son's tolerance of the elixir to a "strong constitution" and the fact that she had recited a novena to St. Martha when he was ill. Likewise 11-year-old Edward Shelby of Chattanooga,

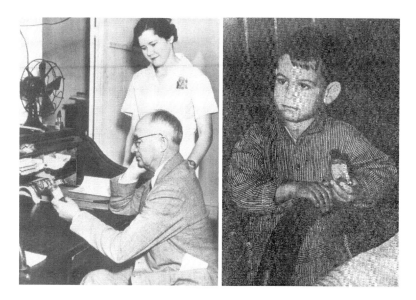

Left, Dr. Archie Calhoun and Nurse Evelyn Sharbrough
(International News Photo. October 24, 1937);
Right, Ecton Terrebonne (*Times-Picayune*. October 24, 1937)

Tennessee, was impervious to more than two ounces of the "red death," as
the city paper described Massengill's elixir on October 26th.[21] "In some
unaccountable manner," the county health officer said, "the boy escaped
the death that overtook the others." Like the Louisiana boy, Edward
remained happily unaware of the elixir's dangers and shrugged off the
attention. "Naw I didn't feel anything," he declared to a reporter.

Yet when symptoms of poisoning and particularly anuria did emerge,
the odds of survival were tenuous. In one of the most complete reports of
the adverse effects of Massengill's product and the status of 1930s medical
diagnosis and attempted treatment, an FDA inspector recorded the
stubborn endurance of an 18-year-old college football player, after he
began taking Elixir Sulfanilamide in early October.[22] The victim was the
son of a physician, who prescribed Massengill's elixir and then diligently
applied whatever limited therapies he could to promote the boy's recovery
from the poison.

This son, a student in the University of California and member of the
football squad, came home from school on the ninth of October with
a sore throat that was diagnosed by his father as of streptococcic
origin. In order to be positive a smear was made of the throat on
Sunday morning, the 10th, and analyses run for the elimination of
diphtheria, which was found to be negative.

Before mass vaccination against diphtheria in the 1940s and 1950s, the chief, suspected causes of pharyngitis in the United States were streptococci and another bacterium, *Corynebacterium diphtheriae.* Writing for the lay press in 1936, Morris Fishbein stressed the importance of distinguishing the two microorganisms:

> Inflammation of [the] tonsils and throat therefore must always be studied to make certain that it is due to the streptococcus and not to the organism of diphtheria, which is of a different character and requires a different type of treatment.[23]

For streptococcus, the prescribed treatment would be the new antibiotic sulfanilamide; for diphtheria pharyngitis, the standard treatment was timely, intramuscular injections of diphtheria antitoxin. Fishbein described the methods for differentiating the two causes of infectious sore throat.

> In cases of doubt, the doctor will always remove a part of the [infectious] membrane [covering the throat] with a swab and examine the germs under a microscope to determine their character.

> He may also send some of the material to the laboratory of the health department, in which they will be grown on a suitable medium, from which it will be possible to determine whether they are diphtheria germs or streptococci.

In the case of Dr. Judson's son, the diagnosis of streptococcal sore throat was established quickly, presumably on the basis of clinical findings in conjunction with the microscopic identification of streptococci or the absence of the *Corynebacterium* species from the throat swab. (Both organisms, after being stained, appear dark blue under the microscope; however, streptococci are reliably spherical and grow in chains, whereas corynebacteria are variably shaped and arrange themselves irregularly.) Because Dr. Judson had previously used Massengill's products, he "decided to administer the Elixir Sulphanilamide orally and a course of three teaspoons at 12:00, 4:00, and 8:00 P.M. in treatment was started at noon on October 10th." The FDA inspector continued his report, outlining the rapid deterioration of the hearty boy and his slow clinical rebound.

> The midnight dosage was reduced to 2 teaspoonsful and on Monday a full course of treatment of two teaspoonsful each was inaugurated. On Monday night early the stomach rebelled and throughout

Tuesday the patient was nauseated but did not vomit. He complained of his head, stating that it did not feel right and that his mind was not clear. The urine on Tuesday was quite scanty.

On Wednesday morning the patient was in an almost comatose condition and Dr. Judson became greatly alarmed because he could not account for these symptoms. He ordered a continuing treatment of hot packs with frequent hot drinks, continuing this treatment throughout Wednesday afternoon and Wednesday night. On Thursday the treatment began to yield satisfactory results and the alarming symptoms cleared up but even up to the time of my interview with Dr. Judson on October 22nd he states that the boy was still in a very weak condition, showing a continued lassitude and dullness. It was also stated that he had lost about 20-lbs. weight and because of the weakened condition was still out of school. Dr. Judson stated that the feeling of nausea continued for approximately one weeks time and that at times the son complained of severe pains in the joints.

In addition to the hot packs and hot drinks, Dr. Judson "thoroughly purged" his son with Pluto Water, a branded mineral laxative, and gave an aspirin-like drug for joint pains. When interviewed by the FDA agent, the doctor believed that his son was "on the road to recovery," but he remained "naturally worried because of the publicity that the Elixir has received in connection with the deaths of certain patients having been treated by it." For his part, Dr. Judson was "firmly convinced" that his son's "alarming symptoms" were the direct result of Elixir Sulfanilamide.[24]

Dr. Massengill, however, would have objected. In an attempt to absolve his company of any blame for the toxic effects of his drug, Massengill issued his first extended public response to the "unfortunate elixir sulfanilamide affair," on the night of October 23rd. It was likely an acute rebuttal to the newly released issue of *JAMA*, which now contained the AMA's October 18th warning in print.[25] Despite the fact that the *JAMA* editorial reaffirmed the suspected toxicity of diethylene glycol, Massengill's strategy was to continue to implicate the "bad effects" of sulfanilamide, while stressing the high standing of his company.[26] He avoided the subject of diethylene glycol altogether. In a prepared statement, the company president declared:

My chemists and I deeply regret the fatal results, but there was no error in the manufacture of the product. We have been supplying legitimate professional demand and not once could have foreseen the unlooked for results. I do not feel that there was any responsibility on our part. The chemical sulfanilamide had been approved for use and had been used in large quantities in other forms, and now its many bad effects are developing.

Perhaps most of the unfair statements have been given out from two sources that are willing to capitalize on this tragic occurrence to further their certain ends.

Massengill refused to identify the "two sources" to the press; however, given the timing of his statement and follow-up comments, he was probably alluding to the AMA, as embodied by Dr. Fishbein, and the FDA, as represented by its chief, Wat Campbell. Both men were more than ready to use the elixir-related deaths to promote stricter drug regulation and the systematic testing of new remedies.

Fishbein continued to provide the national press with a running, elixir-related death tally, which now included fatalities in Laurel, another rural hamlet in southeastern Mississippi. The AMA's Secretary Leech placed a long-distance telephone call to the county health officer on Friday, October 22nd, in an attempt to confirm rumors of at least four deaths in the town due to "kidney complications."[27] But a "hurried check of doctors and death certificates," reported the *Laurel Leader-Call*, "fail[ed] to verify the report heard in Chicago." In its own search at the local health office, the city paper found that death records were "incomplete" and revealed only one fatality within the last week or so. The paper continued its highly provincial investigation by interviewing "Mrs. W. S. Cranford" of nearby Ellisville, the registrar of vital statistics for the county. She said that "no death certificates had been filed with her lately, but that members of an Ellisville family had reported to her that a death in the family had resulted from acute nephritis [...]"

Staff of the local newspaper remained frustrated in their efforts to confirm any elixir-related deaths in the area until after the weekend. Then on Monday, October 25th, a local physician affirmed tentatively, if tellingly, "It is more than possible that elixir of sulfanilamide played a part in the death of five patients here [...]"[28] The 52-year-old practitioner, Dr. Joe Green, found himself, like Archie Calhoun, providing a lengthy defense to the press about his patients' deaths and how he came to prescribe Elixir Sulfanilamide to "some fourteen or fifteen people, all of whom were sick and some desperately sick."[29] In a front-page feature, Green explained that he had been visited by a representative of "one of the large reliable pharmaceutical houses," who gave out samples of the elixir, claiming that it "was the same as the tablet except in liquid form."

Although Green acknowledged that he had indeed prescribed the elixir, he was reluctant to blame it for his patients' deaths. "Only a small amount of the elixir was taken," he rationalized, "and the people that died, with possibly one exception, had diseases that could prove fatal." Green's deceased patients, all men and identified by name in the *Laurel Leader-Call*, had received their elixir prescriptions for a variety of ailments, including venereal disease.[30] All five men had developed the hallmarks of diethylene-glycol poisoning—nausea followed by anuria—and had expired seven to 12 days after first consuming the elixir. Nevertheless Green maintained to FDA agents that one of his patients had probably died of a syphilitic gumma of the brain, an end-stage lesion of chronic inflammation and necrosis. Green floated the idea, despite the fact that the patient had developed kidney failure within a few days of starting the elixir. Green also proposed that another patient had had a "malignant" kidney, and another still had died of carcinoma of the gall bladder and liver; although there were no autopsy data to verify the claims. In a veiled attempt to further acquit Massengill's product and by extension his own role in the fatalities, Green continued his public defense, which drew on the fact that some reactions to the elixir were either neutral or even favorable.

> The other people who took it suffered no ill effects. One small baby about two years old had a rather large amount. Yet she suffered no ill effects and her family was highly pleased with the results obtained. Some five or six people were given the elixir 12 to 30 days ago and none suffered ill effects and are all right at the present time.[31]

But Green was mindful that victims' families suspected drug-induced injury, and he was willing to share information about the fatalities (in an era before patient-privacy laws):

> We want it strictly understood, and have so informed the families where there is a possibility that injury has been done, that my files are absolutely at their disposal. All records are just as they were written and are open to public officials as well as to their families.

> At the present time there is a clouded mystery about the whole affair, yet I believe it will be worked out so that those who feel they are injured will have definite facts upon which to base any complaints.

Green provided an update from the Massengill firm, through a visiting representative. Ignoring or unaware of the fact that Morris Fishbein had publicly declared diethylene glycol to be the fatal ingredient in Massengill's elixir exactly one week ago, Green quoted the detail man:

[U]p to the present time best chemists of the American Medical Association and the company were making a close and thorough investigation, but so far had not been able to determine what poison, if any, caused [the] death of the alleged victims.

The Massengill company, by way of Green, also declared that it "expected to visit every family which felt that the drug had injured their relatives" and now "said the doctors and druggists were not regarded in any way as responsible for any ill effects."

10
NATIONWIDE RACE WITH DEATH

By Sunday, October 24th, the FDA's "nationwide race with death" to recover Massengill's at-large elixir was well underway.[1] More than 700 bottles, wrote the Associated Press, had been distributed throughout the country (most of which were in the lower Midwest and South). Yet "every" FDA agent was "scouring the country" to retrieve them. The agency's Central District chief, Jimmie Clarke, assured a fearful public that all outstanding shipments would likely be recovered within the next 24 hours. The wire service also reported how the AMA had been inundated with inquiries.

> Telegrams and long-distance calls from all over the United States have been pouring into the medical association's office at the rate of one every five minutes. They come from frightened citizens and physicians and officials seeking advice.

Likewise the FDA fielded panicked questions from citizens. In one touching and curious episode, a "lad of about 9 or 10 years of age, dressed in a faded red cotton sweater and overalls," appeared at the FDA's San Francisco station.[2] When approached by agents, the boy pulled out a bottle of greenish liquid from a "tattered newspaper" wrapping. It was his mother's medication, and because the label bore the word "elixir" (one of thousands of tonics that did) he wanted to ensure that the drug was not poisonous. It was not, or at least it was not Elixir Sulfanilamide. The concoction was a popular medley of iron, quinine, and strychnine. The last ingredient, a known poison, was added routinely in miniscule amounts to gastric stimulants of the era.[3]

On Monday, October 25th, Clarke confirmed to the Associated Press that "very few" bottles of Massengill's elixir "remained untraced" and that "practically all" lots at primary distributors and stores had been "cleared up."[4] In addition, "most of the subdistributions, those to individuals purchasers, [had] been traced" and were being confiscated "by court proceeding when necessary." Except, Clarke explained, "[W]e seize it first and go to court afterward." Evidently the legal process for seizing Elixir Sulfanilamide, as commanded by the Food and Drugs Act of 1906, was not always followed to the letter, given that death was a possible result of dilatory court action. And while the agency's efforts to swiftly confiscate Massengill's drug likely prevented fatalities, the death tally continued to rise. In fact, the government's so-called race against death was not so much a dash to prevent the loss of life but a steeplechase to discover it. There were now 46 known deaths due to Elixir Sulfanilamide, reported the United Press on October 25th, and the AMA had received information on "quite a number more."[5] Newly confirmed or suspected victims included additional residents of Mississippi, as well as citizens in Alabama, Texas, Ohio, Georgia, and Florida.

Expounding on wire stories, local newspapers provided more granular, albeit incomplete, coverage. The *Anniston Star* of Alabama publicized five elixir-related deaths in the state: three in Eufaula, one in Headland, and one in Clayton—cotton-milling towns in the far southeastern corner of the state.[6] News of the deaths prompted Alabama's health officer, Dr. James Norment Baker, to immediately wire officials in 64 counties, urging them to "MAKE CONTACT WITH ALL PHYSICIANS AND DRUGGISTS IN YOUR COUNTY" so that further consumption of Massengill's product could be averted.[7] The FDA's chief inspector at New Orleans, Malcolm Stephens, had already alerted Baker by telegraph, stating that there was "NO WAY OF ASCERTAINING WHAT PHYSICIANS OBTAINED PRODUCT FROM DETAIL MEN." The FDA wire continued in necessarily terse prose: "THEREFORE HIGHLY DESIRABLE ALL PHYSICIANS IN STATE BE WARNED OF DRUG IF THERE IS ANY WAY YOU CAN POSSIBLY CONTACT EACH OF THEM." Stephens suggested, perhaps feebly, that Baker might reach the state's doctors through their local medical societies.

The FDA already knew the details of Alabama's five publicly reported deaths, along with the facts of at least one other suspect fatality.[8] In Eufaula, Dr. Paul Salter, a Tulane medical graduate (like Mississippi doctors Calhoun and Green) had prescribed Elixir Sulfanilamide on September 22nd to Syble Gwendolyn Singleton, the infant daughter of a local farmer. At the time of treatment, the ten-month-old girl was desperately ill with streptococcal septicemia (known commonly as blood poisoning). She stopped producing urine 24 hours after the first dose of elixir and died three days later. Notably Elixir Sulfanilamide was dispensed in this case from a two-ounce sample bottle peddled by one of Massengill's detail men.[9] It was a fact that likely prompted Stephens to warn Dr. Baker about the unknown distribution of elixir by salesmen in Alabama. Stephens also discovered that Salter had prescribed the elixir in early October, more than a week after the death of the Singleton infant, to a 68-year-old white widow. Likewise a 47-year-old black "plasterer" had received the treatment from Salter, probably also sometime in early October. Both patients had died in Eufaula, on October 13th and 17th, respectively.[10]

Salter, a locally respected physician and head of the county's only hospital, can be excused for not initially suspecting the toxicity of Massengill's product. His infant patient had been gravely ill, and he had probably assumed—like the elixir-prescribing doctors of Tulsa—that she had succumbed to her raging infection. Nevertheless, at the time of illness, the child's condition perplexed Salter. According to Singleton family history, the doctor and his intern "spent hours reading medical journals in an attempt to find a cure" for the girl.[11] The later deaths of Salter's adult patients were confounded by the presence of a number of longstanding medical conditions—including Bright's disease, a 19th-century eponym for chronic inflammation of the kidneys. Yet Salter came to believe that Elixir Sulfanilamide contributed to or caused his patients' deaths during the FDA's investigation. The complete halt of kidney function, occurring shortly after the treatment was started, preceded all three fatalities.

In Headland, about 40 miles south of Eufaula, the FDA learned that a 63-year-old farmer, Anderson Crews, had abruptly developed the signs of elixir poisoning. Within two days of beginning the treatment, which was prescribed for a traumatic foot injury, the "colored" man became blind and unconscious, and "his kidneys ceased functioning entirely." Nevertheless Crews lasted for another nine days before surrendering entirely to Massengill's product on September 25th. Crews became, along with Dr. Salter's infant patient, one of the earliest known victims of Elixir Sulfanilamide. Crews received his lethal treatment on September 16th—the earliest recorded date for an elixir prescription, the FDA's full investigation would later reveal. It was exactly one week before the first prescription for Massengill's product would be dispensed in Tulsa. The early dates of treatment with Elixir Sulfanilamide in Alabama suggested the possibility, if not the probability, that many victims of the product were yet be recognized in the Southeast, where Massengill's at-large product was liberally distributed.

September 16, 1937, was the same date that a 22-year-old "colored" farmhand from Clayton, a village about 20 miles west of Eufaula, received the first of two prescriptions for Elixir Sulfanilamide from his physician, Dr. George Oscar Wallace. (Wallace was not only a physician and a druggist, he also happened to be the grandfather of George Corley Wallace, Jr., an 18-year-old law student and the future, notorious governor of Alabama.) The FDA learned that Wallace's patient, John Holloway, tolerated his first elixir prescription of four to five ounces; however, he died two days after beginning a second prescription for a "[s]evere case of gonorrhea." Holloway's undeniably elixir-related symptoms, as reported to federal inspectors, were "labored breathing, unconsciousness, deafness," and kidney failure. Wallace admitted to the FDA that Holloway's death, which occurred on September 24th, was "unusual and unexpected," and the doctor believed, at least in hindsight, that Massengill's elixir had contributed to the man's demise. Wallace was, as the FDA's complete investigation would later show, a physician with an unpleasant distinction: He unwittingly caused the nation's first known fatality due to Elixir Sulfanilamide.

During the third week of October, the FDA discovered at least one other elixir-related death in Alabama: that of a two-year-old girl from Guntersville, a provincial ferry landing along the Tennessee River.[12] The daughter of a local farmer, the toddler died on October 16th after drinking three tablespoons of a six-ounce prescription. The treatment, prescribed on October 9th, was intended to cure a streptococcal sore throat. Two days after starting the medication, the girl "seemed much improved," and "was thought to be well." These observations suggested that the antibiotic in Massengill's elixir provided some clinical benefit. However, on the night of October 12th, the girl failed to urinate. The next morning, her doctor observed her face and hands to be "swollen," the probable consequence of widespread edema due to renal failure. Three days later, she died "in convulsions."

Four of at least seven known deaths in Texas were reported by the Associated Press, also on October 25th, and the Texas health inspector wrongly predicted that there would be no more elixir-related fatalities in the state.[13] "I believe the situation is in hand," he promised reporters, referring to a nearly complete statewide confiscation of Massengill's drug. The publicly named victims included a young child and two teenagers. Further details of the deaths were not provided by the wire service, but they were known to the FDA. Federal agents understood that four-year-old Lois Jean Wilkins of Leona died on October 18th, three days after starting Elixir Sulfanilamide as treatment for an infected sore throat. Like the toddler in Guntersville, Alabama, the Wilkins girl initially rallied, presumably because of the antibiotic; but then her condition deteriorated as a result of diethylene glycol. Nineteen-year-old Levy Kelly, a married African-American farmer from Highbank, died on October 12th, 10 days after beginning his elixir treatment for gonorrhea. An autopsy showed "cloudy swelling" of the kidneys. Eighteen-year-old Mollie Mae Schmittou, a student at the East Texas State Teachers College, died at her parents' home in Yantis on October 20th after a brief hospitalization. At first, local physicians thought that the farmer's daughter and recent high school graduate had succumbed to meningitis. The grave diagnosis was entertained despite the fact that the young woman had presented with a relatively innocuous case of "boils," for which Elixir Sulfanilamide was prescribed on October 11th. But Schmittou's hometown physician came to believe otherwise. On the girl's death certificate, he recorded the causes as uremia and "glycoll ethylene poisoning."[11]

The identity of the fourth Texas victim was unknown to the state health officer at the time of the wire report,[15] but FDA inspectors were apparently aware that Robert Montgomery Goode, a married 29-year-old fishing pier operator, had died of "acute toxic hemorrhagic nephritis" and "toxic hepatitis" at a Galveston hospital. His death on October 9th followed five days of progressive vomiting, facial paralysis, vision loss, jaundice, and confusion. The symptoms, unexplainable at the time, were treated with several outpatient remedies, including a mixture of cocaine (presumably for pain or weakness) and a bismuth compound (presumably for gastric distress). When signs of jaundice appeared, two days after beginning Elixir Sulfanilamide, injections of "liver extract" were administered.[16] Regardless the six-foot, 200-pound Texan died within two hours of being admitted to the hospital and eight days after receiving his elixir prescription for an acute gonorrheal infection.

FDA agents knew of at least three other suspect deaths in Texas and anticipated more. Massengill's records showed that 17 gallons of elixir had been shipped from the firm's Kansas City branch and distributed among 96 drug stores and four physicians' offices in 68 communities throughout the then-largest state of the Union. And although some bottles had been sent to major cities, like Fort Worth and San Antonio, the overwhelming majority of supplies were scattered over the state, the various points of receipt looking like so much buckshot on a Texas map. Elixir consignees were located as far east as the Louisiana border, as far south as the Gulf Coast, as far north as the Oklahoma border, and a far west as tiny Wink—a flat, dusty town whose only reason for existence (like so many flat, dusty towns in West Texas) was to capitalize on the discovery of oil a decade earlier. In addition, a staggering number of samples had been shipped into the state.

One salesman, B. H. Hensley of San Antonio, had received 72 one-ounce physicians' samples along with four, two-ounce case samples, for a total of five pints.[17] When confronted by state and federal authorities, Hensley said that he had returned 42 of the one-ounce samples and three of the two-ounce case samples to Massengill's Kansas City branch. He claimed that he had destroyed the remaining case sample and had consumed three of the one-ounce samples without any bad effects whatsoever. (The FDA later commented on the "quite singular" practice of Massengill's reps to self-medicate with the elixir. None of them reported any adverse effects.) If Hensley was being truthful, the tally left 27 physicians' samples at large.[18]

But officials encountered "supreme difficulty" when further dealing with Hensley, who absolutely refused to reveal where he had delivered the toxic drug. For his defiance, the salesman was promptly arrested and locked up. After spending a night in jail, he pleaded guilty to "obstructing an officer in the performance of his duties" and was fined $38.50. The reformed Hensley was then persuaded to assist inspectors with locating and confiscating 12 samples in Waco and 15 in San Antonio. In the process of running down the samples, inspectors were shocked to find that physicians had recklessly tossed bottles into wastebaskets or slop jars. In addition, government agents learned that two of Hensley's samples had been passed onto competitive salesmen, one each to detail men from Upjohn and Abbott. However, none of Hensley's samples was associated with a death.

While continuing to chase down elixir prescriptions in Texas, FDA agents learned that William Taft Parker, a tool dresser for an oil company, died on October 10th at a Wichita Falls hospital. The 27-year-old had obtained Elixir Sulfanilamide "at his own request" from a local physician on September 29th. The treatment was intended as a remedy for gonorrhea. Despite aggressive inpatient therapies, including blood transfusions, for urinary suppression and coma, Parker died of "uremia due to acute nephritis."[19] The man left behind a young widow. The FDA also knew of the death of Alberta Yvonne Howell, the two-year-old daughter and only child of a young couple from the tiny mid-state community of Hatchel. She died of "acute nephritis" on October 13th, after drinking about one ounce of Massengill's elixir, which had been prescribed for her "infected throat."[20]

And nationwide the unbearable pathos continued. The FDA reported a death in Ohio during its accounting of 17 pints of Elixir Sulfanilamide in the state, which had been distributed among nine physicians, five drug stores, and one hospital.[21] The agency determined that the overwhelming majority of these lots, specifically 15, had been returned intact to Massengill's headquarters in Bristol—including one pint from physician Homer Long of Copley. However, Dr. Long had also obtained, on request, a two-ounce sample of elixir from a Massengill salesman. This small amount was used to treat a six-year-old girl from the township, with fatal results.

The daughter of a truck driver and housewife, Jo Anne Cramer died on October 17th at a children's hospital in nearby Akron.[22] The city paper, the *Beacon Journal*, showcased her death in a lengthy feature article, "Roundup of Fatal Remedy Is Too Late to Save Child," on October 26th.[23] The paper reported that, because Dr. Long had successfully treated a mild case of scarlet fever with sulfanilamide tablets in another child, he wanted to use the same remedy for the Cramer girl, who had the same condition. However, Jo Anne could not swallow tablets. As if on cue, a Massengill salesman visited Dr. Long in early October, and the detail man provided a sample of the antibiotic elixir. (According to the *Beacon Journal*, the salesman cheerily replied to Dr. Long's request for a liquid version of the antibiotic, "Why, I have some right here. It's just the thing you want.") Doses of Massengill's elixir were given to Jo Anne for three days, but she rebelled against the drug. "She cried every time she had to take a dose of it," her mother "sobbed" to the local reporter. "She would say, 'Mamma, I hate that medicine, but if you say I must take it, I will.'" After being admitted to the hospital on October 12th, Jo Anne became stuporous; five days later, she died of "uremic poisoning." Her mother was "near collapse," the *Beacon Journal* reported, when she learned that the elixir had caused her daughter's death. The woman's guilt and anguish were captured in a brief statement: "I try to think that I gave it to her unknowingly, but that doesn't bring her back. She might still be alive if I hadn't made her take it." Jo Anne was buried on the date that Dr. Long received Massengill's warning telegram.

* * * * * *

While the nation's recognized death toll due to Elixir Sulfanilamide escalated, the public's general perception of sulfanilamide and its clear distinction from the toxin diethylene glycol remained uncertain thanks to confusing newspaper coverage. Writers for the *New York Times* focused on the properties of the antibiotic, advising, "Sulphanilamide Is Subjected to Attention Following Cures and Some Fatalities."[24] On October 26th, the *Chicago Daily Tribune* declared vaguely, "Warn Surgeons To Be Cautious With New Drug," while other papers offered contradictory headlines like, "Drug Has Life Saving Quality."[25] The write-ups now wove information about sulfanilamide's benefits—including the latest report of cures in meningitis—with the growing death count and general warnings about the antibiotic, including the downsides of self-medication.

On October 27th, the Associated Press reported that the number of deaths due to Elixir Sulfanilamide now exceeded 50 and included a young girl in Arkansas.[26] The FDA recently discovered this fatality as a result of its efforts to locate three pints of Massengill's elixir, which had been shipped into the state from the company's branch at Kansas City. From the FDA's St. Louis station, Chief Lowe directed Inspector Jesse Pitts to track down the bottles in Arkansas and, most important, to account for their contents. The 59-year-old redheaded agent was known within the FDA to drive "like a wild man," and perhaps Lowe thought that if anyone could quickly retrieve the widely distributed elixir, it was Pitts. Pitts was also called an "old timer" by his FDA colleagues, owing to the fact that he was a veteran of the Spanish-American War, as well as being a long-time employee of the agency.[27] Yet Pitts, despite his age and experience, could be surprisingly naïve. He was perpetually astonished that subjects of government investigations could lie to him.

On or about October 20th and 21st, Pitts reached the Arkansas hamlets of Ola and Taylor, about 180 miles apart. At each town's pharmacist, he collected one full, unopened pint bottle of Massengill's elixir. He then sped onto Blevins, another tiny farming town, about 70 miles north of Taylor. At the Blevins drug store on October 21st, Pitts learned that three prescriptions for Massengill's elixir had been dispensed from the pint bottle, and that all three prescriptions had been written by James Gentry, a local physician. One of these prescriptions, the Blevins pharmacist claimed, was for a "Jewell Long."[28] When Pitts interviewed Gentry, the doctor was able to identify two of his elixir-treated patients as local residents: a young white girl and a "colored" woman. However, he denied knowing a Jewell Long and stated that she must have been an itinerant "Negro" laborer whom he had treated for gonorrhea.[29] The doctor then claimed that the young girl had taken her one-ounce prescription without consequence, and Pitts was able to confirm this report by interviewing the child's parents. Pitts learned, however, that the second patient, who had also consumed her entire prescription, was "seriously ill," and her dire condition was contrary to the impression given by Dr. Gentry. Pitts found the woman at home, but he was unable determine if her compromised state was due to an underlying (and undescribed) illness or the elixir. However, he believed that, whatever the cause of her condition, she would "likely not recover."[30]

Pitts was otherwise determined to track down Dr. Gentry's third elixir-treated patient, but he could get no further information about Jewell Long from the doctor or area residents. A visit to the local post office and nearby towns failed to provide any leads on an address. While continuing to make inquiries in Blevins on Monday, October 25th, Pitts learned from a townsman that a girl with the surname of Long "was being buried down the road a few miles." Pitts immediately drove to the house of the deceased girl and looked for an opportunity to interview the grieving parents. Shortly after his arrival, Pitts spotted Dr. Gentry driving up. The inspector walked over and confronted the doctor, who then admitted that he had indeed prescribed the elixir for the girl. As it was revealed, Ruth Jeanell Long, the decedent, was neither an itinerant nor of African-American heritage. On the contrary, she was the seven-year-old daughter of a local white farmer. Furthermore Pitts learned that Gentry had prescribed the medication for a streptococcal skin infection, not gonorrhea. The Long girl had died just the previous day, on Sunday, October 25th—16 days after she began taking Elixir Sulfanilamide and eight days after she stopped taking it. Unmistakably Gentry had lied to Pitts, even as the Long girl was terminally ill. On October 27th, a state paper, the *Hope Star*, reported the fatality and quoted Gentry, who ambiguously suggested that his patient had died "after treatment by elixir of sulfanilamide for [a] streptococcus infection over her entire body."[31]

* * * * * *

Toward the end of October, the AMA warned that "an end to the fatalities was not yet in sight."[32] Fishbein called the tragedy "the most unfortunate incident in the pharmaceutical industry within the last decade." Given the rising number of deaths, Massengill was increasingly anxious to retrieve his outstanding bottles of elixir, a job that required the FDA's vast assistance, but he remained desperate to avoid negative publicity. The bad press included the AMA's running death toll, and Massengill viewed the periodic announcements as unnecessary. When health officials in Puerto Rico confiscated the six pints of elixir that had been shipped from New York to San Juan, the local dealer wrote to Massengill, informing the company of the seizure. The dealer added that a Puerto Rican radio station had just read a cable from Chicago, which provided the latest number of casualties "caused by Elixir Sulfanilamide of the S. E. Massengill Co."[33] The Massengill firm responded on October 26th,

[...] We were sorry to hear that our trouble with Elixir Sulfanilamide has been broadcast in Puerto Rico. Probably if the proper authorities had gotten in touch with you before this was done they would have seen it was not necessary [...][34]

The company added,

> [...] It is our hope that this matter will be cleared up very shortly, and we do not believe it is going to affect our business materially for any length of time [...]

On the same date, the *Atlanta Constitution* reported five elixir-related deaths in Georgia, "as agents of the Pure Food and Drugs Administration spurred efforts to trace down 10 prescriptions remaining in the state."[35]

11
PASSIVE RESISTANCE OR DELIBERATE OPPOSITION

John J. McManus, chief of the FDA's hub in Atlanta, Georgia, was a nearly 30-year career veteran of the Department of Agriculture by the fall of 1937. In fact, McManus's time with the FDA (including its previous incarnations) was almost as lengthy as Wat Campbell's.[1] Shortly after graduating from the Rhode Island College of Pharmacy, McManus joined Campbell's rookie field-inspection team in 1908, and he steadily climbed the ranks of the agency with faithful service thereafter. In his early days as a food and drug official, McManus endured a necessarily peripatetic career. It was the norm for field agents, who focused on the inspection of foods: rotten catsup in Baltimore, moldy cream in Chicago. But the agency's ultimate destination for the Yankee McManus was Georgia. First stationed in the port of Savannah in 1911, McManus found himself, among a variety of duties, inspecting can after can of wormy peaches in the humid Southeast, while struggling to maintain the starched collar of an inspector's unofficial dress code. Years of itinerant government work and loyalty were rewarded with advancement, and McManus became chief of the agency's Savannah office in 1926. When Elixir Sulfanilamide was launched in the fall of 1937, McManus directed a modest staff—including five field agents—out of Room 416 in the fortress-like New Post Office Building[2] in Atlanta, where the FDA station had been relocated.

McManus learned of the nation's first known elixir-related deaths on Tuesday, October 19th, from a brief account in Atlanta's morning paper.[3] The notice prompted him to send Inspector Lewis Smith to survey the state capital. The 56-year-old Smith discovered that several lots of the antibiotic solution had been returned intact by three Atlanta jobbers that very day to Massengill's company in Tennessee, probably as a result of the firm's recall telegrams. Then in the afternoon, Smith learned of a suspect death in the state. Word of the fatality, that of a "Negro baby," and a shipment of Elixir Sulfanilamide to the child's hometown of McDonough, about 30 miles southeast of Atlanta, came to Smith from a drug wholesaler. One of the wholesaler's customers, a young white doctor in McDonough, had sent a gallon bottle of Massengill's product to the vendor for analysis. The wholesaler turned the bottle over to Smith, who discovered that two ounces were missing.[4]

McManus quickly learned that other Georgians wanted Massengill's elixir chemically examined. The following morning, October 20th, he received a troubling report from the state's chief drug inspector. Lawyers from Griffin, about 40 miles due south of Atlanta, had contacted state officials, asking where they "could get some medicine analyzed in connection with a damage suit." The attorneys held the remainder of a prescription for Elixir Sulfanilamide, two-thirds of which had been consumed by Leonard Dees, a 22-year-old African American who had died just two days earlier and had undergone an autopsy. The lawyers possessed "the stomach, liver and kidneys of the victim," which they left with the state official for "safe keeping and possible analysis."[5] The FDA immediately contacted one of the inquiring lawyers at the state inspector's office in Atlanta, and Inspector Smith traveled post-haste to Griffin, where he learned that Dees had obtained a six-ounce prescription for Massengill's product on October 11th. Smith discovered that the prescribing doctor had been motivated to recommend the sulfanilamide solution, instead of tablets, after seeing the newly shipped bottles at his local drugstore.

A half-hour after McManus learned of Leonard Dees, he received an airmailed letter from the FDA's Eastern District office in New York. The letter itemized the elixir shipments to his territory: Georgia, Florida, and the Carolinas.[6] From this communiqué, McManus learned that more than 21 gallons of the product had been distributed among 83 drug vendors or physicians in 60 different communities in Georgia—most of which were small towns in the northwestern part of the state or along the South Carolina border. Nineteen pints had been dispersed among 16 drug vendors and two doctors within six communities in Florida. In South Carolina, bottles representing a total of 11 gallons were scattered among two doctors, nine pharmacies, and one training hospital. Seven of these 12 consignees were located in Charleston, but the others were in one of five small towns in or near South Carolina's Lowcountry. And in North Carolina, more than 14 gallons of elixir had been shipped in various pint or gallon quantities to three doctors and 21 drug stores.[7] A large volume of this elixir, more than six gallons, was concentrated in the area of Rocky Mount, a cotton-milling town within the state's coastal plain. The first shipment to McManus's territory occurred on September 8th; the most recent, October 17th (which consisted of 12 half-pint containers to a physician in North Carolina). Consequently more deaths within McManus's territory were probable, if not certain.

Given the troubling shipment information, McManus organized an immediate plan of action, and his 58-page chronicle of the Atlanta station's investigation of Elixir Sulfanilamide in the US Southeast is possibly the most thorough account of the government's mobilized response to the tragedy. McManus recorded his objectives in order of logical priority: 1) to stop further sale of Massengill's product; 2) to remove outstanding lots from the market; and 3) to investigate related deaths and injury. He divided the tracking of elixir shipments by state, and those consignees who could not be immediately visited by a federal or local official were contacted by long-distance telephone. Owing to the large number of consignees in his territory, 137, McManus hoped for assistance from state and city officials to seize Massengill's deadly product, but he received only patchy support. Georgia's chief drug inspector said he could spare only two of his men to safeguard the state's residents. South Carolina and North Carolina did not employ drug inspectors; therefore the confiscation of Elixir Sulfanilamide in these states was up to the feds, along with whatever merciful cooperation they could get from county or city health officials. However, in Rocky Mount, where shipments of elixir were concentrated in North Carolina, the city health officer "could offer no assistance in the matter," wrote an exasperated McManus. Nevertheless other regional officials were willing to provide much-needed support to the FDA. In Tallahassee, Florida, the agency received notable aid from a supervising state inspector, Phil Taylor. "[T]hough not organized to do drug work," McManus wrote, "[Taylor] gave immediate assistance both personally and through his assistants in checking shipments." The Atlanta station telephoned officials at Charleston and likewise received "[v]aluable assistance" from the city's health officers. In fact, physicians in the southern port had already begun to examine a string of five suspect deaths in the immediate area.[8]

Communicating preferentially by wire (as opposed to the more expensive method of long-distance telephone), McManus mobilized his small, scattered field team and mustered two of the FDA's chemical analysts in Atlanta to augment the government's seizure of Elixir Sulfanilamide. Chief Analyst Arthur Henry, a 49-year-old Floridian, was assigned to northern Georgia, and Analyst Clarence Schiffman, a 34-year-old North Carolinian, was sent to northeast Georgia. These men complemented the investigative efforts of Inspector Smith, a native South Carolinian; Inspector Wiley Simms, a 48-year-old Georgian, who was recalled from downstate; and Allan Rayfield, a 29-year-old seafood inspector and native Alabaman, who was ordered to proceed to Savannah after covering the Jacksonville area in Florida. Also on direct orders, native South Carolinian Monte Rentz, a 31-year-old junior inspector who was investigating insecticide spray residue at Tampa, Florida, proceeded to his home state. To intercept prescriptions in North Carolina, McManus sent Shelbey Grey, a 29-year-old Texan and relative FDA newcomer, from his post in eastern South Carolina to Rocky Mount. The Eastern District's chief inspector, 50-year-old Olaf "Ollie" Olsen arrived in Georgia on October 21st, to fill in on a much-needed ad-hoc basis.

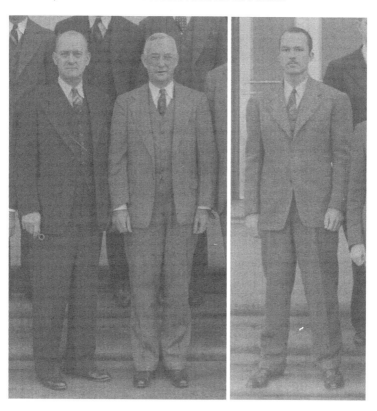

Left, Chief Inspector Olaf Olsen (left) and
Atlanta Station Chief John J. McManus (right), c1939 (FDA);
Right, Inspector Shelbey Grey, c1939 (FDA)

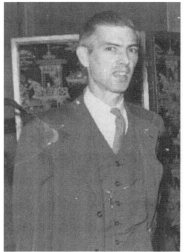 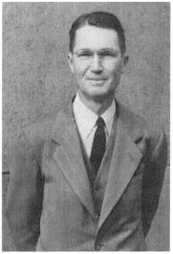

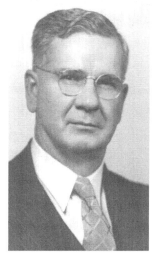

Top left, Inspector Allan Rayfield, date unknown (FDA);
Top right, Inspector Monte Rentz, date unknown (FDA);
Bottom, Chief Analyst Arthur Henry, date unknown (FDA)

Although newspapers, specifically the *Atlanta Constitution*, publicized the FDA's pressing concerns about the distribution of Elixir Sulfanilamide within Georgia and its daily efforts to confiscate the product, these were perfunctory and delayed nods to the agency's workload and troubles.[9] Field agents, who rode hundreds of miles by train and drove over countless dirt roads in government or personal cars, soon discovered that accounting for every last ounce of Elixir Sulfanilamide was irregular, painstaking, and protracted business. Yet within two days of receiving Massengill's shipment records, McManus was able to report to the Eastern District chief that all elixir consignees within his territory had been personally visited or telephoned by a federal, state, or city official. In Florida, Inspector Rayfield and state officials visited all but one of the 18 commercial recipients of Massengill's elixir on a single afternoon, Wednesday, October 20th.[10] In their whirlwind crusade, which extended from the Gulf Coast panhandle to Jacksonville on the eastern seaboard, agents were able to confiscate and destroy three intact pints of the liquid antibiotic.[11] Interviews with pharmacists and physicians led them to believe that another 13 pints had been returned intact to Massengill's headquarters. If the medical professionals were to be believed (which was not always a safe assumption), the quick tally left three outstanding pints, one of which had been shipped to the Gem Drug Store in Jacksonville. When visited that afternoon by Rayfield, the store's African-American proprietor, Dr. Arthur Smith, said that he had just returned two ounces of the product to the manufacturer. The remaining 14 ounces had been dispensed on prescription to two black men: Fred Williams, a 35-year-old merchant tailor, and Emanuel Cauley, a 37-year-old railroad laborer. In fact, Cauley had received two, four-ounce prescriptions for the elixir. It was then revealed that Williams had died on October 12th. The official cause was "acute hemorrhagic nephritis." Cauley had died on October 16th, the cause of which was believed to have been chronic gonorrhea. In neither case did Smith or the men's treating physicians suspect that Massengill's elixir had precipitated or hastened death. (Notably Williams underwent an appendectomy for "acute lower abdominal pains" six days before his death.) Newly aware of the prescriptions and deaths, Rayfield was anxious to retrieve any remaining elixir from the victims' homes. Dr. Smith searched Cauley's residence and found three ounces of the drug, but a hunt for elixir at Williams's home failed to turn up the liquid. At the time, Rayfield's priorities did not allow for a more meticulous investigation of the Florida deaths, when consumption of Massengill's elixir might be interrupted elsewhere. So on orders, he rushed to southeast Georgia to assist with the recovery efforts of five other agents in a state of approximately 58,000 square miles.[12]

Without the same kind of local assistance in Georgia, where a much greater volume of Massengill's product was distributed, the FDA's canvassing efforts in the Peach State were considerably slower than those in Florida. Nevertheless, by the end of Friday, October 22nd, FDA agents, along with limited help from two state officials, had called on 65 (78%) of 83 commercial recipients in Georgia. By the end of Saturday, more than 90% of the consignees had been visited. But during the course of these visits, the FDA became aware of troubling over-the-counter sales of Elixir Sulfanilamide in southeast Georgia and struggled to identify purchasers. On October 21st in Swainsboro, a small farming community, Rayfield learned of direct sales from the Lewis Drug Store to two unknown men. Without any useful information to track down the customers, the inspector advised the county health officer to "be on the lookout for any suspicious deaths in his territory."[13]

The following night, the local doctor found himself examining a 34-year-old farmer at the town hospital. Will Portwood had just been admitted with "acute Nephritis with a picture of Appendicitis." Because of the fresh warning from Rayfield, the doctor specifically asked Portwood about any use of Elixir Sulfanilamide. The patient admitted that he had purchased four ounces of the product without a prescription from the Lewis Drug Store on October 16th. He took the medicine regularly for about two days, he said, until he became severely nauseated. Given the presumed diagnosis of poisoning, the doctor sought directions for treatment through an extended volley of queries: first to Georgia's state health office, then to the FDA's Atlanta and Chicago stations, and finally to the AMA. The medical association gave its best advice, as it had been recently solicited from experts: intravenous glucose (dextrose) and calcium. Despite the therapy—which was probably one of the first attempts to use the AMA's haphazard antidote—Portwood continued to produce only miniscule amounts of urine, and his clinical condition quickly deteriorated. On October 23rd, he complained of "failing hearing and eyesight"; three days later, "he was totally deaf and blind." Likewise "[p]aralysis developed in the throat, arms and hands," indicating a profound and widespread dysfunction of the nervous system. The treating physician officially ascribed Portwood's demise, on October 26th, to Elixir Sulfanilamide poisoning. The next day, the farmer's death was briefly reported by the *Atlanta Constitution.*

A man listed as Will Portwood died yesterday afternoon in Swainsboro, J. J. McManus, chief of the regional office of the United States Food and Drug Administration, said he had been informed. The man had been critically ill for several days after taking four ounces of the elixir, McManus said.[14]

The vigilant county health officer became aware of another suspect death, and he likewise informed Inspector Rayfield. This fatality, perfunctorily reported as that of a "negro of Wadley" by the *Atlanta Constitution* on October 26th, was also traced to an over-the-counter purchase of Massengill's elixir from the Lewis Drug Store. Rayfield, after thoroughly investigating this death, provided McManus with a lengthy account of the last pain-filled days of Seth Durden, which belied the cursory press notice. It was learned that the 28-year-old farmer had purchased eight ounces of Massengill's product, without a prescription, on October 9th. Five days later, Durden presented to his hometown physician,[15] complaining of severe headaches, flank pain, and copious vomiting, which he had treated with crude home remedies of "black pepper tea" and castor oil mixed with a few drops of turpentine. The physician, who was unaware of the sulfanilamide treatment, diagnosed gonorrhea and acute nephritis, and he administered liquids both orally and subcutaneously "to get the kidneys to function." These efforts failed. The physician then sent Durden to a hospital about 30 miles east, where the patient was attended by a resident physician, Dr. R. E. Jones. At the time of admission, on October 20th, Dr. Jones found Durden to be "very ill" but conscious. The physician then relayed his puzzling experience with Durden in a lively note, dated October 21st, to the referring doctor:

> You really handed me something when you sent me that patient. I went over him very carefully and could find nothing organically wrong with him other than his [gonorrheal] infection. As you said, he had almost a complete suppression of urine. I gave him about [four liters] of fluids during the time that he was here, but his kidneys never did open up. I catheterized him last night and got about 1-1/2 ounces of bloody purulent urine.

Jones then described his attempts to examine Durden's kidneys, by obtaining a "flat plate," or x-ray image, of the abdomen. The doctor also injected a radiopaque dye (Hippuran) into Durden's vein. The dye could be seen on the radiographic images of the lower abdomen, and its eventual course through the functioning kidneys—if they were, in fact, functioning—could be observed.

> I took a flat plate of his abdomen yesterday afternoon which revealed no stones nor mechanical blocking of the ureters. I gave him an I. V. Hippuran, took [an x-ray] picture twenty minutes later and there was no dye collected in either kidney.

> From the course that he ran and the general picture that he presented, he undoubtedly had an acute nephritis with almost complete anuria. Just what the cause of this condition I am not certain. Whether the anuria was due to his [gonococcal] urethritis or not I do not know. He had a diarrhea with nausea and vomiting, which to me suggested a possible chemical poison, probably bichloride of mercury.

Dr. Jones also noted that Durden (like Portwood) had developed neurologic symptoms shortly before death—namely facial paralysis. The doctor's succinct and graphic impression of Durden's illness was kidney dysfunction due to "puss poison." Durden died on October 21st. After Rayfield informed Durden's physicians that the patient had taken Elixir Sulfanilamide, both medical men agreed that it was the cause of death.

Identifying citizens who bought Elixir Sulfanilamide without a prescription remained onerous, if not impossible, business, but McManus and his field agents were also stymied in their investigation of known prescriptions. Chief among the difficulties, McManus reported, was "the failure of physicians to keep records of the names or addresses of their patients." Generally McManus's staff "encountered a great deal of indifference on the part of druggists, and even physicians, to the fate of their patients who had been given the Elixir." In addition to a certain clinical laxity, which seemed to be the geographic norm, there was "a definite effort on the part of physicians and druggists to conceal information on this point." The station chief privately ascribed the indifference and deceit, respectively, to the low quality of area physicians and "the fear of injury to their reputation if deaths from their treatment were revealed." Although the native backgrounds of field agents likely facilitated interviews with area druggists and country doctors, stonewalling was common. In particular, physicians' obstructive behavior, like that of uncooperative pharmacists, necessitated repeated, frustrating visits by the FDA to determine the whereabouts of Massengill's outstanding elixir. In some cases, the government's investigation was stalled or nearly so. This was especially true in North and South Carolina, where investigations were performed almost single-handedly by Inspectors Grey and Rentz in their respectively assigned states. In his official report, McManus described several encounters of "passive resistance or deliberate opposition," which rigorously tested the patience of his field staff. The station chief's FDA account directly contradicted his public statements, which were possibly made to encourage local cooperation. "Country doctors and druggists in small towns are aiding us," he told the *Atlanta Constitution* in a charitable lie.[16]

* * * * * *

By Friday morning, October 22nd, Analyst Henry had visited 17 elixir consignees in 13 different communities in northwest Georgia. During his solo, two-day journey of hundreds of miles, Henry discovered four dispensed prescriptions for Elixir Sulfanilamide. After finding the prescribing doctors and instructing them to follow up with their patients and retrieve any residual drug, Henry moved on to find 14 more consignees in 12 different towns before the weekend.[17] Among these yet-to-be-visited recipients was Dr. Samuel West, a "typical country doctor" in the mountain village of Dahlonega. The 69-year-old West had received one pint of Massengill's elixir about a month earlier. On Friday, Henry found the doctor at his country house. When the purpose of the government visit was explained, West "became very excited" and "refused to discuss the matter in his home." So the pair walked to the doctor's office "a little distance" away, where they could continue the conversation. But West remained "very evasive and reticent," reported Henry. In fact, the doctor became so agitated that he was "incoherent"—but not before he admitted to prescribing Massengill's elixir to 19-year-old Robert Parks as treatment for gonorrhea. Henry then learned that the teenager had died on Tuesday, the day that West had received Massengill's recall telegram. West admitted to Henry that he believed the elixir was responsible. Then the "extremely irascible" doctor, who claimed that he had dumped his unused stock of elixir down a sink (and showed the empty bottle to Henry), abruptly ended the interview.

[...] Dr. West forcibly indicated to the Inspector that he wanted the interview terminated, and the Inspector to leave. He was afraid that someone might come in the office and find out that he had been interviewed concerning the death of [Parks] and the administration of the Elixir. Dr. West finally became so excited that Inspector Henry decided it was good tactics to leave him for the time being.

Four days later, Henry revisited Dr. West, at which time the doctor was "still reticent and evasive, but not excitable." At this second interview, West admitted that he had given two ounces of Massengill's elixir to Parks, and when he "began to show bad effects from the medicine," West sent his patient to a hospital about 25 miles southeast of Dahlonega. West then disclosed that the "only other person" to whom he had given Elixir Sulfanilamide was a "white man named Cochran." However, the doctor claimed that he did not know where this patient lived. Perhaps Cochran "worked in a sawmill back in the mountains several miles to the northwest of Dahlonega," West vaguely offered.

Given the limited information, Henry searched local death certificates for the surname of Cochran or "any deaths suggestive of chemical poisoning." Coming up empty and "[i]n view of Dr. West's attitude and several discrepancies," the analyst took to the streets of Dahlonega, where he "gossiped with several natives." From them, Henry learned that Cochran's first name was possibly Joe, and that he was in apparent good health. In addition, the residents confirmed the death of Parks. Moreover they informed Henry of the recent, suspect death of another local man, Jewell Fitts. The 36-year-old had died on October 5th at the same hospital where Parks had expired. Henry circled back to West, but the doctor "denied dispensing or prescribing any Elixir for [Fitts]." The agent then moved on to the hospital, where he interviewed Dr. John K. Burns, who had taken care of both Parks and Fitts.

In his interview with Henry, Dr. Burns described how both young men had been admitted for "kidney lock": Fitts on September 29th and Parks on October 14th. During hospitalization, each had passed only a few ounces of urine, and each had died after less than a week of inpatient care. At the time of the older man's death, October 5th, Burns ascribed the fatality to "Edema of the Lungs, Suppression of Urine and Gonorrhea," because he (like the rest of the nation) was unaware of the toxicity of Elixir Sulfanilamide. The hospital physician admitted to Henry that he was now willing to attribute this death to Massengill's product, as he had done for Parks. Dr. Burns also divulged that he had recently discussed both deaths with Dr. West and had urged the prescribing doctor to relay the probable cause of death to the victims' families. But West refused, Burns said, because such an act would "ruin his practice."[18]

* * * * * *

As it was for Analyst Henry, Friday, October 22nd was a busy day for Inspector Shelbey Grey, who scouted for bottles of Massengill's elixir in the middle of North Carolina. In Rocky Mount, Grey visited eight drug stores and was able to account for a major volume of the elixir that had been shipped to the city. However, he also discovered that 10 elixir prescriptions had been written there, nine of which had been provided by a Dr. Perry. Grey was able to personally track down at least three of the doctor's elixir-consuming patients that day and found that none had been adversely affected. However, in four cases, "Dr. Perry claimed he did not know [the patients'] names or make any inquiries as to their identity." When interviewed by Grey, the doctor explained that he treated "many patients for venereal diseases [but] that they pay cash and that he keeps no record as to their names or addresses," despite the fact that Perry was obligated by state law to report cases of venereal disease. Moreover Perry "did not appear to be unduly concerned about his patients or worried about any possible publicity which might result if they died."[19]

Grey's frustrating encounter with Dr. Perry, which clearly mandated follow-up, was surpassed by his interaction the next day with Dr. John H. Martin of Red Oak, an approximate ten-mile hike from Rocky Mount. Martin had received five pints of Elixir Sulfanilamide directly from Massengill's Bristol headquarters and had returned only four pints to the manufacturer on October 19th, the date of the company's warning telegram. What happened to the fifth pint? Grey wanted to know on his Saturday visit. The 69-year-old physician admitted that he had dispensed three prescriptions for Elixir Sulfanilamide, as treatment for gonorrhea, but he also confessed that "he kept no records of the names of Gonorrheal infection patients and had no knowledge of their identities." Furthermore Martin "made no inquiries, since this class of patients with venereal infections try to keep their troubles secret and hide their identities." Martin further explained the anonymous nature of regional care to Grey, of which the FDA agent was becoming painfully aware.

> Many such patients do not go to their own family doctors, but do go to out of town doctors where they are not known. In some cases fictitious names are used, and in other cases friends of the person wanting the medicine are used as messengers.

Martin, whom Grey found "very feeble" and "in poor mental condition," went on to declare in stunning fashion that his elixir-treated patients "must be all right as he had not heard from them." Certainly FDA agents like Grey and Henry had to weigh, with some intangible judgment, the odds that continued pressure on prescribing physicians would produce the names of vulnerable or dead citizens against the possibility of intercepting Massengill's elixir elsewhere. In the case of Dr. Martin, Grey apparently decided, or was instructed, to move on to other elixir consignees, while planning a repeat visit to Red Oak.

During the next several days, the FDA became aware of at least 20 prescriptions for Elixir Sulfanilamide in North Carolina; although the fates of several consumers could not be verified, largely because their names had not been recorded by treating doctors or dispensing pharmacists. Nevertheless Grey assured the Associated Press on October 27th that nearly all of Massengill's outstanding elixir had been collected in the Rocky Mount area.[20] The wire service, citing a local hospital, also reported "as 'unimproved' the condition of a man listed as James Thomas Tanner, 60, who attaches said was suffering from elixir of sulfanilamide poisoning."

The next day, Grey revisited Dr. Martin in a renewed attempt to identify his three elixir-treated clients and to specifically ask about Tanner. At this second interview with Grey, Martin admitted that he had, in fact, sent Tanner to the Rocky Mount hospital on Monday, October 25th, when the patient presented to his office with a seven-day history of anuria. Tanner, as Martin further revealed, had consumed all of a four-ounce supply of elixir, which Martin now admitted to prescribing on October 10th. Because of the drug's publicized toxicity, a fact certainly stressed by Grey during his first interview with Martin, the doctor advised Tanner to go to Rocky Mount for inpatient care. Tanner, a logger, did so with heroic effort, walking the approximate 10 miles from Martin's office to Rocky Mount unassisted. Martin obviously failed to alert the FDA agent of Tanner's dire condition, until Grey followed up in person.[21]

* * * * * *

Outside of Charleston, Inspector Rentz was largely on his own in South Carolina, tasked with the job of visiting five inland communities where a total of eight gallons and two pints of Massengill's elixir had been shipped. On Friday, October 22nd, he met Dr. Johnston Peeples of Estill, a village near the Georgia border. The white 50-year-old doctor, who had received one gallon of the liquid antibiotic on September 16th, told Rentz that he had "telegraphed and telephoned the three white patients and two negroes to whom he had dispensed the drug," after receiving Massengill's recall wire. But Rentz found Peeples "very evasive and indefinite" about the identities of his elixir-treated patients, and the doctor "kept reiterating that he had had no deaths as a result of this Elixir." Moreover these patients were not from Estill, Peeples said, implying that they might be difficult to track down (despite the doctor's claim that he had telegraphed and telephoned them). At Rentz's continued insistence, Peeples reluctantly gave only general descriptions of the patients to whom he had dispensed Massengill's elixir. They were "a white woman [...] whose name he does not know"; a "white man who works for the State Highway Department"; and a "white man who operates a large battery station." All resided outside of the town, the doctor hedged. In addition, Peeples admitted that he had given several ounces of elixir to "two negroes" whose names he did not know. The doctor then claimed, paradoxically, that he had seen at least three of these patients within the last few days. They were well, he implied. The two black men, in particular, were "in good health," Peeples stressed. Rentz did not accept the doctor's rambling and inconsistent story.

Assured that Dr. Peeples had destroyed his remaining elixir, Rentz moved on with his investigation, which included a "considerable" amount of independent work to identify the doctor's vulnerable patients. Part of this investigation, like that of Analyst Henry, included conversations with local residents about recent deaths in the area. In a town of approximately 1,400 residents, where everyone seemed to be related to everyone else, Rentz probably had little difficulty locating Dr. Bertie Johnston, a cousin of Dr. Peeples, and Dr. Marion Peeples, an uncle of Dr. Johnston. In addition, Rentz found another, very informative doctor in Estill, Dr. Jack Wertz, and another physician in nearby Fairfax, Dr. John Folk (who may have been related to the wife of Dr. Johnston Peeples). Collectively the physicians described four suspect deaths in the area: those of a white teenage girl, a 25-year-old black man, a 34-year-old white laborer, and a 35-year-old black lumber-mill worker. All had seen Dr. Johnston Peeples at some point during their recent care, the doctors revealed. With respect to the two white patients, the treating doctors could attest to the use of Massengill's elixir, which had been supplied by Dr. Johnston Peeples.[22] Dr. Bertie Johnston was also certain that he had briefed his cousin about the death of the lumber-mill worker, J. J. McDaniel.

Rentz returned to interrogate Dr. Peeples on October 27th, and the doctor denied—astonishingly and in direct contradiction to his previous statement—that he had given Elixir Sulfanilamide to "any negroes." Rentz must have been flabbergasted. The FDA agent then specifically asked Peeples about McDaniel, and the doctor reiterated that he had not given McDaniel any Elixir Sulfanilamide. The patient had died of "Hemorrhagic Fever," Peeples declared, and he had signed the death certificate "as such." Rentz persisted: Was Dr. Peeples the last physician to have seen McDaniel? No, the doctor replied, but he "felt like the negro was his patient and [...] he knew Dr. Bertie Johnston would not object to him signing the [death] certificate."[23] Despite Rentz's presumed frustration, he was determined to uncover the fate of the doctor's elixir-treated patients.

Rentz proceeded to the home of the other deceased black man, 25-year-old Willie Badger, in nearby Scotia. There in the tiny, poor, and largely African-American hamlet, Rentz found Badger's widow. Yes, her husband had seen Dr. Johnston Peeples. When? Rentz asked. October 2nd, she replied. And when he came home from the visit, she continued, "he began taking some red liquid medicine and some pills," which he had gotten from the doctor. Four days later, her husband "went to bed sick." Twelve days later, he died.[24] What happened to the medicine? Rentz asked. Badger's wife replied that "all the medicine had been thrown out in the weeds and grass away back of the house." Rentz then dutifully searched the overgrown field, where he eventually found a four-ounce bottle containing about two-and-a-half ounces of a red liquid, resembling Elixir Sulfanilamide. The bottle's label showed the name and address of Dr. Johnston Peeples and directions for use. Rentz secured the bottle as an official sample.[25]

Rentz then traveled a few miles toward the Georgia border to Cohen's Bluff, a landing along the Savannah River. There he found the lumber-mill camp where McDaniel had died on October 14th. Rentz interviewed the superintendent. McDaniel "had been sick only a short time," the superintendent recalled; but if Rentz wanted more information, he should talk to McDaniel's brother-in-law, his sister, and his boss, the man advised. McDaniel's boss was called over, and he confirmed that McDaniel had seen Dr. Johnston Peeples sometime during the first week of October. The employment records were reviewed. Yes, McDaniel had quit work because of illness on October 8th. The boss then revealed that, after McDaniel's death, he had packed up the items in McDaniel's "shack" and sent them with the body for burial. It was the local custom among African Americans "to send all medicines, glasses, spoons, etc. with the body at death." Yes, maybe there was a vial of red liquid, the boss dimly recalled. Rentz searched McDaniel's cleaned-out hovel. There were no medicine bottles. Rentz then interviewed McDaniel's brother-in-law at the camp, who said that McDaniel "was buried in Dixon's Graveyard" several miles north, and he confirmed that "the medicine, dishes, etc. that went with the body was put on the grave." Rentz and the brother-in-law proceeded "over dirt roads" to the cemetery, stopping on the way at the home of McDaniel's brother-in-law and sister. Rentz also met another sister of McDaniel, visiting from Detroit, and a brother.

McDaniel's sister in South Carolina confirmed the story that Rentz had learned at the lumber camp. Moreover, she added, Dr. Johnston Peeples had visited the camp on October 4th and had given "some red liquid medicine" to her brother, who became "very ill" a few days later. She also recalled that Dr. Bertie Johnston had been summoned more than once to the camp to attend to McDaniel, perhaps alternately with Dr. Peeples. McDaniel's sister told Rentz that "the doctors changed medicine practically every time they came," and that the remaining bottled drugs had been placed on her brother's grave. Rentz wrote of his continuing journey, with McDaniel's relatives, to the gravesite.

Together with the four negroes I began the trek to the grave a-foot. We walked over fields and finally came upon a little wooded knoll with the single grave with fresh earth on it. It was stated others of the family were buried here, but there was no sign of tombstone or grave.

The fresh grave, instead of flowers had bottles, dishes, spoons and a part bottle of tomato catsup on it. The Detroit sister picked up the bottle of catsup and said "You know that's no way to do" -- modernistic!

Upon examination of the several bottles of liquid medicine on the grave one 4 oz. bottle containing about 1 oz red liquid resembling the fatal Elixir was collected and identified as Inv. 43875-C, as check for Elixir Sulfanilamide. Three other bottles containing some liquid but not appearing to be the Elixir were also taken, but will not be submitted unless the above sample shows that it is not Elixir Sulfanilamide.

The sample (Inv. 43875-C) had a label on it which was badly weatherbeaten but it can clearly be seen that it is the label of Dr. Johnston Peeples, Estill, S. C. The bottle as submitted for analysis still shows some of the dirt from the grave around the cork. The bottles were inverted with the necks stuck in the soft dirt on the grave.[26]

* * * * * *

By October 29th, FDA agents had completed their first-time visits to all of the commercial recipients of Massengill's elixir within McManus's territory. Follow-up visits, some of them painstaking and heartbreaking, were nevertheless necessary to ensure the whereabouts of the outstanding product and to learn of its effects. In addition to over-the-counter purchases and prescriptions of the elixir, samples handed out by Massengill's detail men had to be tracked down. Publicly McManus appealed to the company's sales reps through the *Atlanta Constitution.* "We are finding it difficult to reach these salesmen who may have distributed samples among physicians," he confessed to the paper on October 27th.[27] Privately McManus disparaged the detail men. In his FDA report, he wrote that, when they were located and contacted, they "did not exhibit much concern about the matter." "[I]n many cases," McManus continued, "their information as to the amount of samples distributed and to whom they were given was indefinite. In only a few instances did they volunteer information as to where the product had been sold."

Accounting for Massengill's errant elixir remained pesky business into the first week of November and beyond. Inspector Smith, who was described by McManus as "one of our older inspectors" and "not in good health," volunteered to personally track down and retrieve one missing prescription in the rural Piedmont of Georgia. The FDA first learned of this prescription on October 22nd, when Analyst Henry visited a drug store in Ellijay, some 80 miles north of Atlanta, where one pint of elixir had been received on September 23rd. At Ellijay, Henry learned from the druggist that two prescriptions for Elixir Sulfanilamide had been dispensed, but Henry was only able to account for one of them (which, it was learned, had caused no ill effects). Henry's continued efforts to discover the whereabouts of the second prescription, which had been written by Dr. Luke Foster for a "Mrs. Weeks," included visits to several families in the area with the same surname. However, the agent could get no leads on the Mrs. Weeks in question. Henry proceeded with his other investigations in northern Georgia, but he returned to Ellijay a week later and found the prescribing doctor. The FDA agent admonished the young physician to "make every effort to locate this woman and secure the return of the prescription." Dr. Foster tepidly replied that he hoped Mrs. Weeks "might come in some week-end and he would check up on her condition and report."[28]

On November 4th, McManus personally telephoned Dr. Foster to follow-up on the prescription for Mrs. Weeks, but the doctor merely replied that he did not know where Mrs. Weeks lived and that he had not seen her since he had given her the prescription for Elixir Sulfanilamide. Dr. Foster's continued passivity toward the matter evidently prompted an irritated Inspector Smith to procure "the government car on a drizzly fall day" and drive immediately to Ellijay. Smith's sole aim for the impromptu road trip was to recover the prescription for Mrs. Weeks—that is, if she had not already consumed the elixir.

Arriving at Ellijay, Smith "made numerous inquiries in and around [the town] without success." He then visited Dr. Foster's office, where he encountered the District Nurse for North Georgia. As a representative of the state, she was pursuing an independent search for Mrs. Weeks.[29] Perhaps motivated by simultaneous visits from two government officials, Dr. Foster suddenly remembered that the first name of his patient's husband was Kelly. From local townspeople, Smith was then able to determine that Kelly Weeks "lived back in the mountains in a place known as Cherry Log," nine miles north of Ellijay. So Smith and the state nurse drove over "the dark mountain road" to the country hamlet, where they promptly learned from its few residents that the Weeks family had just moved several days ago. Undoubtedly frustrated, Smith nevertheless found a Cherry Log neighbor who knew where the Weeks family now lived. This neighbor offered to direct Smith and the nurse to the new location. So "just over the next ridge" the group traveled and ultimately found Mrs. Weeks (whose first name was Lula) living in a backwoods cabin. She was obviously alive and apparently well.[30]

Thinking that the state nurse "might be the better person to see Mrs. Weeks and secure the return of the prescription," Inspector Smith held back his own interrogation of the country woman. When questioned by the nurse, Mrs. Weeks said that she had discontinued the medicine "a short time" after receiving it, because it "did not appear to do her any good"; however, she could not remember what she had done with the bottle. Hearing this news, Inspector Smith intervened and engaged in an "hour's talk" with the woman. He, no doubt, stressed the importance of locating the prescription bottle during their extended conversation. Finally Mrs. Weeks "suddenly recalled that when they had moved, they put a lot of bottles in an old black bag." The bag was promptly located in a corner of the cabin and opened. There, among several prescription bottles, Smith found Massengill's elixir. One ounce of the three-ounce prescription remained. He secured the bottle and drove back to Atlanta, where he personally delivered the missing prescription to his boss. Smith's odyssey to the Georgia mountains for a few tablespoons of Elixir Sulfanilamide was thereby concluded.

* * * * * *

To confirm the whereabouts of every ounce of Massengill's elixir, exact quantities from field reports had to be reconciled with volumes of the drug returned to Bristol. These checks were performed through a series of volleyed reports to the FDA's station chiefs from Inspector Ford, who continued to rely on the begrudging hospitality of Massengill and his employees. If Ford calculated a difference of even a few ounces between the amounts received at Massengill's headquarters and the field reports of returned elixir, inspectors had to revisit the recipient pharmacists or doctors to define the nature of the difference. In such cases, which were disturbingly common, the extra legwork delayed the FDA's investigation of Elixir Sulfanilamide and, as McManus reported, "usually revealed the dispensed prescriptions, and in some cases disclosed additional deaths." For instance, when a Florida inspector visited a pharmacist in Tallahassee and a physician in nearby Quincy, on October 20th, both declared that they had returned their respective pints to the manufacturer intact and unused. Yet a later reckoning at Bristol revealed that the pint bottle from Tallahassee was missing two-and-a-half ounces; the physician's bottle contained only 14 of 16 ounces. Inspector Ford wired his findings to the Atlanta station in early November, which prompted Inspectors Rayfield and Olsen to immediately revisit the Florida establishments. Directed interviews by the federal men, who now exerted informed pressure, revealed that three prescriptions had, in fact, been dispensed from the missing ounces, and that one of these prescriptions was associated with the death of a four-year-old "colored" boy on October 16th.[31] Likewise when Rayfield visited a drug store in Millen, Georgia, on October 22nd, he was told by the store manager that no sales of Elixir Sulfanilamide had been made, and that the full gallon bottle had been returned to Massengill on October 18th "via express." Examination of the store's records supported the manager's contention that no sales of the deadly product had been made. At Bristol, however, Inspector Ford found that only seven pints and 10 ounces had been returned from Millen, leaving six ounces unaccounted for. The discrepancy required Rayfield to conduct an extensive investigation in the area and to make repeated trips to the drug store to discover the truth of the matter. But not until November 4th did the store manager finally admit to Rayfield that he had surreptitiously supplied Massengill's elixir to a local man who had died on October 16th.[32]

On November 11th, McManus submitted his comprehensive, but still preliminary, report on the confiscation and investigation of Elixir Sulfanilamide in his territory to the chief of the FDA's Eastern District. Although McManus's staff, like FDA agents throughout the country, would remain in the field for weeks, if not months, chasing down outstanding elixir prescriptions and samples and reviewing state and county records for suspect deaths. The *Atlanta Constitution* provided its final coverage of the elixir investigation in Georgia on October 28th. The paper assured a worried public, "Fears Subsiding," thanks to a nearly complete recovery of Elixir Sulfanilamide in the state by the FDA.[33] In the same write-up, the AMA's Secretary Leech projected a national death toll of "between 60 and 63," and FDA Chief Campbell reiterated his disgust with the current drug law: "It is unfortunate that under the terms of our present inadequate federal law the Food and Drug Administration is obliged to proceed against this product on a technical and trivial charge of misbranding." Citing unidentified Washington sources, the journal forecasted that more stringent drug bills would be introduced at the next session of Congress.

12
PURSUING A TIGER WITH A FLYSWATTER

It was a macabre Halloween for readers of the *Chicago Daily Tribune*, when the paper mapped the locations of 58 deaths due to Massengill's Elixir Sulfanilamide on October 31st.¹ The national tally included victims in Oklahoma (9), Missouri (1), Illinois (7), Texas (5), Arkansas (1), Tennessee (1), Mississippi (16), Alabama (7), Georgia (6), and South Carolina (5). However, the graphic, labeled "Where Elixir Has Claimed Victims," was far from complete, given that the FDA knew of yet-unpublicized deaths and suspected more. The *Tribune*'s annotated map was a complement to news that a citation would be issued against The S. E. Massengill Company by the FDA's district headquarters at Cincinnati, Ohio. The basis of the citation: mislabeling. Elixir Sulfanilamide was not a true elixir, the FDA maintained, because the product contained diethylene glycol, not ethyl alcohol, and the use of diethylene glycol in an elixir defied the drug trade's understanding of it, the agency patently concluded. The reported maximum penalty for the citation, as far as the Food and Drugs Act allowed: $100. (Although press coverage didn't clarify whether the fine was per shipment of Massengill's elixir or for its entire distribution. Sensational headlines implied the latter.) Massengill's public response to the citation was one of regret and denial. He was sorry for the drug-related fatalities, but he also defended the reputation and innocence of his company. "We have been supplying a legitimate professional demand," he offered, "and no one could have foreseen the unlooked for results. I do not feel there was any responsibility on our part."

Officials at the FDA and specifically Chief Campbell were giving "a great deal of thought to the procedure to be followed in the criminal prosecution of those responsible for the shipment of Elixir Sulfanilamide in interstate commerce."[2] It was decided within the agency that "[a]ll citations," such as they were, should be confined to The S. E. Massengill Company, along with Massengill personally and his chemist Harold Cole Watkins. Campbell specifically rationalized the pursuit of Watkins and "our purpose to recommend to the Solicitor [General] that prosecution of the chemist Watkins be based on all shipments involved in the citation." He continued,

> His intimate connection with the acts preceding the interstate shipments suggests that he should be held accountable. If for any reason he is relieved of responsibility for some of the shipments, we should be in a position to show his connection with the first batch of 40 gallons [...] which Mr. Watkins prepared himself.

Campbell believed that, if necessary, Inspector Ford could testify to certain admissions made by Watkins and Massengill during their interviews with the FDA agent on October 18th and later.

Massengill's legal worries weren't confined to federal actions. Announcements of civil claims were a sign of things to come for his beleaguered firm. On November 2nd, the father of Bobbie Sumner, Tulsa's first victim of Elixir Sulfanilamide, was appointed administrator of the two-year-old's estate by a county judge.[3] The appointment was made in conjunction with the father's wrongful death claim against The S. E. Massengill Company for $6,000. The same judge set a date for a hearing in the wrongful-death case of Earl Beard, the 25-year-old air-conditioning engineer who had died on October 16th in Tulsa. The case was being pursued by his mother. In anticipation of more damage suits against Massengill in Oklahoma, the father of five-year-old Millard Wakeford and the father of six-year-old Michael Sheehan were appointed administrators of their sons' respective estates on November 3rd.[4] Relatives of other victims seemed to be arming themselves with evidence of injury for civil damages. In Laurel, Mississippi, the families of five victims (all adult men, three white and two black, and all of whom had been treated by Dr. Joe Green) met, according to local news coverage.[5] The reasons for the conference were not specified, but they were presumably to discuss the victims' common cause of death and perhaps share information. After the session, an autopsy was performed on one of the deceased, James Vick, by order of a local judge. Vick had died on October 20th, and Dr. Green had attributed his death to carcinoma of the gall bladder and liver without postmortem support. After the court-ordered autopsy, Vick's organs were shipped to a Vicksburg pathologist for examination.

* * * * * *

On November 2nd, the United Press updated the nation's "authenticated" death tally to 61.[6] The wire service cited the latest issue of *JAMA*, dated November 6th. The prereleased edition of the medical journal contained a "Special Article from the American Medical Association Chemical Laboratory."[7] The multi-part feature offered a chronicle of the AMA's investigation, including the herald case reports from Drs. Ruprecht and Nelson in Tulsa and Dr. Hagebusch in St. Louis. In addition, the journal printed the AMA laboratory's chemical examination of Massengill's elixir (which was based, in part, on Dr. Childs's forwarded sample from Tulsa) and preliminary results of toxicity experiments on rats, rabbits, and dogs at the University of Chicago. These experiments—in which Elixir Sulfanilamide, pure diethylene glycol, pure sulfanilamide, and a synthetic version of Massengill's product were administered to laboratory animals—were necessary and useful. Foremost among the rationales for the experiments: The toxic and lethal doses of diethylene glycol, when given in small, repeated doses, were not well established (despite the fact that the adverse effects of diethylene glycol in laboratory animals had been reported in two previous, albeit small, studies). The overriding conclusion of the Chicago pharmacologists was that diethylene glycol was indeed the toxic ingredient in Elixir Sulfanilamide. All of the animals reacted similarly to pure diethylene glycol and Massengill's elixir—whether the elixir was from the manufacturer or concocted on site. Initial lassitude and diuresis (excess urine production) were consistently followed by anuria, coma, and death. When diethylene glycol or Massengill's elixir was taken in divided doses that produced toxic effects,[8] approximately 20% of the animals died. This mortality rate was similar to the emerging death rate among human victims who had consumed some or all of their prescriptions for Massengill's product. Moreover the scientists found that sulfanilamide by itself was not deadly, although when the antibiotic was given in very high doses, several animals experienced "convulsions." But anuria, importantly, was not seen. Among the more intriguing, although preliminary, observations: Massengill's elixir, especially if administered in "large doses," was more lethal than pure diethylene glycol. The pharmacologists proposed an explanation for the curious finding.

[I]t is possible that if the kidneys and the liver are rapidly injured by a large critical dose (10 cc.) of diethylene glycol, the sulfanilamide, especially in large amounts, may not be eliminated or detoxified and may have an injurious action on the other tissues. In this way sulfanilamide may then be regarded as having an additive toxic effect.

The postmortem findings in animals that died of poisoning were remarkably similar to the changes seen in human victims of Elixir Sulfanilamide. The most significant abnormalities were confined to the kidney and liver, although evidence of "congestion" or edema, the probable consequence of renal failure, was noted in the heart, lungs, and brain. In particular, the convoluted tubules of the kidneys, an essential portion of the organ's microscopic filtering system, were strikingly damaged, with evidence of necrosis and obstruction. The changes undoubtedly explained the anuria and uremia seen during the end stages of life. But how diethylene glycol damaged the renal tubules, whether directly or indirectly, was unknown. Notably the gastrointestinal tract was completely unaffected, in contradistinction to what might be expected with poisoning due to mercury bichloride. The lengthy *JAMA* report concluded by tabulating the confirmed nationwide deaths due to Elixir Sulfanilamide, and the AMA explained its methods for verifying these deaths. On the basis of seminal reports from "various press services" or physicians and "chiefly clues from" the FDA, "[e]ach suspected case of death was then checked by the American Medical Association by telephoning or telegraphing physicians or other medical authorities," the medical group explained. The AMA also warned, "There are many additional reports not confirmed as yet."

Drawing on the tragedy, an editorial in the same *JAMA* issue excoriated "many smaller and unenlightened groups of pharmacists and pharmaceutical manufacturers [who] fail to recognize the importance of high standards in all the professions concerned with health."⁹ The anonymous writer, possibly Fishbein given the autocratic tone, then called out the Massengill company specifically. It remained possible "for such manufacturers to place on the market semisecret preparations, untested as to either toxicity, potency or therapeutic value," the editorialist charged, because of the inadequacies of current drug regulation. The FDA, in its role to protect the American public, was "as inefficiently armed as a hunter pursuing a tiger with a fly swatter." The scolding continued,

> Under our present laws there is nothing to require the S. E. Massengill Company or any other firm to divulge the formula or to make adequate pharmacologic or clinical tests before placing a hazardous "patent medicine" or proprietary preparation on the market. Ironically the label for Elixir of Sulfanilamide-Massengill carried the recommendation "continue at this dose until recovery"!

Public and private responses from Massengill himself, who deflected blame for the "unlooked for action" of his elixir, were particularly galling to the writer, who charged factually that the firm had "done essentially nothing to contribute to the knowledge of medicine" and had merely capitalized on the discoveries of others. However, the finger pointing was not confined to Massengill. Pharmacists (particularly those who were willing to sell medicines over the counter) and especially physicians "who will not heed the warnings concerning the use of proprietary, unstandardized, semisecret remedies" were complicit in the tragedy, the writer alleged. The reproach concluded,

> Sixty persons have been sacrificed simply because the toxicologic observations now reported were not determined in advance by a manufacturer who had no hesitancy in importuning physicians to use the elixir. Both chemical and medical literature contain references to the toxicity of diethylene glycol in the amounts recommended by the manufacturer. Diethylene glycol, administered in doses comparable to the dose recommended by the manufacturer of Elixir of Sulfanilamide-Massengill, acts as a cumulative poison. Surely there has been no blacker picture of the inadequacy of our present food and drug laws or the lack of common scientific decency in drug manufacture than that illustrated by this tragic disaster.

In a separate *JAMA* editorial, "adequate legislation" for the regulation of drugs was demanded, either by amendment to the 1906 law or, preferably, completely new legislation.[10] The writer asserted that the current Food and Drugs Act failed to provide "adequate standards of purity, potency, wholesomeness and labeling of food and drugs," and that the penalties for violating the existing, minimal standards were feeble slaps. Furthermore there was virtually no regulation of medical devices or cosmetics and "no potent weapon against false or fraudulent advertising." The editorial, presumably speaking for the AMA, described the current version of a bill championed by Senator Royal Copeland (the latest version of a drug-reform bill that had been slogging its way through Congress) as "weak."[11] Chief among the bill's shortcomings was "the failure to set up adequate legal standards for drugs and diagnostic and therapeutic devices or to establish machinery by which such standards can be established." If such standards had existed, along with sufficient penalties for their violation, the author argued, the Elixir Sulfanilamide tragedy would never have occurred. The editorial then expressed general animosity toward the Wheeler-Lea bill, separate legislation that gave control of drug advertising to the FTC and not the FDA. The division of responsibility for drug oversight between the two government bodies was considered by the medical group as "dangerous." Yet of first and foremost importance was the creation of "obligatory legal standards for drugs and other materials used in the human body" and "sufficiently severe" penalties for violating them, the editorial concluded. Otherwise "there will be possible disasters such as the deaths from elixir of sulfanilamide, which for more than a fortnight have continued to shock the nation."

Joining the public chorus for reform was the highly vocal League of Women Voters. Despite repeated pleas for new drug legislation, the influential group believed that Congress had persistently recognized "special interests" at the expense of public safety. In the *St. Louis Post-Dispatch*, the local chapter chastised legislators for their historical ineptitude.

> For four years the league has been vainly urging on Congress adequate regulation of food, drug and cosmetic products. In the face of opposition of special interests, one measure of protection after another has been whittled away from pending bills. The bill that passed the Senate at its last session and was pending in the House had been shorn long since of original provisions that would have protected the public against the tragedies of this elixir.[12]

In his official capacity as FDA chief, Wat Campbell agreed that Senator Copeland's latest drug-reform bill would not have prevented "this wholesale tragedy."[13] Although the bill, despite being recently watered down by a House subcommittee, could have provided a more powerful basis for seizing Massengill's drug. Instead of tenuous misbranding charges, the government could have confiscated Elixir Sulfanilamide on the basis of its lethality alone (that is, when the drug was used according to the label's directions). But to seize toxic drugs after the fact was not sufficient for the FDA leader. Campbell wrote,

> It is our view that legislation should be enacted to require a license from the Government preliminary to the distribution of all drugs containing any potent ingredient or combination of ingredients, the use of which has not become well established in medical practice.

FDA officials and medical pundits argued that the original Tugwell-Copeland bill of 1933 (S. 1944) might have averted the elixir-related deaths, but the proposed legislation had "long been pulverized by lobbyists and their congressional sympathizers," charged Washington journalist Rodney Dutcher.[14] Even so, the original bill provided "no certain assurance that inadequately-tested drugs might not be sold." At the time of the bill's original submission to Congress, the FDA did not have the "political temerity" to demand the premarket testing of drugs, admitted an anonymous official to Dutcher. "We thought we would have trouble enough getting the less drastic provisions of the Tugwell bill adopted," the official explained, "And we did." Accusatory fingers pointed at Senators Josiah Bailey of North Carolina and Joel Bennett Clark of Missouri for "the final emasculation of such shreds of the Tugwell bill as remained when it was last heard of." In Dutcher's write-up, Campbell called the marketing of Elixir Sulfanilamide "an exceedingly thoughtless act." Dutcher rejoined that there was "apparently no question of legality, the law being what it is today." He furthermore found it "questionable" whether the Elixir Sulfanilamide incident would revive congressional efforts to pass "some version of the Tugwell bill" or "further drastic preventive and protective laws."

State drug laws, if they existed, were scattershot and apparently difficult to enforce. Many were faint echoes of the 1906 federal law. Among state laws enacted in 1935 and 1936, some focused on the regulation of specific drugs, like barbiturates, narcotics, and cannabis, and others addressed the sale of contraceptives and "venereal prophylactics."[15] A few states prohibited or otherwise controlled the distribution of established poisons, like arsenic, mercury, and strychnine. During the government's investigation and confiscation of Massengill's drug, the president of Louisiana's board of health wrongly claimed that his state's "model" pure food and drug law had prevented Elixir Sulfanilamide from entering Louisiana.[16] In fact, 14 pints of the elixir had been shipped directly from Bristol, Tennessee, to 13 Louisiana retailers, and four prescriptions had been dispensed in the state (including the publicized prescription to four-year-old Ecton Terrebonne of Westwego). The state law, which had been passed more than a year earlier, included a licensing provision, the only one that existed in the Union. The provision directed companies to submit every food, drug, and cosmetic product or prophylactic device to the board of health for examination before sale. Campbell himself praised Louisiana's law (if not its lackluster enforcement) and publicly urged all state health officials to "acquaint" their congressmen with the need for such drug-licensing provisions at the federal level.[17]

Even industry groups recognized the need to intensify government oversight of drug manufacturing in the wake of so many deaths. Editors of the trade journal *Drug and Cosmetic Industry* wondered, "Why a comparatively small manufacturer should, in ignorance or carelessness, believe that he alone had suddenly discovered a proper answer to a problem which the entire industry was trying to solve is beyond comprehension."[18] The only way to prevent a similar "accident" was through external regulation—by default, from the federal government. Perhaps government oversight of the drug industry was preferable to what was perceived as the sanctimonious, but impotent, piety of the AMA (and specifically that of Morris Fishbein, by inference). The trade journal criticized the medical organization for "throwing out its chest and trying to impress everyone the desirability of the association having full power over all drugs and how they shall be marketed." The editorial continued, "This is so despite the fact that the association has been unable to control its own members as is evidenced by the fact that physicians failed to follow the Council of the association and prescribed or dispensed this 'Elixir' even though it had not been accepted by the Council."

Likewise the *Oil, Paint and Drug Reporter* found Massengill's sale of the elixir "appalling for its evidence of ignorance or greed on the part of some who seek to be entrusted with ministration to the needs of the sick."[19] The trade journal was particularly stunned by the use of diethylene glycol, declaring, "Why a pharmaceutical manufacturer would use an industrial solvent of unknown pharmacologic activity in the making of a medicine for internal use is beyond comprehension." For the drug industry, it was recognized:

> Experimentation is as desirable in pharmacy as it is in medicine. Improved or more acceptable dosage forms of valuable drugs are helpful to the medical profession. It is an important function of pharmacal [sic] manufacturing to provide these. But experimentation with drugs in every connection should be scientific. Empirical trial and error is dangerous, especially when concerned with potent drugs of complex chemical composition and inestimable potential chemical reactivity.

The journal predicted, given the FDA's anemic misbranding charges against Massengill, an "inevitable" arousal of public sentiment to revise the Food and Drugs Act.

> There will be no great difficulty in calling up a pending bill in the special session of Congress. It cannot be denied that revision of the law has been too long deferred. It must be realized that the delay had to be attended with the possibility of increasing demand for still more rigorous prohibitions.

> It is to be expected that the public demand for protection will not be satisfied with making it possible to catch a poisonously adulterated drug in commerce, or with classifying the undisclosed presence of a dangerous ingredient as misbranding. The cry will be for formula disclosure and for factory inspection. The drug industry must expect attacks more severe than any it has known.

In its truncated coverage of the national tragedy, *Time* magazine agreed with Wat Campbell that the latest, failed drug-reform bill would not have subjected Massengill to stiffer federal prosecution. Regardless, the magazine assured, Massengill—who was described as a compounder of "veterinary medicines in a good-sized factory at Bristol, Tenn."—remained vulnerable to significant civil damages.[20] To that end, wire services reported on November 13th that the widow of C. W. Miller was suing the Massengill company and a Memphis drug store for $50,000, a substantially greater civil penalty than any threatened to date.[21] Miller, a filling-station attendant, had died on October 20th after taking several ounces of Massengill's elixir, which he had obtained without a prescription.

Public sympathy for the elixir victims and near-victims was maintained by *Life* magazine. In the issue dated November 8, 1937 (with a cover portrait of Greta Garbo), a dedicated one-page spread featured a photograph of a somber Dr. Archie Calhoun of Mississippi and a separate picture of his unfazed nurse, Evelyn Sharbrough, using a candlestick telephone.[22] Shown also was a picture of one of Calhoun's surviving patients, a young black woman who reportedly consumed a "whole bottle" of elixir, "swole up," and then quickly rebounded. Snapshots of the fresh graves of three of Calhoun's less fortunate patients were a sobering coda to the heart-tugging pictorial.

Similarly the drama created by Elixir Sulfanilamide and its possible legislative aftermath did not go unnoticed by Hollywood. Writing for a "motion picture" news service, gossip columnist Louella Parsons advised her readers, "Never let it be said that any crusade is ignored by our movies." She revealed that two separate films would dramatize the "shocking elixir deaths and the furor that has resulted." Warner Brothers had evidently bought the rights to *The Clarion*, a muckraking novel by journalist Samuel Hopkins Adams. The book, published in 1914, was an exposé of the fraudulent advertising of patent medicines. Screenwriters would incorporate the recent elixir-related deaths into the film adaptation, Parsons revealed, which was to star Dick Foran and newcomer Ann Sheridan as "the romantic leads." The working title for another anticipated film, also in preproduction, was *Permit to Kill*, with Edward Arnold in a starring role.[23]

Moviegoers were otherwise treated to a short documentary of the elixir story in a contemporaneous "News of the Day" newsreel. While attending the movies in Flushing, New York, a pleasantly surprised FDA chemist saw the "well conceived" "dramatic presentation" and praised the "clear and distinct voice" of Wat Campbell.[24] The chemist described the newsreel scenes from memory to his FDA boss: a shot of Massengill's plant; images of Dr. Calhoun and his nurse; and a short sequence of distillation experiments at the AMA laboratory. The newsreel concluded with a scene showing the FDA chief on the phone, "instructing all agents to immediately stop all other work and to concentrate on locating the Elixir, [which was] to be seized wherever found."

* * * * * *

On November 15th, FDA officials publicly declared that "every traceable quantity of elixir sulfanilamide [...] had been removed from the public's reach"; although there were "a few ounces obtained by itinerants and others who could not be located."[25] At approximately the same time, Massengill's in-house counsel and son-in-law, Frank DeFriece, wrote Morris Fishbein, requesting "a complete list of the recent fatalities alleged to be attributable to Elixir Sulfanilamide" and "the addresses of the parties in question." Fishbein referred the matter to Secretary Leech, who declined the lawyer's request for "obvious reasons." Leech then offered to DeFriece, "Whether or not the Federal Food and Drug Administration would care to supply you with their list is a matter about which this Laboratory is not informed." Copies of DeFriece's letter and Leech's terse reply were forwarded to Wat Campbell.[26]

Whatever legal defense or settlements Massengill's chief counsel was in the process of making, Massengill and his rogue chemist attempted to undermine their public disgrace. In addition to the brief statements made by Massengill, Watkins had evidently penned a flabbergasting letter to a professional journal, *Drug Trade News*, defending his creation. The letter, published originally in the November 8th issue, was picked up by at least two newspapers, which reprinted choice excerpts.[27] The implicit intent of the news editors was to shock readers, which evidently accomplished. Watkins's dispatch, possibly written in rebuttal to the *JAMA* issue of November 6th, stated that the Massengill company had performed its own animal experiments after news of the first elixir-related deaths. "We gave forty times the human dose of the elixir to [guinea] pigs and they liked it," he alleged, adding, "Then we shot it into them, and they still lived with no harm done." Watkins quickly offered that the animals had not "of course" been taking other medicines with the elixir.

In addition to suggesting that the elixir-related deaths were due to interactions with other drugs, like Epsom salts or other sulfates, Watkins floated the idea that the casualties were caused by sulfanilamide and not diethylene glycol. Patients may have overdosed on the antibiotic, he proposed. Watkins went on to charge, "The solvent itself [diethylene glycol] had nothing to do with the deaths," despite mounting and compelling evidence to the contrary. Watkins boasted that he had taken the elixir himself, without consequence, after the first public warning from the AMA. "On Monday [probably October 18th] I started taking the elixir, one ounce a day, in two doses, and am still here and writing to you, though I have taken four ounces in four days." Alluding to the official visit of Chief Medical Officer Klumpp and Inspector Ford at Bristol on October 18th, Watkins claimed, "Federal men and our men saw me take it." (Although Klumpp patently denied that he had ever seen Watkins consume the elixir and doubted that the chemist had ever done so.) Stunningly enough, Watkins also cited a recent animal study by Haag and Ambrose ("Studies on the physiological effect of diethylene glycol" in the *Journal of Pharmacology and Experimental Therapeutics*), which showed that diethylene glycol, while less toxic than ethylene glycol, was still sufficiently lethal. Watkins attempted to bolster whatever specious argument he was weaving by noting that the AMA's laboratory had reported no apparent chemical reaction between diethylene glycol and sulfanilamide in its distillation experiments of the company's elixir. This finding was raised by the chemist despite the fact that scientists at the University of Chicago had reported in the same *JAMA* issue that pure diethylene glycol and Massengill's product were similarly toxic, and that sulfanilamide was relatively safe. Last Watkins noted that the use of diethylene glycol in consumer products was not unprecedented. The substance—which Watkins inexplicably wrote was "manufactured exclusively by the Carbon and Carbide Chemicals corporation" and derived from "casinghead gas taken from oil wells"—was incorporated into cigarettes to prevent throat irritation.[28]

If some measure of public sympathy for Massengill and his company could not be obtained nationally, Massengill's hometown paper, the *Bristol Herald Courier*, was willing to oblige locally. On November 21st, the beginning of Thanksgiving week, the publication took particular umbrage with the brief coverage of the elixir-related deaths in *Time* magazine. In a front-page opinion piece, the paper—while giving a passing nod to the tragedy of the deaths—defended the ample size of the Massengill company and its reputable history.[29]

It is deplorable, of course, that any deaths have occurred. But had there been many more deaths, and could they have been traced to the sulfanilamide elixir, the fact would not have warranted Time in publishing an article containing an intimation that the Massengill Drug Company is a small and irresponsible firm. The company is domiciled in a large group of modern buildings, it employs an army of men and women, and it has branch houses in New York, Kansas City, and San Francisco. And thousands of physicians and druggists all over the country will bear testimony to its responsibility.

The article in Time quoted a Federal agent as saying the Massengill Company lacks testing facilities and is careless in the manufacture of drugs. Not by practices of that kind did Dr. Massengill, who holds the degree of M. D., become one of the leading manufacturing pharmacists of the country. He has built up an enviable reputation over a period of forty years, by patient and persevering effort, by sound business judgment and capable management, by close personal attention to the affairs of his company, and by turning out honest products.

In a show of general ignorance or willful misrepresentation, the pseudonymous writer ("Old Timer") then minimized the extensive field work of numerous FDA agents to retrieve the at-large bottles of Massengill's elixir and failed to note that Massengill's explicit recall telegrams of October 19th (which warned that the product was "dangerous to life") were sent at the direct urging of Inspector Ford in Bristol.

The Time article stated that Federal men "confiscated every last flask of the Massengill 'elixir' upon which they could lay their hands." That publication may not have known that with the first report of a *death from sulfanilamide* [emphasis added], which came from Oklahoma, Dr. Massengill deluged the Western Union office in Bristol with telegrams to his salesmen and others to take every ounce of the elixir off the market. Probably there were few flasks left for Federal men to confiscate.

While the writer reserved judgment about the "lethal quality" of Elixir Sulfanilamide, Massengill's "six registered chemical pharmacists" were summarily acquitted of any mistakes in the manufacture of the product. The writer then boldly parroted the defense of Watkins, by implicating adverse reactions between the antibiotic component of Massengill's elixir and other drugs: "All the evidence seems to be that the fatalities caused by sulfanilamide were due to the use of other medicines in connection with the elixir." Moreover while "this product has been fatal in a few cases," the writer brazenly offered, "it has been beneficial in many— though the fatal results are not, of course, offset by the beneficial effects." The inane scribbling concluded,

> One unacquainted with Dr. Massengill and unfamiliar with the history of his company would gain a false impression of both from the Time publication. We say what we have said with a view to correcting, as far as possible, the injustice and the false impression.

Misinformation about the cause of the elixir-related deaths—whether propagated by Massengill, his employees, the Bristol press, or generally lazy reporting—continued to be sufficiently widespread to prompt the AMA's Secretary Leech to respond in a *JAMA* update.[30] In the journal issue dated November 20th, he acknowledged that there had been "considerable confusion" in "newspapers and elsewhere" about the cause of the elixir-related deaths, many of which had been attributed to sulfanilamide. But the antibiotic was "not the causative factor," Leech wrote in no uncertain terms. He then reiterated unequivocally that diethylene glycol "was the harmful agent." In addition, the journal provided an updated tally of the nation's elixir-related deaths. The official count, as of November 11th, was 73. Fatalities were now acknowledged in Mississippi (21), Oklahoma (10), Georgia (8), Illinois (7), South Carolina (7), Alabama (6), Texas (6), Tennessee (3), Arkansas (1), California (1), Missouri (1), Ohio (1), and North Carolina (1). It was emphasized, however, that the newly charted deaths had not occurred recently, but had merely been recognized recently. The fact that no elixir-related deaths had occurred within the last few weeks was attributed to the "wide publicity initiated by The Journal," as well as "the excellent work of the government in removing the product from the market." The information in *JAMA*'s update would be underlined and expanded considerably in a landmark report to Congress.

13
THE BABY I GRIEVE FOR DAY AND NIGHT

In response to resolutions passed sequentially by the Senate and House in mid-November, Secretary of Agriculture Henry Wallace submitted his 34-page report on "Elixir Sulfanilamide-Massengill," complete with appendixed exhibits, to Congress on Thanksgiving morning, November 25, 1937.[1] The contents of the plain-speaking "Letter of Transmittal," although submitted officially by the Secretary, were heavily, if not exclusively, informed by FDA officials.[2] The report's raison d'être, if not to unpack the details of the Elixir Sulfanilamide tragedy for America, was to use the catastrophe as a springboard for urging new drug legislation. Wallace's report revealed not only the known extent of elixir-related casualties in the United States (even as the FDA continued its multi-state investigation), but it laid out for the first time the sequence of events that led to the deaths. Details included the incentive for creating Massengill's elixir, its recipe, the company's failure to conduct a "few simple and inexpensive tests on experimental animals" before marketing the elixir, the wide distribution of elixir shipments, the evasive wording of Massengill's first recall telegrams, and the FDA's yeoman efforts to confiscate the poisonous medicine—despite considerable barriers.

There were now 93 deaths due to Elixir Sulfanilamide (73 confirmed, 20 probable), ranging from California to Virginia, Wallace revealed. Yet most were in the Southeast and Midwest (as shown in the report's appendixed map [p 141]), where the bulk of the elixir had been shipped. Of the 240 gallons manufactured by The S. E. Massengill Company, 228 gallons and two pints (95%) had been "seized under federal and state laws, destroyed, collected as laboratory samples, or wasted by spillage and breakage." The remaining 11 gallons and six pints had been dispensed by prescription or sold over the counter. Of this amount, the FDA reckoned, about half had been consumed and was responsible for the deaths; the rest had been retrieved from patients.

Through the efforts of "[p]ractically the entire field force of 239 Food and Drug Administration inspectors and chemists," the agency had tracked down 633 commercial shipments and 671 sample bottles, the report claimed. And despite the fact that the FDA had received only sporadic help from local officials, Wallace lauded "the wholehearted and effective cooperation of State and local food, drug, and health authorities." The Secretary explained how federal agents had accomplished their objectives. It had not been sufficient to examine Massengill's shipping and consignees' records. To account for every parcel of Massengill's elixir, the firm's approximately 200 salesmen had been contacted for their records of sale and distribution, as well as any samples they might have given out. In addition, Wallace revealed, the FDA had cross-checked the accuracy of Massengill's distribution lists by making random inquiries at major drug houses throughout the country for any possible unrecorded shipments. To add color and to further define the FDA's efforts, the report gave examples of the many impediments faced by the agency's field agents. There was the examination of 20,000 sales slips at "one establishment" (the drug wholesaler, Meyer Brothers, in St. Louis); the difficulty of tracing over-the-counter sales (particularly in Georgia); the vaguely written prescriptions in East St. Louis; the obfuscation of a "South Carolina doctor" (Johnston Peeples); and the subsequent discovery of a weather-beaten elixir bottle on the fresh grave of an unnamed "Negro" (J. J. McDaniel) by an unnamed inspector (Monte Rentz).

The composite effects of Massengill's elixir were then described. Victims were ill from one to three weeks with "very much the same symptoms": "stoppage of urine, severe abdominal pain, nausea, and vomiting." Stupor and sometimes convulsions preceded death. But symptoms and death were not predictable. There were individuals who experienced "unfavorable symptoms" but recovered after stopping the product. Others completely tolerated the elixir, taking up to nearly eight ounces. Conversely one child died after taking less than two ounces, the report offered. And if this information did not sufficiently convey the random waste and nonsensical pain of the tragedy, the full contents of a letter written by the mother of victim Joan Marlar to President Roosevelt were provided as an agonizing coda.

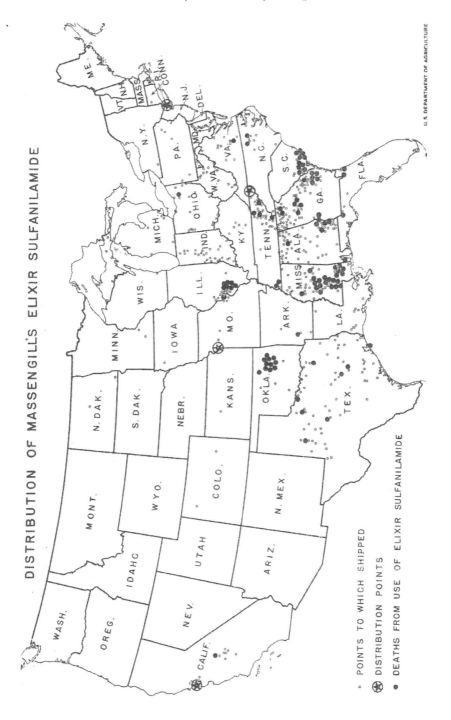

DISTRIBUTION OF MASSENGILL'S ELIXIR SULFANILAMIDE

U. S. DEPARTMENT OF AGRICULTURE

∘ POINTS TO WHICH SHIPPED

⊛ DISTRIBUTION POINTS

● DEATHS FROM USE OF ELIXIR SULFANILAMIDE

Tulsa, Okla., November 8, 1937.

President Roosevelt:

Dear Sir: Two months ago I was happy and working taking care of my two little girls, Joan age 6 and Jean age 9. Our byword through the depression was that we had good health and each other. Joan thought her mother was right in everything, and it would have made your heart feel good last November to have seen her jumping and shouting as we listened to your reelection over the radio.

Tonight, Mr. Roosevelt, that little voice is stilled. The first time I ever had occasion to call in a doctor for her and she was given the Elixir of Sulfanilamide. Tonight our little home is bleak and full of despair. All that is left to us is the caring for of that little grave. Even the memory of her is mixed with sorrow for we can see her little body tossing to and fro and hear that little voice screaming with pain and it seems as though it would drive me insane. During her 9 days of illness as we sat by her bed only once did those little eyes lose their dull and unknowing look. Jean and I begged her to look and know us. A smile broke over her face and she laughed aloud with us and as quickly it vanished, never to smile and know us again.

Tonight, President Roosevelt, as you enjoy your little grandchildren of whom we read about, it is my plea that you will take steps to prevent such sales of drugs that will take little lives and leave such suffering behind and such a bleak outlook on the future as I have tonight.

Joan's distraught mother continued, relaying her knowledge of and contempt for Dr. Spann's attempted deception.

Surely we can have laws governing doctors also who will give such a medicine, not knowing to what extent its danger, and then lying and stealing the prescription they wrote supposedly from a reliable drug store. I don't believe such a doctor has taken his oath in all sincerity. Our lives are not safe entrusted in the hands of such a doctor, for that was my experience to my sorrow.

In my confidence in you I am writing you and hope that you can realize a little of what I am suffering and that you will take steps to prevent such in the future for I realize also there are other homes where hearts are broken such as mine.

It is easy for people to say "Try to think that she died that others might live." It is easier to say when it doesn't strike in your own home.

Enclosed is a picture of the baby I grieve for day and night.

Thanking you and
   Sincerely,

(Mrs.) Maise Nidiffer

Although the included photograph of six-year-old Joan Marlar—an impish-looking girl with Shirley Temple curls—was not printed in Wallace's report, it was filed and kept in the FDA's official records on Elixir Sulfanilamide for posterity.

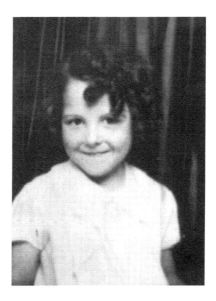

Joan Marlar, daughter of Maise Nidiffer, c1937 (FDA)

Wallace revealed that 25 federal seizures of Massengill's elixir had been made under the Food and Drugs Act, but that many lots had also been seized or embargoed by state or city officials.[3] The federal seizures were based on the fact that the product had been described as an elixir

(Wallace's report repeatedly printed the term elixir, when referring to Massengill's drug, in quotation marks). "Had the product been called a 'solution' [...] no charge of violating the law could have been brought," Wallace advised. The message to Congress was plain: Federal charges were based on tenuous semantics, and there was little in the way of legislation to prevent a similar tragedy. In fact, the American public relied on whatever moral fiber and savvy existed among drug manufacturers, some of whom had "considered making a solution of sulfanilamide in diethylene glycol before the 'elixir' was put on the market," Wallace divulged, "but abandoned the idea on investigating the toxicity of the solvent." Limitations of the existing law, thanks to the "spectacular" "'elixir' incident," were axiomatic. Nevertheless the tragedy was "but a repetition of what has frequently happened in the past in the marketing of such dangerous drugs as dinitrophenol, cinchophen, and other substances," Wallace added.[1]

The Secretary offered four minimum recommendations for new drug legislation.

1. The "license control" of new drugs (with provisions for defining "new drugs"). This measure, which went beyond the reach of the Tugwell-Copeland bill, was proposed by Wallace to ensure that experimental and clinical safety tests were conducted on drugs before their distribution. It was now the position of the Department of Agriculture (and by definition, the FDA) that no other mechanism would sufficiently protect the public from dangerous drugs: not stiffer penalties for violations; not full disclosure of ingredients (which was also recommended). The licensing of drugs, and by default their manufacturers, was justified by the fact that licensing provisions existed for physicians, pharmacists, and even tradespeople, like plumbers. "But there is no such control to prevent incompetent drug manufacturers from marketing any kind of lethal potion," Wallace proclaimed. For those who countered that the professional education of drug manufacturers should offer sufficient and informed protection against dangerous drugs, the rebuttal was easy. "It should be remembered," Wallace advised, "that Dr. Massengill and his chemist, Watkins, are far better equipped from the standpoint of technical training than many other persons now engaged in the manufacture of drugs." And yet Massengill and Watkins had produced Elixir Sulfanilamide.

2. The prohibition of drugs that are dangerous when used according to the manufacturer's directions. This provision, included in the latest, albeit diluted, version of Senator Copeland's drug-reform bill,

provided a more compelling basis for seizing Massengill's drug than the flimsy misbranding charges. Moreover, Wallace warned, "A number of dangerous drugs are now on the market against which not even a trivial charge of violation can be made."

3. The requirement that drug labels provide sufficient directions for use and information about misuse, such as overdose and the risk of addiction (particularly in an age when alcohol was a significant ingredient in many medicines, and opiate use was minimally regulated, if at all).

4. The prohibition of secret remedies, with the label disclosure of all ingredients. It was a paradox that labels of exported US drugs had to conform to this requirement (on the basis of foreign laws), while labels for the same medicines sold in America did not. The upfront disclosure of diethylene glycol in Massengill's elixir might have alerted some informed physicians to the toxicity of the product and others to more easily pinpoint the cause of adverse symptoms after the product had been taken.

In contradistinction to the spotty national coverage of the elixir-related deaths, Wallace's report received widespread attention. In a full-column write-up, the *New York Times* marveled at the "[u]nusually outspoken" document that told a "graphic story" of "the greatest man-hunt in the history of the Federal agency," "without attempting dramatization."[5] The *Washington Post* found the report "[c]rammed with dramatic details."[6] Wire services focused on Wallace's proposals to strengthen drug regulations.[7] Senator Copeland, in response, vowed to introduce a bill that would "embody" Wallace's recommendations.[8] (A few days later, he proposed a ban on the interstate shipment of drugs unless they were approved by the Secretary of Agriculture as "not unsafe for use.")[9] On its editorial page, the *St. Louis Post-Dispatch* declared, "Reform the Drug Law!" and warned, "Battle lines are forming for a showdown fight in Congress on the long-needed strengthening of the Food and Drugs Act."[10] And while the paper acknowledged, "Drug interests have made valid objections to previous bills on the ground that they were unduly drastic," it was concluded that the scores of elixir-related deaths "[outweigh] all the arguments advanced by the obstructionists at previous sessions of Congress."

On the other hand, news coverage of Wallace's report in Sullivan County, Tennessee, the home of Massengill's company, was perfunctory at best. The *Kingsport Times* buried a brief version of a wire story on page three, with the diminished headline, "Legislation Favored Control New Drugs."[11] The two-paragraph write-up, which was hidden beneath a pictorial of Cleveland's labor rackets, mentioned "recent deaths attributed to the use of an 'elixir sulfanilamide' in treating infections" but not the Massengill company. The *Bristol Herald Courier* was mum on Wallace's report until Saturday, November 27th, when a front-page headline charged, "Massengill Avers False Statements Made About Elixir," and "Charges Food and Drug Officials Are Trying to Stampede Congress." In addition, subheads claimed, "Product Tested" and "Several Hundred People Took Sulfanilamide With Good Results."[12] Massengill's lengthy, printed rebuttal to Wallace's report was, in essence, a countercharge that the FDA was exploiting the elixir-related deaths in an effort to widen its powers. In detail, the doctor's response was an unfocused, head-spinning tirade that defended the use of the term elixir, the relative safety of diethylene glycol, the often-beneficial nature of his product, and stringent drug regulation.

Massengill proclaimed that he had never contacted (and thereby had not attempted to influence) his congressman, Republican B. Carroll Reece, who led a successful opposition campaign in the summer of 1936 against an earlier version of Copeland's drug-reform bill (S. 5). The doctor added that he was "heartily in favor" of the current bill pending before Congress. To defend the label of elixir for his diethylene glycol–containing drug, he cited the *National Formulary*, which included two nonalcoholic formulas for elixirs. And while curiously "not defending the preparation," Massengill claimed that his elixir had not been "rushed on the market by us before it was tested." He cited the "several hundred patients who took it with good result" to demonstrate its "unpredictable effect." Last he supported the choice of diethylene glycol as a solvent, "which is much less toxic than the ethylene glycol which is used as an anti-freeze mixture." As support for the use of more toxic glycols in medicines, he cited the AMA Council's recent approval of two products containing ethylene glycol.

Massengill was correct on this final point. In fact, during the last year the AMA Council had accepted Luminal, a brand of phenobarbital, in a solution of ethylene glycol.[13] The product was intended to be injected subcutaneously (underneath the skin) or intramuscularly (into muscle) and was advertised by Winthrop Chemical as a treatment for intractable epileptic seizures, acute psychosis, drug addiction, and the "vomiting of pregnancy."[14] In 1935, the AMA Council had also accepted a bismuth compound (iodobismitol) in a solution of ethylene glycol.[15] The product, manufactured by E. R. Squibb and Sons, was intended as an intramuscular treatment for syphilis.[16] (It is unknown if the administration of either of these advertised products ever resulted in adverse outcomes because of ethylene glycol. Regardless Squibb replaced the ethylene glycol in its product with propylene glycol, to avert any systemic toxicity of the former solvent.[17] Winthrop likewise changed up its Luminal formula.[18])

* * * * * *

At the end of November 1937, the gaping disconnect between the sadness and anger generated by Elixir Sulfanilamide on a national scale and the defense and denial of Massengill in East Tennessee could not be more apparent. The polar views were epitomized in two, nearly simultaneously penned letters. On November 30th, Wat Campbell drafted a reply to Mrs. Nidiffer, the grieving mother of Joan Marlar.[19] The job was left to the FDA chief by the White House. Twenty-four hours later, the Sullivan-Johnson County Medical Society, Massengill's local professional chapter, met at the General Shelby Hotel in Bristol to extend a letter of confidence to the drug manufacturer.[20] Massengill's small empire undoubtedly hung in the balance because of deaths like Joan Marlar's. The FDA chief began,

My dear Mrs. Nidiffer:

Your letter of November 8 was received and read at the White House and immediately referred to the Food and Drug Administration, which was even then trying by all means in its power to trace down every possible ounce of the poisonous Elixir Sulfanilamide. In sending your letter to me there was transmitted the President's request that your letter be answered.

Believe me when I say, Mrs. Nidiffer, that in the course of my thirty years in the Government service I have never had a more difficult assignment than the President's request to reply to you. Your letter was laid before me during the weeks that we were desperately following up outstanding lots of the Elixir. I have looked at the lovely smiling face of your little girl and I think I realize in some measure your unending sorrow at a needless sacrifice [...]

In its resolution, Massengill's local medical society responded with seemingly bureaucratic indifference,

Whereas, Dr. S. E. Massengill is a member of this organization in good standing, and has always enjoyed a reputation for professional integrity and all-round good citizenship.

Whereas, Dr. S. E. Massengill, as owner of the company known as The S. E. Massengill Company, has a reputation for honest business dealings, and has supplied to the medical professions for over 40 years pharmaceutical products that are used by many of the leading physicians and hospitals [...]

Campbell's note of condolence to Mrs. Nidiffer continued,

The President and the Department of Agriculture, and many enlightened legislators as well as representatives of the public, have been urging with the utmost earnestness for the past four years the passage of a food and drug law which will give more ample protection than our present statute. One of the first actions of both the House and the Senate when they convened for the present special session was to pass resolutions calling upon the Secretary of Agriculture for a report on the Elixir Sulfanilamide tragedy, together with recommendations for legislation which would prevent such catastrophies [sic] in the future. The Secretary's report was delivered to both Houses of Congress on Thanksgiving morning. Your letter was included as a part of the report in the belief that it would impress upon our national legislators, more forcibly than any official recital, the horror of this tragedy and the absolute necessity for national legislation which will make its repetition impossible [...]

Evidently unmoved by national sentiment, the Tennessee physicians concurrently volleyed,

Whereas, The S. E. Massengill Company is one of the large companies manufacturing pharmaceutical products in America, employing over 500 persons.

Whereas, we have knowledge of and acquaintance with the many fine citizens and high class workers connected with The S. E. Massengill Company.

Whereas, the products of the company are supplied only through the professions and are not advertised to the laity, and its formulas are widely used with known satisfactory results.

Whereas, neither Dr. Massengill nor The S. E. Massengill Company has ever, previous to the regrettable Elixir Sulfanilamide occurrence, been subjected to the serious criticism of its products or methods of doing business [...]

Campbell concluded by attempting to reassure Mrs. Nidiffer.

> I agree with you it should not have been necessary for your baby to die to arouse public sentiment to the point that proper legislation will be enacted. If it is enacted—and I sincerely believe that there are strong and good men in both the House and Senate who have resolved that laws will be passed which will make a repetition of this tragedy impossible—it may be of some small comfort to you to know that your letter has had a real influence in bringing about this result.
>
> With the most sincere sympathy, I am
>
> Sincerely yours,
>
> W. G. Campbell, Chief

The medical group concluded its disposition toward Massengill and "the unfavorable publicity,"

> Be it resolved that we, the members of the Sullivan-Johnson County Medical Society, deeply regret the unfortunate occurrence and unfavorable publicity to which The S. E. Massengill Company has recently been subjected, and extend to Dr. Massengill and his employees a sincere vote of confidence in their integrity and honesty towards the medical profession and to the public, and our assurance of our continued complete confidence in his products.

14
DRAFTING A SANE, SENSIBLE, WORKABLE BILL

Proponents of stricter drug regulation, like Senator Copeland of New York, now had the "political temerity" to ask for, if not demand, the premarket testing of new drugs. On December 1st, Copeland introduced S. 3073 to emend the current version of his drug-reform bill, S. 5 no. 2.[1] The new measure, informally dubbed the "sulfanilamide bill," called for the license control of new drugs to ensure that animal tests and human trials for safety were conducted before the interstate distribution of pharmaceuticals. Specifically S. 3073 required that any manufacturer seeking to market a new drug must submit a list of the drug's components, testing records, an explanation of the manufacturing processes, labeling examples, and drug samples (if requested) to the Secretary of Agriculture— or really the FDA, the decisions of which would be guided by an expert advisory committee. The drug could only be marketed if and when the Secretary determined that it was "not unsafe for use."[2]

This time Copeland could expect the passage of an effective drug law. Massengill was right. Proponents of reform, and specifically the FDA, could use the "unfortunate" affair with Elixir Sulfanilamide to their political advantage. It was the grand tragedy—beautifully narrated in Secretary Wallace's report to Congress—that generated popular outrage, and popular outrage was what was typically needed to prompt Congress to act in any bold, meaningful way. For four years Copeland had championed new legislation, in one version or another, to replace the inadequate 1906 Food and Drugs Act, and now was the time to expect tangible results for his longstanding cause.

A physician[3] and the former Health Commissioner of New York City, Copeland became enamored with the FDA and its cause for legislative reform during a special hearing before the Senate Agricultural Committee in the summer of 1930. Wat Campbell was called before the committee to answer charges that the FDA had been lax in its enforcement of the 1906 law, and Campbell effectively rebutted that his agency could only do so much under the existing act. By the end of the inquiry, Copeland, who was asked to participate in the acrimonious hearings, was so outwardly sympathetic to the FDA that he was described by the press as the "counsel for the defense."[4]

In 1933, Copeland became the congressional sponsor of the so-called Tugwell bill—a measure drafted largely by FDA officials and sponsored by then-Assistant Secretary of Agriculture, Rexford Tugwell, to reform the food and drug law. Senate Bill 1944, as the Tugwell bill was officially labeled, was something of a hot potato, primarily because FDR was ambivalent, at best, about stricter food and drug regulation. His overwhelming priority was to approve measures that hastened the country's economic recovery from the Great Depression, and the stricter oversight of foods, drugs, and cosmetics could be viewed as stifling commerce. Moreover Roosevelt believed that passing a bill to replace the Food and Drugs Act was a Sisyphean task. He anticipated correctly that industry groups would aggressively lobby to defeat any revision of the 1906 law. Consequently Tugwell and Campbell had a hard time finding a necessary congressional backer for S. 1944. In search of a sponsor, they "literally peddled the thing up and down the halls of Congress," wrote one FDA staffer; but they found no takers, only advice to loosen the bill's stiffer provisions.[5] Finally the pair recruited Copeland, who offered his steadfast, if initially naïve, support. Described as "blythe and debonair" by the press, the senator was distinguished at the time not so much by his personality as by his appearance. By Senate standards, Copeland was a natty, modern dresser, and his suit-coat lapel featured a fresh, red carnation, pinned on daily by his wife. But time would show that Copeland was not a dandy pushover. He would prove himself at critical moments to be a shrewd legislator, a maverick freethinker, and an unwavering advocate for public safety. Copeland's adoption of the Tugwell bill and his commitment to drug reform, to paraphrase historian Charles Jackson, would shape much of the senator's remaining years.

For its time, S. 1944 was a remarkable and arguably drastic measure. Among the bill's more radical and broad stipulations: Misbranding was defined as any therapeutic claim on a drug label that was contrary to general medical opinion (as nebulous as that might be), and the charge of adulteration was applied to any medicinal product that was dangerous when used according to the manufacturer's directions. S. 1944 also removed the government's burden of proving a drug manufacturer's intent to defraud. In addition, the bill required drug makers to disclose all of their products' ingredients and to distinguish palliative claims from curative ones. Tugwell's strategy with S. 1944, at the time of its drafting, was to propose aggressive regulation of the drug trade and its advertising, in anticipation of inevitable legislative compromises.

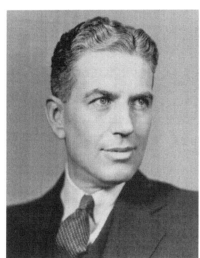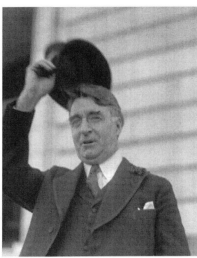

Left, Rexford G. Tugwell, c1935-1942 (Library of Congress, US Farm Security Administration); Right, Senator Royal S. Copeland, c1923 (Library of Congress, National Photo Company Collection)

In June of 1933, Copeland introduced the measure in the Senate at the close of an emergency congressional session (which had been called by the newly elected FDR in March to address the country's economic crisis). However, it appears that Copeland presented the bill in relative haste, without thoroughly reviewing its contents. Consequently the senator was blindsided on the floor by S. 1944's vague language and overreaching militancy—particularly with respect to the regulation of advertising. At the time, Copeland was ill-equipped to defend what could be viewed as alienating demands on the part of an obtrusive government. After he got around to carefully reviewing the bill (months later, according to historian Jackson), Copeland came to believe that S. 1944 was sorely in need of clarifying revisions. "There are a number of changes that ought to be made," he admitted to the *New York Times* in December of 1933, "but I don't want to discuss them yet," he cryptically added.[6]

Independent of Copeland's ambivalence toward S. 1944, general support for the bill was mixed. Not to anyone's surprise, most of those affiliated with the drug and advertising industries wanted the bill quashed. Trade representatives argued repeatedly and effectively that the measure gave far too much discretionary power to the government and would stymie business and thereby national economic recovery. The AMA's response to S. 1944 was curiously guarded, perhaps because the organization hadn't been consulted in the bill's drafting. The group publicly stated that it was "wholly behind the principles" of the bill but implied that S. 1944 itself was not yet "suitable" for ratification.[7] The AMA apparently believed that the measure was not sufficiently rigorous, stating in *JAMA* that the bill "seems in some parts to fall short of [its] purpose," particularly with respect to the regulation of advertising.

Perhaps also, AMA leaders weren't particularly fond of Copeland. The senator, although educated in allopathic medicine, was a cheerleader for homeopathy (an alternative, unscientific form of medical treatment that was condemned by the AMA as quackery). Copeland also had a number of commercial relationships with drug manufacturers that represented potentially significant conflicts of interest.[8] Through his syndicated radio program, *The Dr. Royal S. Copeland Hour*, or by direct promotion, Copeland had received or was receiving financial remuneration from the makers of Pluto Water (a branded laxative), Eno's Fruit Salt (essentially sodium bicarbonate), and Phillips' Milk of Magnesia. Consumers' Research, an influential nonprofit group and frequent critic of the FDA, likewise called S. 1944 anemic and voiced its doubts about Copeland as a properly disinterested sponsor of drug reform. The group went so far as to demand Copeland's resignation from the Senate subcommittee in charge of the Tugwell bill. "We do not believe it is possible to receive fair dealings, not only in the hearings but in the committee's deliberations, when the chairman we are informed is receiving pay for broadcasting in behalf of a nationally-advertised product," the group charged.[9] Reliable support for S. 1944 and Copeland, however, was found among women's groups—particularly the difficult-to-ignore League of Women Voters.

To counter industry's unrelenting attack on S. 1944, the FDA engaged in a coordinated campaign to promote the bill through public speeches by agency personnel, government posters, the Department of Agriculture's "National Farm and Home Hour" radio show, and the shocking "Chamber of Horrors" exhibit. But opposition to the bill, specifically from trade groups, charged that the FDA's open enthusiasm for S. 1944 violated the 1919 Deficiency Appropriation Act, which prevented government agencies from lobbying their causes to Congress. Checks within the Department of Agriculture confirmed the legal breach, and the FDA thereby shut down its open sponsorship of S. 1944 during the last months of 1933. The resulting, unconstrained opposition to new drug regulations, and specifically S. 1944, told Copeland and other reformers that concessions to industry would have to be significant if there were to be any hope of revamping the old Food and Drugs Act. A backlash against government regulation generally and S. 1944 specifically was also informed by the failure of Prohibition and its ultimate repeal at the end of 1933. Opponents of the Tugwell bill saw it as the food and drug equivalent of the now-defunct National Prohibition Act, a law originally championed by former Congressman Andrew Volstead. As one editorialist argued,

> It is admitted that the food and drugs situation can and should be improved upon, but if we are chumps enough to follow Tugwell sentiment like we followed the Volstead sentiment we will run into a similar impasse just to create jobs for a new and numerous batch of bureaucrats. When trade regulations become too intricate trade will outwit them as surely as the prohibition bureau was outwitted.[10]

Undaunted, Copeland introduced his major rewrite of the Tugwell bill, called S. 2800, in the Senate in February of 1934.[11] This "sane, sensible, workable bill," as Copeland described it, provided four major concessions to industry, three of which directly affected drug manufacturers. First, full disclosure of ingredients would no longer be required on drug labels; instead the manufacturer need list only specified components of his product. This allowance was made "on the complaint that patented formulas would be revealed to chiseling competitors."[12] Second, publishers of false advertising would not be held legally liable; however, they would be required to identify those manufacturers who produced the false copy to the Department of Agriculture. And in response to concerns that previous bills had given unrestricted regulatory power to the government, the revised bill allowed for the creation of advisory boards to appeal alleged violations. But as is the case with most compromises, no one was particularly happy with S. 2800. Trade groups, while appeased to some extent on the issue of advertising, predicted continued economic gloom with so much regulation of their business. Tugwell himself, despite the fact that the revised bill still carried his name, was unhappy with the industry concessions—to the point of publicly calling the bill "very disappointing" and losing interest altogether in its passage.[13] Disappointment in S. 2800 was echoed by consumer lobbyists, who described the new measure as "emasculated" and a godsend to quacks. The FDA's leadership favored passage of S. 2800, while harboring reservations about the bill's concessions to trade groups. This sentiment was generally shared by the AMA, which warned, "There are indeed some aspects of this bill which could not be supported by the medical profession and these have been called to the attention of Senator Copeland."[14] Nevertheless the medical group urged its members to support the bill's passage by contacting their congressmen. Influential women's groups also backed S. 2800, while continuing to lobby for restoration of the original components of the first Tugwell bill.

Unfortunately Tugwell's sour opinion of S. 2800 informed FDR's apathy for the measure. Tugwell was a conspicuous and influential member of the President's liberal inner circle, or "brain trust," and without FDR's good opinion of S. 2800 to champion it through Congress, the bill died a death of indifference at the end of the second congressional session, in June of 1934. FDR's coolness toward S. 2800 was also likely political, given that Copeland was not always in lockstep with the administration's New Dealers. Moreover the President's ambivalence toward the bill probably had something to do with the FTC's struggle with the FDA over the control of drug advertising. The President generally sided with the FTC and its desire to retain purview over drug advertising (although FDR could vacillate on this issue). In the ensuing years, contention between the FTC and the FDA would become a major obstacle to the passage of any food and drug reform measure.

* * * * * *

After his November reelection (with little thanks to FDR), Senator Copeland began drafting yet another food and drug bill, this time without the input of Tugwell or the FDA. In January of 1935, Copeland introduced his new reform bill, S. 5, in the Senate. Concessions made to industry in this measure were even heavier than those in S. 2800. "[T]he great objection to the Tugwell bill," Copeland explained to the press, "was that it gave arbitrary life and death power to the Secretary of Agriculture."[15] Requirements for drug labeling in S. 5 were considerably more lenient. Formulas merely had to be filed with the Secretary of Agriculture, a stipulation that averted the public disclosure of ingredients on a drug's label. Constraints on drug advertising (which would be overseen by the FDA) were also loosened, and the agency's seizures of misbranded items were limited to three actions on a single product. Drugs that varied from the recognized standards of the US Pharmacopeia were also allowed.

Once again, FDA leaders recognized that Copeland's latest draft was a general improvement on the 1906 law and a realistic, if unsavory, compromise. Copeland's new measure, like his previous bills, gained the reluctant support of all-important women's organizations, as well as professional pharmacy groups. However, the AMA found S. 5 inadequate, charging, "On the whole, the Copeland food, drugs, devices and cosmetics bill is disappointing in its weakness."[16] Likewise consumer activists were unhappy with the new bill. For contrary reasons, proprietary drug manufacturers—whose congressional lobbyists became instrumental in the bill's fate—were also dissatisfied with S. 5. FDR, ever capricious in his views toward the government's stricter oversight of food and drugs, publicly asked Congress to tighten the regulation of industry's "evaders and chiselers"; however, he curiously failed to endorse S. 5 specifically.[17]

Regardless of the uneven support for S. 5, public hearings in the Senate forecasted its early passage. The bill was reported out of committee on March 22nd, despite opposition efforts from Democrats Josiah Bailey and Joel Bennett Clark. The two senators' objections to S. 5 were likely guided by vital business interests in their respective states. Bailey's North Carolina was the home of the Vick Chemical Company, maker of Vick's VapoRub. The firm's vice-president was a leading member of a patent-medicine trade group and a vocal critic of Copeland's bill.[18] He was particularly concerned about S. 5's provisions allowing for multiple seizures on the basis of false or misleading advertising. The Lambert Pharmaceutical Company, maker of Listerine, was located in Clark's home state, Missouri. On April 1st, S. 5 came up for Senate debate, and Copeland expected a speedy vote. However, Bailey and Clark had other ideas. In an attempt to gain oppositional support, the senators extended the debate on the bill for eight days, arguing for 1) modified definitions of misbranding and adulteration that eroded the FDA's right to seize products and 2) the FTC's continued regulation of drug advertising. Bailey grandstanded,

> I understand the department of agriculture was created to foster agriculture and not to govern advertising. It is inconceivable to me that it should take charge of medicine, cosmetics, and advertising. There might be an argument that the department has made such great triumphs in agriculture that it is seeking new worlds to conquer.[19]

Copeland denounced the opposition on the Senate floor, charging "that every slimy serpent of a vile manufacturer of patent medicines is working his wicked way around this capital."[20] Notwithstanding Copeland's protest, limits on the FDA's seizure of dangerous medicines were carried in a bill amendment (the Bailey amendment), which—to Copeland's frustration—was passed by the Senate on April 8th. Bailey then aimed a personal shot at Copeland and his crusade to regulate drug advertising, while the doctor simultaneously endorsed several health-related products in public ads. The North Carolinian mocked,

> The distinguished senator from New York has spoken not unfavorably of some of these articles over the radio, including Fleischmann's yeast and Phillips' milk of magnesia. I had never assumed that there was anything poisonous about yeast or milk of magnesia.[21]

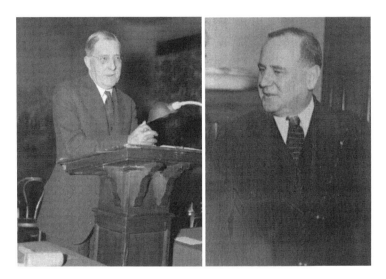

Left, Senator Josiah W. Bailey, c1940 (Library of Congress, Harris & Ewing Collection); Right, Senator Joel Bennett Clark, c1936 (Library of Congress, Harris & Ewing Collection)

S. 5 was at a critical juncture in its journey through the Senate. To avoid further compromise on the bill, Copeland wanted to call for a Senate vote. Bailey and Clark wanted to return the bill to committee to attack the advertising issue. To the relief of reformists, the flash point was defused by a calculated procedural maneuver on an unrelated bill, and S. 5 was put back on the senatorial calendar. There it was placed in the relatively safe harbor of limbo. The maneuver aborted a Senate vote on S. 5 and any hope for its imminent passage, but at least the bill was out of the hands of a dickering committee. The next month, a compromise on the Bailey amendment—instigated by FDR at Tugwell's urging—was reached between Copeland and the opposition. Multiple seizures of a product by the FDA would be allowed, if there was "probable cause" that the product was "imminently dangerous to health." But the FDA and women's groups remained disheartened by the compromise, because the 1906 law stipulated no such restrictions. (Before the compromise, Copeland publicly lamented, "With the Bailey amendment attached, the bill is worse than the present law.")[22] Nevertheless reformists continued to support the passage of S. 5, while hoping to strengthen the seizure language before the measure was enacted. On May 28, 1935, Copeland's S. 5 was brought to a "sudden and surprising" vote in the Senate and passed without dissent.[23] The bill was now at the mercy of the House. Copeland wrongly predicted that S. 5 would prevail easily in the Lower Chamber.

In the summer of 1935, the House conducted lengthy public hearings on S. 5. Chairing the proceedings was Democrat Virgil Chapman, a Kentucky lawyer (like Wat Campbell) and a newcomer to food and drug reform. Chapman, however, was quick on the uptake. He perceived the power and guile of industry lobbyists and the chief issues impeding S. 5's passage—particularly the conflict between the FTC and the FDA for advertising control. In August, at the end of extended and often hostile testimony, Chapman concluded that the bill's best chance for survival lay in a discrete campaign among his fellow congressmen, until sufficient House support could be assured. Yet the public impression was that S. 5 was finished, primarily because FDR had given the measure only "a left-handed endorsement."[24] The "controversial bill [...] ran into the hearing doldrums and powerful lobby in the House and died there," concluded the *New York Times* on August 28th.

During the next congressional session, from January to June of 1936, interest in S. 5 ran from tepid to hot, as FDR's fickleness toward a new food and drug law inexplicably swung in its favor. In early April, the President requested that S. 5 be placed "on the 'must' list for legislative action."[25] Chapman strategically held the bill in subcommittee, where efforts were made to strengthen the clauses on drug standards and seizures. To bolster a complementary public campaign for legislative reform, the FDA renewed its educational efforts to expose the inadequacies of the 1906 law (while avoiding the specific endorsement of S. 5).[26] Likewise outspoken women's groups voiced their independent support of the bill, while hoping to correct its "present weaknesses."[27] But the chief question remained: Who would control drug advertising, the FTC or the FDA? On this point, the President offered little in the way of decisive input or direction. His abstruse leadership favored the status quo—that is, the FTC.

On May 22, 1936, the House version of S. 5 was reported out of committee, with a minority dissent (led by Virgil Chapman) on the FTC's control of drug advertising. On June 19th, the penultimate day of the congressional session, "certain Senate leaders" (and FDR, according to

Jackson) pressured a House vote on the revised bill.[28] S. 5 was "unexpectedly" brought up for consideration, and after a mere 40 minutes of debate, the House measure was overwhelmingly passed by a vote of 151 to 27. The passage likely disappointed the AMA, consumers' groups, and even FDA leadership. The AMA had recently voiced its sour opinion of the latest iteration of S. 5 in *JAMA*. "[I]t will probably be better for the public if in the end the bill is not enacted," the director of the AMA's Bureau of Legal Medicine and Legislation opined, because the bill had been debased in House committee and would "almost certainly retard the passage of needed laws" to adequately regulate drugs.[29] Consumers Union succinctly dubbed the House version of S. 5 a "legislative monstrosity,"[30] and FDA Chief Campbell wished that the bill had died in the Lower Chamber, believing that a tougher measure could be passed in the coming year.[31]

Regardless of dissenting views toward the latest version of S. 5, Senate and House conferees met in a flurry of last-minute activity to hammer out a compromise on the bill's amendments—specifically the issue of advertising oversight. After considerable wrangling on June 20th, a Saturday, Copeland announced a split compromise: All health-related advertising would be regulated by the FDA, and the FTC would oversee the marketing of food and cosmetics. The Senate accepted the compromise, but fierce opposition to the advertising agreement was led in the House by Tennessee lawyers B. Carroll Reece, a Republican from Massengill's district, and Democrat Samuel D. McReynolds, also from East Tennessee. Their opposition to S. 5 was likely motivated by important political allegiances in the House to the FTC. In addition, Tennessee was the home state of Ewin Lamar Davis, a highly influential member of the FTC and a former chairman of the agency.[32] The Tennesseans' arguments, which drew heavily on FTC loyalty and persistent fears of the radical Tugwell, were persuasive. Twenty-four hours after S. 5 was revived by the House and seemingly on its way to ratification, the bill was killed by a decisive 190-to-70 vote. The death of S. 5 was the "final salute" of a disbanding Congress, reported the press.[33] Privately Copeland offered a succinct postmortem of his latest food and drug measure: "Tugwell and Tennessee beat us," he concluded.[34]

* * * * * *

In his relentless pursuit to pass a new food and drug law, Copeland announced on June 30th that he was drafting yet another bill, "entirely independent" of Tugwell and the FDA.[35] At the beginning of the new congressional session, on January 6, 1937, Copeland introduced his second version of S. 5 (confusingly called S. 5 no. 2 or S. 5-1937).[36] In some respects, S. 5 no. 2, like its predecessor, was weaker than the existing law, because it placed limits on multiple seizures. Without publicly defining his specific objections, FDR expressed his unmistakable disappointment with Copeland's latest bill at a February press conference. The President's "first impression of the bill," reported the *New York Times*, "was that it weakened the law passed thirty two years ago."[37] Whatever the bill's shortcomings, the President's open disapproval of S. 5 no. 2 was also likely a personal attack on Copeland, as part of an ongoing tit-for-tat political dispute. The senator had boycotted the 1936 Democratic Convention in Philadelphia, "in an expression of his protest against Mr. Roosevelt's nomination."[38] But FDR's unhappiness with the new food and drug bill may have also been due to his wife. In a roundabout strategy to strengthen Copeland's measure, women's groups had appealed to the First Lady to exert her influence on the President. Regardless of FDR's reasons for publicly maligning Copeland's latest bill, the President's open scorn prompted Copeland to immediately return the bill to committee, where he consulted the FDA and fortified the misbranding and seizure clauses. S. 5 no. 2 was finally brought to a Senate vote on March 9th and passed unanimously.[39] Copeland's bill was then forwarded to the House, where the FTC had historically exerted its influence to retain advertising control. In fact, the chief obstacle to enacting a new food and drug law remained the ongoing feud between the FDA and the FTC over drug marketing. Although industry representatives had traditionally favored the FTC's continued supervision of advertising, they were increasingly willing to acquiesce to the FDA's control— particularly if it meant that some kind of federal law would override the increasing tangle of state drug laws.[40] Regardless of the bending interests of industry, political advocates of the FTC continued to wield their influence in the House.

The power struggle between the FTC and the FDA was further complicated by the simultaneous introduction of the Wheeler-Lea bill in Congress. This measure (S. 1077), spearheaded by Democratic Senator Burton Wheeler of Montana and Democratic Representative Clarence Lea of California, was drafted to expand the FTC's general authority over advertising, including food and drug advertising. The bill removed the agency's burden to prove fraudulent marketing by showing harm to competitors (as the Supreme Court had ruled in 1931 in the case of *FTC v Raladam*). After passage of the Wheeler-Lea bill by the Senate on March 29, 1937, the measure was sent to the House. The timing meant that both S. 5 no. 2 and the Wheeler-Lea bill would be debated in House committee at the same time—namely mid-May of 1937. Extended political maneuvering between supporters of the FTC and those of the FDA, and specifically between Representative Lea and Representative Chapman, trapped both measures in a kind of congressional purgatory when Massengill's Elixir Sulfanilamide hit the market in the fall of 1937.

* * * * * *

The scores of deaths caused by Massengill's drug mobilized a previously indifferent press and public to demand an overhaul of the 30-year-old federal statute. The principal House opponent of Copeland's first S. 5 bill, Congressman Reece, was particularly stung by the fact that Massengill's company was headquartered in his district, and reformists were only too happy to point out this detail. Congressional opponents of stiffer drug regulation, particularly Southern legislators, must have also been chagrined by the high volume of elixir shipped to their states and the related deaths among their voting public. But passage of S. 5 no. 2, while facilitating the FDA's ability to seize bottles of Elixir Sulfanilamide, would not have prevented the disaster. The bill—and any previously considered bill, for that matter—contained no licensing provision to ensure that new drugs entering the market were safe for human consumption.[11] This fact was verified by Representative Lea with the FDA, and the California legislator requested an appropriate amendment to the current bill to rectify the omission. But Copeland, primed by years of legislative wrangling, was way ahead. On December 1st, he introduced his bill amendment, S. 3073, to S. 5 no. 2.

Easy forecasts were made about the amended bill's passage, and industry interests—if not embracing drug licensing—now seemed resigned to its inevitability. Lee Bristol, vice-president of the Bristol-Myers Company, urged "government action to prevent 'such calamities as that resulting from the sulfanilamide elixir concoction.'"[12] The general counsel of the Vick Chemical Company, the commercial interest of Senator Bailey, predicted that drug licensing would be "pushed in Congress at its current session or at the regular session in January."[13] Although favoring less stringent oversight than that included in the latest Copeland measure, drug interests generally acquiesced to the license control and premarket testing of drugs. Yet they feared that the FDA's slow deliberation to approve new drugs would upend their quick-to-market business model. The trade journal *Drug and Cosmetic Industry* correctly predicted the adjustments that drug manufacturers would have to make for decades to come.

> After having spent a large amount of time and money, research and formula work on a new product, the manufacturer might be required to wait a year or more before marketing the same, pending

[Department of Agriculture] approval. Meanwhile his capital is tied up and other research work and plans hinging upon the first work along that line would be subject to delay. Meanwhile also his competitor might come forward with a similar product and beat him to the market, because one product might take longer than another to be checked by the Department.[44]

To reinforce the view that new regulations of food, drugs, and cosmetics remained necessary, the FDA reported on December 9th that diethylene glycol was being used in the manufacture of "foods and other items for human consumption."[45] To determine if the solvent existed in other consumed products, the FDA had obtained sales records from Union Carbide and found that diethylene glycol had been purchased and used by a candy maker in Nebraska. Although the volume of diethylene glycol in the candy "was not sufficient to cause fatal results or cause illness," publicly assured FDA Station Chief William Hartigan, he nevertheless advised, "Diethylene glycol has no place in any food or drug product." Hartigan also warned that the solvent "was used in many products which were beyond the jurisdiction of the food and drug administration," specifically cosmetic creams. The next day, the FDA seized "'considerable' quantities of flavoring extracts containing diethylene glycol" in Denver, Kansas City, Baltimore, Pittsburgh, and Cleveland; although the amount of poison in the extract was not considered life-threatening (unless consumers drank the solutions as beverages, an unlikely event).[46]

It was also notable that the FDA continued to discover and report previously unrecognized deaths due to Elixir Sulfanilamide in the South.[47] For example, while checking up on outstanding physicians' samples in the Rocky Mount area of North Carolina in early December, Inspector Grey learned of the death of Charles Richardson at a local sanatorium. Grey discovered that the 28-year-old African-American farmer, who officially died of "acute appendicitis" and "acute urinary suppression" on October 17th, had obtained four ounces of Elixir Sulfanilamide from the "very feeble" Dr. Martin of Red Oak on October 6th.[48] Consequently one more patient, forgotten or concealed by the elixir-prescribing doctor, was identified. Another inspector, 28-year-old Roland Sherman, working out of the agency's New Orleans station, was on a one-man crusade in December to detect more elixir-related casualties in Mississippi. While reviewing death records in the state, he uncovered five suspect fatalities: those of a 33-month-old boy, a seven-year-old "colored" girl, an 11-year-old "colored" boy, a 32-year-old "colored" cotton farmer, and a 38-year-old "negro" sawmill worker. Through painstaking and protracted interviews with pharmacists, doctors, and the victims' relatives, Sherman confirmed the deaths as being due to Elixir Sulfanilamide. He then moved on to rifle through death certificates in east Texas, where he uncovered yet more victims.[19]

* * * * * *

On December 15th, simultaneous federal citations were issued in Kansas City (Missouri), Cincinnati, and New York City for Dr. Massengill to appear before FDA officials on Monday, December 20th. The explicit charge for the company president was to show why the FDA's information on the elixir-related deaths should not be turned over to the Department of Justice for prosecution. The agency's citations in the cities covered 32, 52, and four cases, respectively, of interstate elixir shipments.[50] Ruby Garrett, Massengill's outside counsel in Kansas City, told the Associated Press that the company had settled "about a dozen cases and will continue to settle others purely on a basis of good faith." However, the attorney admonished, "[W]e will continue to deny all liability and responsibility for deaths of persons whose relatives claim they took the sulfanilamide compound."

The Massengill company had recently paid out less than $300 each in two Mississippi cases and had given another $2,000 to the widow of St. Louis resident William Schroeder, the obstinate brewery employee who had refused to give up his remaining elixir to the FDA.[51] In a lengthy statement to the *St. Louis Post-Dispatch*, Garrett declared that Massengill intended to dispose of all "justified" claims before they could make it to court. The attorney added that the company, which was solely owned by Dr. Massengill, had no insurance to cover death claims resulting from the use of its products. The firm's assets consisted entirely of its drugs, some real estate, and its revenue-generating sales force. Garrett added that "a number" of elixir claims were unjustified. Some were presented by people whose deceased relatives did not even consume Elixir Sulfanilamide, he alleged; in other cases, the decedent would have died anyway. Garrett punctuated his charges with brief anecdotes:

> Several doctors told me and my investigators that deaths had been attributed to sulfanilamide erroneously, due to the widespread publicity regarding the fatal cases. One woman took an elixir which she thought was sulfanilamide because she developed *all the symptoms of sulfanilamide poisoning* [emphasis added]. Later it was found that she had taken a harmless cough medicine and she had recovered.

In no case, Garrett asserted, could Massengill's product be proved conclusively as the cause of death. Claimants would probably receive greater financial compensation by settling, he threatened. Bad publicity from the elixir-related deaths had reduced the company's income and would thereby limit the firm's ability to pay off high-dollar court rulings.

Shortly after the first out-of-court settlements were publicized, The S. E. Massengill Company distributed a lengthy question-and-answer statement to its "friends and customers." The document was intended "to correct the false statements that have been circulated" about Elixir Sulfanilamide. However, "[f]or legal reasons," the company hedged, "we cannot at this time give some information that we would like to give."[52] Among the 29 questions that the firm asked of itself and answered were several concerning the inclusion of diethylene glycol in Elixir Sulfanilamide. Massengill defended his use of the substance on the basis of its properties as a solvent and, perhaps unbelievably, its relative lack of toxicity when compared with the common antifreeze ingredient, ethylene glycol. While attempting to dissociate diethylene glycol from ethylene glycol, Massengill indicated, nevertheless, that the former substance, if ever used as an antifreeze, "should not reflect unfavorably upon it." Both ethyl alcohol and glycerin had been used for the same purpose, he argued. Moreover he reiterated that ethylene glycol was a solvent in hypodermic injections that had been approved by the AMA.

Massengill then endorsed his control department, claiming, "[W]e have six graduate pharmaceutical chemists in our employ who spend their entire time in the control and testing of our products before they are placed on sale." It was specifically denied that Elixir Sulfanilamide had been rushed into the marketplace. Massengill was unable to say, however, why the company's tests did "not show any bad results." "[U]ndoubtedly," he responded, "we will have the answer when it can be shown why many using the identical lots sold had most excellent results." Massengill suggested that the reason for the elixir-related fatalities may never be known.

Is your company making an effort to ascertain what did happen to cause the ill effects?

Yes, our own chemists are continually working on the problem, and we also have independent sources doing similar work. After working on the problem for several weeks, one body of scientists makes the statement: "It is probable that no chemist or pharmacologist will ever be able to determine exactly what happened," and added, "Theory and guess work on the part of all who are working on this problem is all that has developed at the present time." The latest report of another one of our connections is as follows: "We are making an effort to determine the exact cause of the present trouble, and shall keep you advised of the progress of the work as soon as it has advanced to the stage where any reasonable interpretation of the results obtained can be made."

The company continued to maintain that deaths due to its elixir were caused by adverse drug interactions with sulfanilamide. The only drug that could be safely taken with the antibiotic was sodium bicarbonate, Massengill claimed, and a number of drugs—saline cathartics, Epsom salts, many laxatives, and some analgesic drugs (like Bayer's Phenacetin)—were contraindicated with the antibiotic.

By the end of December, Massengill had settled at least seven more Elixir Sulfanilamide claims for a subtotal payout of $8,250.[53] The father of eight-year-old Kathleen Hobson, from Tulsa, received $1,000. Another Tulsan, Mrs. Maise Nidiffer—who had written the heartbreaking letter to FDR about the death of her daughter Joan Marlar—received $1,250 from the company. Public settlements were also made with relatives "of five Negroes who died in East St. Louis." While continuing to deny liability, the Massengill company claimed that "it was to the advantage of both parties to make some settlement" in these cases. Compensation in the amount of $1,000 each was paid for the deaths of five-year-old George Nixon, four-year-old Maurice Slaughter, and 70-year-old Alexander Brooks (who had no dependents). Separate payments of $1,500 each were given to the families of Gertrude Black, a 38-year-old housewife and mother, and 60-year-old Joseph Henry.

15
SIMPLE PERSECUTION

On January 12, 1938, at a closed federal hearing in Cincinnati, attorneys for The S. E. Massengill Company denied that the firm's Elixir Sulfanilamide was adulterated or misbranded.[1] Massengill's outside counsel, Ruby Garrett, along with attorney Robert Burrow of Bristol, submitted a written denial to the federal charges at the truncated hearing, which had been postponed twice to permit the company "to gather all facts" before its response. A transcript of the proceedings, which entailed "only minor discussion," said an FDA official, was sent to Washington, where a "prompt decision" was expected.

After about a month of busy preparation, the FDA then forwarded its records on the interstate shipment of Elixir Sulfanilamide to the Department of Justice.[2] Campbell specifically urged the Solicitor to engage in an "expedited" prosecution of Massengill and his chemist Watkins, "first, because of the extensive public interest in this matter and, second, because of the gravity of the offense." The FDA chief justified that Watkins, along with Massengill, was a fair-game defendant. The chemist had a responsibility to ensure that the firm's antibiotic elixir complied with the Food and Drugs Act because his employer's business was "largely interstate." However, with respect to the shipments of elixir from the firm's Kansas City hub, Campbell recommended that Massengill be named as the sole defendant. Campbell reasoned,

Although 5 of the 30 samples shipped from Kansas City bore code numbers of two batches made at Bristol, the remaining 25 samples were taken from Kansas City shipments representing a batch made at

Kansas City with which Harold C. Watkins had no connection in the actual manufacture. It is accordingly felt that Watkins should not be included as a defendant on the Kansas City shipments.

The FDA chief presumably believed that the preponderance of the evidence did not sufficiently incriminate Watkins in the alleged infractions out of Kansas City. This conclusion thereby left only Massengill in the government's crosshairs.[3] Campbell described the FDA's support for federal prosecution, while modestly adjusting the proposed definition of "elixir" (the original basis for the government's seizure of Massengill's product). "To both the physician and pharmacist," the term meant "that the drug is dissolved in a palatable, aromatic, harmless solvent" and not a poisonous medium, like diethylene glycol. Campbell offered,

> We will be in a position to adduce medical and pharmaceutical testimony to the effect that the term "Elixir Sulfanilamide" means a solution of the sulfanilamid[e], having the medicinal properties of sulfanilamid[e] alone. We will be able to adduce clinical testimony that the principal effect of this product, "Elixir Sulfanilamide", when administered to patients, was due to the highly toxic ingredient, diethylene glycol, as a matter of fact.

The FDA could now implicate Massengill's product in "nearly 100 deaths," Campbell revealed. He argued to the Solicitor that Elixir Sulfanilamide "fell below the professed standard under which it was sold" and was thereby adulterated. The product was not, as it should have been, "a solution having the therapeutic action of the drug sulfanilamide," but one having the deleterious action of "an acute poison."[4] The misbranding charges, Campbell continued, were "practically restatements of the adulteration charge, and are based on the same considerations." In the anticipated prosecution of Massengill, the FDA chief believed that it was "highly important" to use the testimony of doctors whose patients died of poisoning due to Elixir Sulfanilamide. Such testimony would allow the introduction of evidence that implicated the toxicity of diethylene glycol—a charge that Massengill and Watkins continued to refute. Moreover the prescribing physicians could give their common understanding of the term "elixir," which was presumably in agreement with the FDA's definition.[5] Campbell believed that most physicians who lost patients to Elixir Sulfanilamide would be perfectly willing to testify for the government owing to their "sufficiently public service attitude." To that end, the FDA was preparing a complete list of attestants and was ready to undertake the mammoth task of locating (or relocating) every one of them.

In addition to these putative, independent witnesses, at least one former employee of The S. E. Massengill Company offered his corroborating services to the FDA.[6] Thirty-year-old Clarence Falstrom had worked from 1925 to 1933 as an assistant chemist in the company's Kansas City "laboratory," a word he placed in quotation marks in a January letter to the FDA. Falstrom, who had been impressed with Wat Campbell's appearance on the "National Farm and Home Hour" radio program, claimed that he had seen "many abuses which were in violation of the laws" at Massengill's plant. He exclaimed, "They don't even have a registered pharmacist in Kansas City!" He further predicted, "You will see the day again when they violate the law." Falstrom went on to describe how the company had prepared for government inspections, by fixing up special batches of products to ensure their passage or by temporarily hiding away disallowed products. The chemist submitted, "I would like to appear as a witness against them but I am afraid it would actually hurt me on future jobs." Campbell was intrigued by Falstrom, but he ultimately believed that the man's testimony would not be useful in the government's case against Massengill, particularly since Falstrom had been terminated from the company at least four years earlier.

* * * * * *

With the progression of the new calendar year, circumstances for Massengill went from bad to worse, as he braced for more repercussions from his company's colossal blunder. In his insular Tennessee home, Massengill must have believed that he was the target of a concerted three-pronged assault: first, from the federal government and its impending prosecution; second, from Congress (or at least certain members of Congress), who were ready to use the Elixir Sulfanilamide tragedy as a catalyst for the passage of a new drug law; and third, from multiple personal-injury attorneys and their palpable threats of lawsuits. Ongoing civil litigation from numerous parties loomed for the company president. Throughout the winter and spring of 1938, the FDA received regular correspondence from lawyers of victims' families, who requested samples of the seized elixir and testimony of field agents.[7] On March 11th, the *Kingsport Times* reported that Massengill was now preparing to contest a suit for more than $120,000 brought by the mother of Oklahoman Earl Beard.[8] The case was scheduled for argument in the federal court at Greeneville, Tennessee.

Simultaneous developments in Congress ensured the passage of some kind of new drug law, but the issue of advertising oversight continued to frustrate the FDA and its supporters. In January, the Wheeler-Lea bill—which was designed to give the FTC sole, expanded control over the advertising of food, drugs, and cosmetics—came up for debate in the House. The minority protested, arguing that the FDA was infinitely more capable of overseeing drug promotion than the FTC. Nevertheless, after a heated argument, the House passed the measure in an overwhelming vote on January 12, 1938 (the same date of Massengill's federal hearing). According to historian Jackson, the FDA was "apoplectic"—but not just because the agency would be stripped of any control over drug marketing.[9] The Wheeler-Lea bill also required the government to prove fraudulent intent on the part of the drug manufacturer—like the ever-vexing Sherley Amendment of 1912. The FDA, along with women's and consumers' groups, lobbied the White House to veto the measure, but their protests were lost in the prevailing winds. On March 14th, the Senate approved a conference version of the bill, with Copeland as the lone dissenter.[10] "The consumers of this country are being raped," he charged with notable heat.[11] FDR signed the measure into law on March 21st.[12]

Notwithstanding the power of the FTC and its backers, supporters of the FDA still had S. 5 to usher through Congress. Comparable versions of the measure, each with a new drug-licensing provision, were being championed by Copeland and Chapman, respectively, in the Senate and House; although, as historian Jackson wrote, "the FDA came to favor the Chapman version, presumably because of its greater legal clarity."[13] During the spring of 1938, the congressional drama surrounding food and drug reform was chiefly generated by the House version of S. 5. As chairman of the Commerce Committee, Representative Lea had the leverage to bring S. 5 out of committee and up for consideration on the House floor, but he conspicuously stalled the measure, even after his own favored Wheeler-Lea bill was ratified. Perhaps he hoped to suspend S. 5 in committee until the end of the congressional session, when the bill would inevitably die of neglect. Yet the dilatory Lea was compelled to bring up the measure for open debate by a number of sources. Copeland led the appeals, impugning, "Dear Brother Lea, I feel like urging you again to push the matter, because of the shortness of the time. It would be a great pity to delay the matter until it's too late."[14] Women's and consumers' groups were also unrelenting in their mission to breathe congressional life into the latest hope for drug reform. Others warned of the growing number of conflicting state drug laws, which would generate innumerable headaches for interstate dealers.[15] And an increasingly impatient public asked directly and through the press: Why has Congress still done nothing to prevent another Elixir Sulfanilamide tragedy?

In fact, other episodes of harm had occurred, although they were not as dramatic or wide in scope. Most recently, at least 10 Floridians had died after consuming "Ensol," an experimental cancer therapy contaminated with tetanus toxin. As the *Washington Post* advised on April 4th,

> It is not certain whether this tragic but doubtless inadvertent impurity could have been prevented if the revised food and drug bill sponsored by Senator Copeland had been in effect. But certainly the manufacturers of the serum, as all others, would under such a law have been under greater pressure to exercise caution than they have been. As it is today, they have only to avoid deliberate misrepresentations and adulteration to satisfy the Federal code. And even if they slip, the penalty is a mere $100 fine.
>
> Their regulation would be considerably tightened under the terms of the pending bill. It is to be hoped that, with the Florida fatalities before it, the House can be moved to pass what the Senate approved many months ago.[16]

The House or more specifically Representative Lea *was* moved. He finally brought S. 5 out of committee in mid-April, but not before he slipped in—without the support or advice of conferees, it appears—a whopper of a provision. A new section of the bill, ostensibly drafted at the last minute by Lea, now required the court review of any rebuttal suits brought by alleged violators, before the law could ever be enforced against them. Furthermore the provision permitted numerous appeals by the commercial parties in any one of the 85 federal districts. Lea's rationale was to check the Secretary of Agriculture's regulatory power, but reformists saw the provision as a ploy to nullify S. 5 generally and the bill's gatekeeping authority specifically. They argued that Lea's provision would indefinitely tangle up the federal court system and set an ugly precedent for undermining the government's power to regulate pretty much anything the bill was otherwise designed to regulate. The League of Women Voters was incensed, declaring that Lea's version of S. 5 was "so devitalized" that they would have to oppose it.[17] Secretary Wallace essentially threw up his hands, saying that he would rather rely on the old Food and Drugs Act, as impotent as it was. "It is the Department's considered judgment that it would be better to continue the old law in effect than to enact S.5 with this provision," he publicly submitted.[18] Nevertheless Lea's version of S. 5 prevailed in the House, probably because of the congressman's deft skills at open debate. House representatives were also under increasing pressure from a voting public to get some form, perhaps any form, of a new food and drug bill passed. The House measure, dubbed the Copeland-Lea bill (to Copeland's probable irritation), succeeded in the Lower Chamber on May 31st.

Copeland's remaining parry was to hammer out a compromise on S. 5 in a joint conference, given the major differences between the Senate and House versions of the food and drug bill. (Copeland's complete version of S. 5, with its drug-license provision, had been unanimously passed by the Senate on May 5th.) Consumers' and women's organizations remained outraged at the House version of S. 5 and bombarded the President through their vast membership with pleas to intervene. FDR did so, although again cryptically. Publicly he gave no indication that he would sign S. 5 if Lea's appeal section remained, but privately he informed congressional members of a forthcoming veto if the codicil was left in. The Presidential threat was apparently enough to force a major compromise on Lea's provision during the Senate-House meeting. Industry's appeals to the Secretary of Agriculture would now be significantly restricted by circumstance and confined to the 10 federal circuit courts. Continued machinations in the joint conference otherwise strengthened S. 5. The final bill, which was reported out of committee on June 11th, adhered to or even exceeded stipulations in the Senate measure. Specifically conferees accepted stronger language on the subjects of label disclosure, standard variations, and seizures. The consensual version of S. 5 was quickly ratified by both chambers and sent to the White House on June 15th. Ten days later, FDR signed the bill into law—which became known as the Federal Food, Drug, and Cosmetic Act of 1938.

But Copeland did not live to see the law go into effect (in its entirety, one year from its Presidential endorsement), nor did he even get the satisfaction of seeing FDR sign the landmark measure—a truly historic law for which Copeland was largely responsible. Copeland, at the age of 69, collapsed on the night of June 16th at a Washington hotel, after prematurely leaving the Senate floor. He died 24 hours later, with his wife and physicians at his bedside. The cause of his sudden death was unclear, but it was publicly ascribed to "a general circulatory collapse complicated by a kidney ailment."[19] Copeland's doctor said that the illness may have been precipitated by overwork at the end of the congressional session, but he also admitted that "the senator hasn't really been well in a long time." Others were convinced that Copeland's unceasing efforts to reform the regulation of the food and drug trades specifically "shortened his life."[20] Thanks largely to Copeland's tireless efforts over five years, federal law required, for the first time in the history of the United States, that manufacturers demonstrate the safety of their drugs before they could be sold. For the short time that he was able to, Copeland viewed the successful bill as "the crowning achievement of his Senatorial service."[21]

* * * * * *

Meanwhile the government could only use the old 1906 law to prosecute Massengill. On June 3rd in Kansas City, Missouri, a federal complaint from US District Attorney Maurice Milligan alleged that Samuel Evans Massengill, trading as The S. E. Massengill Company, had violated the Food and Drugs Act on 93 counts.[22] Five days later, US District Attorney James Frazier, Jr., confirmed to news sources that the government had also filed criminal charges against Massengill in the US District Court in the Eastern District of Tennessee at Greenville.[23] Despite Wat Campbell's argument to the Solicitor, there were no charges in either federal district against chemist Watkins. The Tennessee complaint alleged violation of the Food and Drugs Act on 166 counts, each relating to an interstate shipment of adulterated and misbranded Elixir Sulfanilamide.[24] In essence, Frazier took 56 interstate shipments of Massengill's elixir from Bristol and charged that each shipment had violated the Food and Drugs Act on multiple counts. In the case of 54 shipments, Massengill was charged on three counts. First, the elixir was adulterated, because "its purity fell below the professed standard or quality under which it was sold." In a paraphrase of Wat Campbell's argument to the Justice Department, Frazier wrote that the drug was billed as "sulfanilamide in a non-poisonous solvent, whereas, in truth and in fact, the said article of drugs was sulfanilamide in a poisonous solvent, to wit, diethylene glycol and water." Second, Elixir Sulfanilamide was "misbranded within the meaning of said Act of Congress." Here the product's label was "false and misleading," because the antibiotic was not contained in an innocuous medium, but a poisonous one. A second misbranding charge was applied to individual shipments of Massengill's drug because each bottle stopper was affixed with a sticker declaring, "Quality Pharmaceuticals." The label was misleading, charged Frazier, while drawing on specific text in the 1906 law:

[T]he said statement represented that the article was an article of drugs of a superior grade, that is to say, that it was a mixture of substances intended to be used for the cure, mitigation or prevention of disease of either man or other animals, and was suitable and appropriate for said purposes, whereas, in truth and in fact, said article of drugs was not of a superior grade and did not consist of a mixture of substances suitable and appropriate to be used for the cure, mitigation or prevention of disease of either man or other animals, in that it was a poisonous mixture.

Notably the shipments cited by Milligan and Frazier in the federal complaints were not necessarily tied to deaths (which, by reckoning of the FDA on May 10th, totaled 104).[25] While the Food and Drugs Act allowed for the condemnation of drugs "as being adulterated or misbranded, or of a poisonous or deleterious character," it did not stipulate violations on the basis of personal injury, including the ultimate injury. Massengill was not being charged with murder or even manslaughter. Mass death was only the subtext of the federal complaint—the indirect result of adulterating and misbranding Elixir Sulfanilamide as a therapeutic, not poisonous, product. Shipping the lethal drug across state lines was apparently sufficient to incur the federal charges, without showing a direct link between the contents of a specific bottle and physical harm. Nevertheless, to bolster the federal complaint, each count against Massengill was affixed with the charge that he had been found guilty of a prior infraction—namely a shipment from Bristol to Ohio of adulterated and misbranded Tincture of Aconite tablets in 1935. Frazier explained to the Associated Press that the federal complaint was equivalent to an indictment and recommended that Massengill be placed under arrest, with a $25,000 bond. On June 13, 1938, Massengill was indeed arrested in Bristol by a Deputy US Marshal and brought before the US Commissioner in nearby Johnson City, where he pleaded not guilty and quickly posted the bond. He was scheduled to appear for his defense against the US government at the federal court in Greeneville, Tennessee, on September 19th.[26]

Massengill's general counsel was indignant. Frank DeFriece charged that, if the government prevailed, the doctor could be fined a total of $261,000 and sentenced to 261 years in prison.[27] "This ridiculous situation is made possible in a simple misdemeanor offense," DeFriece continued in a lengthy and rambling statement made in July, "because [the] alleged offense is the second one" (the first offense being the adulteration and misbranding of the Tincture of Aconite tablets). DeFriece predicted the fallout for his father-in-law, which he likened to "simple persecution." In a misguided attempt to counterbalance the approximately 100 dead from his boss's elixir, the lawyer invoked the destruction of income for Massengill's employees and their dependents.

> So far as Massengill is personally concerned perhaps the Department [of Agriculture] figures he hasn't suffered enough, but there is another angle. Continuous gouging at the business will, of course, eventually kill it. When that is done it may be that Massengill's financial ruin would be pleasing to some, but to do it destroys the source of living for 350 families all over this country, and also destroys a substantial business in Tennessee-Virginia, of which the entire South may be justly proud. Is such animus fair to these people, who had absolutely nothing to do with it, and who are paying for houses and subsistence, all of which may be suddenly wiped out! There are limits to financial existence under such proceedings [...]

DeFriece estimated that the Massengill company "may have been worth" $2 million before the "catastrophe," but, he added, "that [amount] included good will, much of which was lost." Perhaps revealing his own animus toward the recent enactment of Social Security (or more generally FDR's policies), DeFriece curiously offered that the firm had remitted about $18,000 in taxes for the new federal program in 1937. The S. E. Massengill Company "has paid its part in support of the government," he declared, "and it expects to do so if permitted to exist."

Speaking for Massengill, DeFriece claimed that the company president had "taken no sides in the passage of any legislation regulating its business" and had always fully complied with the law. Massengill had, in fact, "favored" Copeland's bill "with few exceptions," but the doctor resented the "unfair use of the Elixir Sulfanilamide catastrophe to hammer the bill through Congress." DeFriece added, "[T]he bare facts would have been just as effective in the absence of the extra grilling to which he was subjected." Alternatively the chief counsel shockingly offered that Massengill should be viewed as some kind of martyr to the cause of legislative reform, by ensuring "the safe use of a very fine drug"—that is, sulfanilamide.

It might be well said that through becoming the goat [...] he has helped to bring about a more intelligent and safe use of a very fine drug, has really saved hundreds of lives of those who might have taken the drug without proper caution, and, through it all, and by reason of his misfortune, furnished the strongest force leading Congress to enact an amended Drug Bill, curing many defects in the old one and making the Federal Drug Department more effective in rectifying the wrongs of irresponsible manufacturers. It does seem a little unfair.

The FDA's campaign against Massengill had also become an expanding witch hunt, DeFriece implied. The lawyer alleged that inspectors had entered drug stores or physicians' offices and requested one of Massengill's products for testing. When offered similar products by other manufacturers, the inspectors had declined the offers and ostensibly growled, "We are after Massengill and expect to get him sooner or later." DeFriece stated that Massengill had expended a total of $148,000 in settling damage claims due to Elixir Sulfanilamide and "not less than $300,000.00" in "profits [and] loss of prestige," among other losses. "All claims," DeFriece explained without indicating their absolute number, "have been compromised except two, and negotiations are in progress for their settlement." He further revealed that only two unnamed civil suits had been filed, but that one of these had been settled. The settlements, however, were by no means admissions of guilt.

Dr. Massengill has tried to compensate for injuries suffered, looking not so much to his legal liability, but rather to the unfortunate results, from no matter what ultimate cause provided the elixir was administered with no other complications, and in spite of what other additional drug was taken.

DeFriece's statement was a clue to the company's ongoing, insistent defense: That sulfanilamide, not diethylene glycol, was to blame for the adverse effects of the antibiotic solution. That sulfanilamide, not Massengill's elixir, "had been rushed on the market," and now the "many bad effects" of the drug, including "many deaths," were becoming apparent, DeFriece argued. Moreover sulfanilamide "is so responsive to the influence of other simple drugs and body conditions, being converted into a deadly poison. For example, common salts, magnesium sulfate [Epsom salts], will render small doses of sulfanilamide deadly," the attorney floated.

Conversely the Massengill company had "on file over 300 case reports where [Elixir Sulfanilamide] proved to be beneficial to the users." DeFriece doubted that any fatalities would have occurred if the antibiotic had not been "grossly overdosed" or "if some food or other drug had not been erroneously taken in connection." In its own investigations, the company had determined that deaths were due to "other causes" or that some had occurred in connection with the use of sulfanilamide tablets from another company. Nevertheless, DeFriece acknowledged, "[T]here has been so much publicity attached to this whole procedure that it is felt that, if possible, for the welfare and best interest of the company, further litigation should be avoided." While Massengill had offered $9,000 to the government, or about $100 per shipment itemized in the two federal indictments, DeFriece believed that the charges against Massengill were not rock solid, and he was conceivably right, given the limitations of the 1906 law.[28]

During the same month, the FDA learned of Massengill's elaborated defense strategy through a "confidential source."[29] A government informant had obtained details from a pharmaceutical chemist who was a "close friend" of Massengill. Reportedly the company had "procured either 660 or 680 affidavits" from people who had used Massengill's elixir with "entire satisfaction." The company president would further contend that the deceased consumers of Elixir Sulfanilamide had "used the medicine recklessly and in excess of the dosage recommended." When given under "competent medical supervision" in the recommended dosages, Massengill argued, the elixir had caused no harm. Massengill was also ready to propose that the use of sulfanilamide alone "caused adverse results, including deaths, in some 15 percent" of consumers. This number compared favorably with the firm's calculated elixir-related death rate of 13%. The latter statistic was acquired by dividing the estimated number of elixir-related deaths, approximately 100, by (according to the Massengill firm) the total number of people who had consumed the product, 760 (100 + 660). The FDA also learned that Massengill's personal wealth totaled $11 million, and that he had expended less than 5% of this value on the tragedy. And while Massengill certainly regretted the deaths, the informant relayed that the doctor also believed himself to be "blameless." Massengill's virtuous self-image was supported by other Bristol residents, who considered the doctor to be a "public benefactor." Finally Massengill's anonymous friend told the FDA informant that he had "no respect" for Harold Cole Watkins. The creator of Elixir Sulfanilamide was an "unreliable individual."

16
TO SECURE JUSTICE FOR THE PUBLIC

The FDA certainly was "after Massengill," but not necessarily in the manner charged by the doctor's chief counsel. Campbell specifically refuted DeFriece's allegation that inspectors were homing in on the firm during their random audits of marketed drugs. The allegation had reached the executive office of the Department of Agriculture, and Campbell rebutted the charge in an internal inquiry. He clarified that inspectors were instructed to collect samples "as to cast no reflection on any manufacturer's products." But Campbell promised, "If sufficient facts are submitted to make it possible to conduct an appropriate investigation, such an investigation will be promptly made."[1]

Yet the FDA was committed to providing vital aid to the Justice Department in its federal case against Massengill. During the summer and early fall of 1938, agency officials were busily arranging incriminating testimony. "[S]ome of the most eminent scientists in this country," Campbell wrote to the Department, "will state their opinion, contrary to that expressed by Mr. [sic] Massengill, that the fatal consequences of the administration of elixir sulfanilamide were due to the solvent rather than to the sulfanilamide."[2] To that end, the FDA was lining up deponents and witnesses, including the University of Chicago scientists who had conducted animal experiments with Massengill's elixir and an expert pathologist from the South Carolina Medical College.[3] The Chicago doctors, Eugene Geiling and Paul Cannon, were preparing to publish their final report on the pathologic effects of Massengill's elixir on rabbits, rats, and dogs in *JAMA*.[4] They would reiterate that diethylene glycol was the unmistakably fatal ingredient in Massengill's elixir, and that the solvent appeared to damage the cells lining the microscopic, convoluted tubules of the animals' kidneys. Furthermore, when the solvent was given to animals in a dosage approximating that of human victims, the fatality rate was similar to what had been seen nationwide. Sulfanilamide, to the likely disappointment of Massengill's defenders, was summarily dismissed by Geiling and Cannon as a cause of the pathologic changes. These conclusions were "[b]ased on more than 100 necropsies and a considerably larger number of [animal] experiments." After examining the internal organs of 12 human victims of Elixir Sulfanilamide, the physicians were ready to proclaim that "[t]he similarity between the clinical course and the pathologic picture of the fatal human cases and that observed by us in the experimental animals affords conclusive proof that the chief toxic agent in Elixir of Sulfanilamide was diethylene glycol." On microscopic examination of the victims' kidneys, there was "an unusual type of chemical nephrosis," and the cells lining the convoluted tubules of the organ appeared "'ballooned,' as if the cytoplasm of each cell were a bag of water," the doctors observed. They further noted,

> This profound swelling leads to complete obliteration of the lumens [of the tubules], and the anuria and uremia are most reasonably explained on the basis of mechanical stoppage of the flow of urine [...] The general picture suggests a "water-logging" of the cells rather than an effect of an extremely toxic protoplasmic poison.

In other kidneys, the cells looked "collapsed," as if they "had ruptured and had liberated their contents." In these cases, the lumens of the tubules "were open but seemed to be functionless." Despite the consistent pathologic changes caused by Massengill's elixir and diethylene glycol in animals and humans, Geiling and Cannon could not state exactly how the solvent exerted its toxic effects. Moreover the physicians would have to acknowledge that many people had consumed substantial quantities of Massengill's elixir without suffering "serious effects."

The South Carolina pathologist, Dr. Kenneth Lynch, had performed autopsies on several elixir victims and published his findings in the February issue of the *Southern Medical Journal*.[5] Like the University of Chicago scientists, Lynch did not hedge on the cause of death. The article, "Diethylene Glycol Poisoning in the Human," described the clinical course and pathologic findings of four "Negro" residents of Charleston, including two children, who died after consuming Elixir Sulfanilamide for various reasons. The poison's degenerative effects on the organs, specifically the kidney and liver, were consistent with those observed in other published cases.[6] Again the cells lining the microscopic, convoluted tubules of the kidneys were noted to be remarkably swollen—some to the point of blocking the lumen entirely. The changes undoubtedly explained the anuria observed shortly before death. In return for Lynch's testimony against Massengill, the government would provide an expert-witness fee of $25 per day.

On September 7th, attorneys for Massengill filed a demurrer, or formal objection, to each of the 166 charges of adulteration or misbranding in a federal district court in Greeneville, Tennessee.[7] The demurrer overtly capitalized on the inadequacies of the Food and Drugs Act of 1906. Massengill responded that the government's charge of adulteration did not violate the law, because the term "is not anywhere so defined under said Act, nor by any interpretation thereof." Massengill's defense drew on the loose and arguably irrelevant definitions in the act, which stated that a drug was adulterated if it "differs from the standard of strength, quality, or purity as determined by the test laid down in the United States Pharmacopoeia or National Formulary official at the time of investigation" or "its strength or purity fall below the professed standard or quality under which it is sold."[8] On the counts of misbranding, specifically with respect to the use of the name "Elixir Sulfanilamide," the government charged that Massengill had used the term in a misleading fashion. Instead of dissolving the antibiotic in an innocuous liquid, the company had used a poisonous medium. The defendant, however, rebutted that the law did not specify any such definition for misbranding—an argument of legal merit. A misbranded drug was merely an "imitation of or one offered for sale under the name of another article." Alternatively a misbranding charge might apply if the contents of an original package were replaced by other contents or if the package failed to specify "the quantity or proportion of any alcohol, morphine, opium, cocaine, heroin, alpha or beta eucaine, chloroform, cannabis indica, chloral hydrate, or acetanilide, or any derivative or preparation of any such substances contained therein." Given the legislative wording, the federal misbranding charges were conceivably a stretch. Certainly Massengill's lawyers were ready to argue that they were.[9] Last Massengill countered against the government's misbranding charges on the basis of the "Quality Pharmaceuticals" sticker, which had been pasted across the stopper of each elixir bottle. The defendant rebutted that the sticker's words had "no reference to the contents of the bottle to which it was attached." The phrase "referred solely and alone to the S. E. Massengill Company as pharmacists, and is a sort of slogan."

Massengill's lawyers presented their oral arguments in Greeneville on Monday, September 26th. Three days later, Judge George Taylor rendered a mixed decision.[10] He sustained Massengill's demurrer on the second misbranding charge, which was based on the "Quality Pharmaceuticals" sticker. This decision wiped out nearly every third count lodged by the government against Massengill. Taylor then carefully considered the government's first misbranding charge, particularly as it applied to the use of "elixir." The US attorney contended that the term denoted a "nonpoisonous vehicle or solvent," whereas Massengill argued that the word had no such meaning. On this issue, Taylor offered a measured and carefully worded verdict. When Massengill used "elixir" with "sulfanilamide," the judge considered, Massengill represented his product as something that did not contain a counteractive or harmful ingredient. In other words, Elixir Sulfanilamide, by its very name, should not offer a substance that would "counteract the effect of the active drug sulfanilamide, or kill or seriously injure the patient." Taylor rendered, "If this construction clearly be correct, the charge clearly presents an issue of fact to be determined, and if determined in favor of the Government's contention, an offense against the act exists."[11] Massengill was therefore required to "plead the merits" of the remaining 112 federal counts in Tennessee.

To that end, the FDA and the Justice Department prepared for the only two practical outcomes: a dramatic and potentially lengthy trial or Massengill's admission of guilt. Subpoenas were issued. Scientific experts and field agents were prepared for the witness stand. But the topic of plea bargaining was a consistent thread in ongoing FDA correspondence, even before Massengill's demurrer. Writing to Station Chief Hartigan at Kansas City, Missouri, in September, an FDA leader wired that the "DECISION AS TO ACCEPTABLE PENALTY IN CASE OF PLEA OF GUILTY SHOULD BE LEFT TO [...] DEPARTMENT JUSTICE."[12] Hartigan was also advised:

> YOU SHOULD MAKE NO RECOMMENDATION AS TO SIZE OF PENALTY. RESTRICT YOURSELF TO POINTING OUT SERIOUS RESULTS OF OFFENSE, THAT IT IS SECOND OFFENSE, MAXIMUM PENALTY AS PROVIDED BY STATUTE FOR SECOND OFFENSE AND THAT IN OUR OPINION A SUBSTANTIAL PENALTY SHOULD BE IMPOSED

On October 3rd, the federal case against Massengill was concluded. There would be no sensational court proceedings: no tearful accounts from family members of the deceased who drank Elixir Sulfanilamide; no damning testimony from leading scientific experts. Massengill pleaded guilty to the remaining 112 counts of adulteration or misbranding in the US District Court of the Eastern District of Tennessee at Greeneville.[13] The penalty, as recommended by US District Attorney Frazier, was $150 per count, for a total penalty of $16,800. Despite the fact that no jail time was handed down, the fine was five times larger than any that had ever been imposed under the 1906 Food and Drugs Act, newspapers reported. Massengill was allowed to pay down one-third of the penalty, with the remainder due in 30 days. Wire services indicated that Massengill would also plead guilty to the 62 federal counts pending in Kansas City, and he did so on October 19th.[14] A similar fine was levied there for a total penalty of $9,300. The cumulative payback for the cited interstate shipments of Elixir Sulfanilamide totaled $26,100. For those who considered the fine a substitute for a murder sentence, the penalty was less than $260 per death. The final outcome, although relatively costly to an individual citizen, even one of considerable means, was almost certainly a relief to Massengill, who wanted the experience unequivocally behind him. The plea was also desirable to the US attorneys, who were keen to avoid the real risk of an embarrassing acquittal solely because of an anemic, outdated law. For the contemporary spectator and today's historian, the verdict was and remains the typically dissatisfying compromise of opposing parties who were less eager to achieve victory than to dodge the tangible threat of defeat.

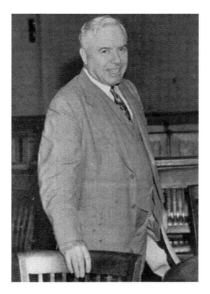

Samuel Evans Massengill after pleading guilty to federal charges of
adulteration and misbranding in Kansas City, Missouri
(Acme News, October 20, 1938)

A *JAMA* postmortem of the entire incident, published on October 22nd, empathized with federal officials in their "attempt to secure justice for the public."[15] They "were miserably handicapped by the weak law in existence at the time of the offense," the editorialist lamented. But the journal forecasted that a "similar incident would not be dealt with so lightly under the new laws." The admonishing coda to physicians: Restrict your prescriptions to "those brands accepted by the Council on Pharmacy and

Chemistry and [...] use them as described in New and Nonofficial Remedies."

It is always hazardous to prescribe unstandardized and uncontrolled remedies, or drugs sold under catchy names. Any pharmaceutic house which desires to market its products honestly and in accordance with the rules of the Council may have its products considered.

For its part, "the Council had consistently refused to accept, and to this day has not accepted, any liquid preparation of sulfanilamide, as there has been no evidence of usefulness and stability." Certainly Massengill's elixir had not been submitted to the AMA, and in fact, "no product of the S. E. Massengill Company ever stood accepted for inclusion in New and Non-official Remedies," the journal affirmed. Within the FDA, there had been reports of an "identical" liquid sulfanilamide marketed by the William S. Merrell Company of Cincinnati, although there was apparently no follow-up evidence to support the rumor.[16] In addition, at the height of the investigation and seizure of Massengill's elixir, the AMA Council and the FDA had become aware of a "solution of sulfanilamide with citra-lactate," sold by Donley-Evans and Company of St. Louis. Responding to a letter from a St. Louis physician in November of 1937, the Council said that it had accepted none of the products from Donley-Evans, let alone the sulfanilamide preparation that the doctor reportedly had in his possession.[17] The advisement continued,

[F]or the Council to recognize a solution of sulfanilamide, the product must be stable and, at the same time, the solvent must be nontoxic in the doses given. Possibly a satisfactory solvent has been developed. However, there is no evidence to indicate that this is the case.

In an internal report, dated December 14, 1937, an FDA chemist described his examination of the liquid sulfanilamide from Donley-Evans.[18] The concentration of the antibiotic, in a solution of potassium citrate and sodium lactate, far exceeded its solubility in water, the chemist noted, and he was curious about the possible formation of "some double salt" to explain the composition. However, no legal action would be taken. The product's labeling accurately conveyed the drug's ingredients and did not bear any therapeutic claims. Also the product was not, at least on its face, lethal.[19] The contention by Secretary Wallace in his congressional report that other drug firms had tried to create a liquid sulfanilamide (but had abandoned the idea on the basis of the toxicity of ready solvents) is supported by a contemporaneous US patent submitted in August of 1937 by Walter Christiansen.[20] Working for E. R. Squibb and Sons of New York, Christiansen had proposed solutions—which were specified for intravenous injection and not oral consumption—that used pure or diluted glycols, including ethylene glycol and diethylene glycol. However, no evidence of the marketing or use of these solutions has been found.

* * * * * *

Three months after Samuel Evans Massengill pleaded guilty to 174 federal counts of adulterating or misbranding Elixir Sulfanilamide, he was elected president of the Bristol Chamber of Commerce in a show of municipal confidence.[21] The front page of the January 10, 1939, issue of the *Bristol News Bulletin* featured a two-column portrait photograph of Massengill. The accompanying write-up described him as "prominently identified with the industrial and civic growth of Bristol since 1899" and made no mention of the Elixir Sulfanilamide affair or the doctor's admitted federal crimes. Massengill was merely cited as the "president of the S. E. Massengill Company, manufacturing pharmacists," and the Bristol company was touted as "one of the largest plants of its kind in the South, with branches in many of the larger cities of the nation."

Exactly one week later, chemist Harold Cole Watkins, a man for whom recurrent death and transience were ways of life, shot himself in the heart with a .38-caliber automatic pistol in the kitchen of his brick bungalow.[22] The act was committed approximately two blocks from Massengill's mansion. The 58-year-old creator of Elixir Sulfanilamide was found dead on January 17th at 7:30 in the morning by his wife. He was lying face down, the pistol about a foot from his head, his spectacles lodged beneath his body. Watkins had left the Massengill company about six months earlier, presumably after Dr. Massengill's June indictment. The circumstances of Watkins's departure from the firm, whether voluntary or by request, were not publicly acknowledged by the company or the suicide's widow.[23] At least for some period of time during his recent unemployment, Watkins had remained oblivious to the damage caused by Elixir Sulfanilamide. Shortly after leaving the firm, Watkins asked Inspector Ford to think of him, if the FDA agent "heard of anyone wanting a man."[24] In addition to his widow, Watkins was survived by his two sons. At the time of the suicide, the oldest child was attending an aviation school in St. Louis. The youngest, a teenager, was presumably away at a military academy.

In conjunction with news of Watkins's death, Massengill's sales manager reported that the company had paid out more than $500,000 in claims because of Elixir Sulfanilamide. Chief Counsel DeFriece had spent and would continue to spend months on the road in an effort to directly settle civil suits with family members of elixir victims. Per company history, the lawyer traveled incognito, carefully avoiding claimant's lawyers and local officials, who had reportedly issued arrest warrants for top executives of the firm.[25] In the company's questionable account of its negotiations, DeFriece "actually made friends with most of the bereaved"—a claim that, if true, says as much or more about the graciousness of Southerners than it does about the lawyer's skills at mediation. In one particularly dubious anecdote, the brother of an elixir victim recognized DeFriece at a gas station and invited the lawyer to dinner. He declined.

If more than $500,000 was in fact paid out by Massengill in civil claims for the deceased, then the average individual settlement exceeded $4,600. However, it is doubtful that the firm paid on all deaths, or if claims were even made in every instance of death. This alleged amount of cash to settle claims is also likely exaggerated, given known individual settlements. As of January 1939, the highest, reported civil settlement offered by Massengill to a single family was $3,000.[26] The lowest individual payout did reach $300.[27] In addition, the company's efforts to avoid the courtroom appear to have been relatively successful. A survey of archived court records reveals that only six civil complaints were submitted to the District Court of the Eastern District of Tennessee at Greeneville—the same court where Massengill pleaded guilty to federal charges of adulteration and misbranding.[28] Most notably, five of these suits, which were submitted between September of 1938 and March of 1940, were dismissed. In at least two cases, dismissals were made because out-of-court settlements had been reached. However, the case of *Norris T. Beard, Administratrix of the Estate of Earl Lee Beard, Deceased, v S. E. Massengill* was argued before Judge Taylor (the same judge who presided over the federal case against Massengill).[29] After Taylor considered the "statements [...], pleadings and proof" of counsel, he awarded the mother of the Oklahoma air-conditioning engineer an unprecedented $8,500, $7,500 of which was for "loss of support and other pecuniary loss." The remaining $1,000 was intended to allay her "conscious pain and suffering." The judgment was made, in part, on the basis of Earl Beard's lifetime earning potential (with a life expectancy of 38.81 years) and the dependency of Beard's mother on her son's potential income (quoted at an anticipated $500 per month). The settlement was also intended, per the plaintiff's argument, to compensate Beard's estate for funeral expenses ($596.43), hospital bills ($127.00), and "the services of physicians, surgeons and nurses" ($500.00).

Most civil plaintiffs cited Massengill's violation of federal law, a count routinely denied by the defendant as "immaterial, impertinent, and scandalous." Some civil complaints also cited the violation of state drug laws, which typically mirrored the tepid stipulations of the 1906 Food and Drugs Act. At considerable issue in one case, that of Mississippi farmer John Gibbons, was the proximate cause of death. Depositions of his treating physicians indicated that Gibbons's sudden demise was most likely due to acute coronary thrombosis, or a fatal heart attack. However, there was much discussion over whether the patient had shown any signs, like urinary suppression, that might have been due to diethylene glycol and not prostatic hypertrophy or infection. The hospital urologist could not state whether Gibbons's urine production had been compromised, owing to the fact that the man's bladder had been regularly irrigated with an antiseptic solution during hospitalization. "[It] made the measuring of the urinary output difficult, or impossible," the doctor acknowledged. Notable also was the fact that, during discovery, there was no discussion of pertinent blood tests, such as BUN or creatinine levels, which might have indicated kidney damage. Moreover no autopsy was performed, a fact that the urologist regretted. After depositions were completed in April of 1939, the suit was "dismissed without prejudice," when the plaintiffs moved for a "voluntary non-suit." Gibbons's widow and adult children were required to pay the balance of the court costs ($15.25), which remained outstanding at the end of the calendar year. The plaintiffs were also evidently saddled with the costs of the farmer's funeral expenses ($456.00), hospital bills ($65.00), and physicians' and nurses' fees ($60.00).

In at least two civil cases, the expired statute of limitations for damage claims was strenuously argued by Massengill. The statute of limitations in Tennessee, where out-of-state claimants were evidently obliged to try their cases, was limited at one year; whereas in Florida and South Carolina the statutes were two and six years, respectively. Judge Taylor ruled in favor of Tennessee's shorter statute on March 18, 1940. This ruling effectively ended the civil claim of the widow of elixir victim Emanuel Cauley. The complaint had been filed against Massengill two days before the two-year anniversary of Cauley's death in Jacksonville. The same ruling by Judge Taylor in August of 1940 would have likewise stifled the claim of the administrator of Pearl Locklair's estate. The original complaint had been submitted to the Tennessee court more than two years after the death of the "Negro" domestic worker and resident of Charleston. But the plaintiff immediately appealed Taylor's ruling to the Circuit Court of Appeals for the Sixth District in Cincinnati, Ohio. Nearly 17 months later, Taylor's decision was reversed, and Locklair's cause was "remanded for trial upon its merits." Massengill's determination to maintain the shorter Tennessee statute was demonstrated by his response. He petitioned the US Supreme Court to review the appellate court's decision. However, the writ of certiorari (or record of the case) from the appellate court was denied by the ultimate court on May 25, 1942. Several months later, Massengill settled with the Locklair family for $1,500, plus $150 for expenses and court costs.[30]

In only one of the six discovered civil suits against Massengill did the elixir-consuming patient escape death. The father of Jack Voorhees, the Tulsa boy who survived treatment with Elixir Sulfanilamide, submitted a complaint against Massengill on September 8, 1939. The plaintiff, who was represented by Tulsa attorney Austin Gavin, the uncle of another elixir victim (eight-year-old Jack King), requested $55,000 in damages and a jury trial. At considerable issue during the discovery stage of the suit was whether the boy had, in fact, exhibited the typical signs and symptoms of diethylene-glycol poisoning and whether there were any lasting repercussions. Ironically the suit's weakness appeared to be the relative lack of harm, either at the time of treatment with Elixir Sulfanilamide or during the child's extended convalescence. In other words, the plaintiff was at a disadvantage because the child survived, ostensibly without permanent injury. Notable among the many facts laid out during several depositions, including that of Dr. Ivo Nelson (the pathologist who performed autopsies on Tulsa's elixir victims), was the revelation that the boy had received treatment at home despite being considerably ill. Consequently the boy's medical records (meaning those filed among public court records) are limited and fail to clarify whether the child had indeed suffered diethylene-glycol poisoning. The detection of liver enlargement by the boy's examining physician at the time of illness suggested the toxic effects of Massengill's product. However, the child, who was originally treated for a strep throat, did not experience complete anuria, and a very limited, contemporaneous study of the boy's urine revealed, at most, nonspecific findings (eg, "amorphous carbonates" on microscopic examination).[31] To demonstrate the rudimentary nature of the child's medical workup and care, circa 1937, apparently no blood work was performed to directly assess his renal or liver function.[32] This information, positive or negative, would have provided essential information about the toxic effects or lack thereof of Massengill's elixir. Likewise these tests were evidently not performed at later dates. As a result, both the plaintiff's and the defendant's medical experts, who failed to comment on the remarkable absence of these medical tests, could not testify to any bodily harm. One of Massengill's expert witnesses, pathologist Ferdinand Helwig, stressed the unpredictability of Elixir Sulfanilamide by emphasizing the survival of at least 100 consumers (as the fact had been acknowledged by Drs. Geiling and Cannon in *JAMA*).[33] Moreover on physical examination, the boy appeared healthy, if not a little plump, more than a year after consuming the antibiotic solution.[34] In April of 1940, after depositions of the boy's parents, teachers, and doctors, as well as the boy himself, the suit was voluntarily dismissed by the plaintiff, presumably because definitive evidence of injury was lacking. A settlement was not stipulated in court documents.

* * * * * *

The Massengill company survived the Elixir Sulfanilamide tragedy of 1937, a fact that is astonishing to anyone who is familiar with the scale and scope of personal-injury litigation in America during the late 20th and early 21st centuries. According to the company's own history, however, the short-term losses were substantial.[35] During the next two years, the firm lost more than 60% of its customers. By the end of 1937, the company—which had realized a nearly 25% increase in sales during the first 10 months of the year—experienced an 18% loss. In 1938, sales were down nearly 12%. Notwithstanding this "bruising effect," the firm actually experienced a "modest profit" during both years by "muscularly reducing or dropping entirely every nonessential expenditure"—one of which was, of course, the continued employment of its chief chemist, Harold Cole Watkins. Another company response was to potentially indemnify the sole proprietor Massengill from future litigation by incorporating the various branches of The S. E. Massengill Company in 1938.

The firm continued to sell tablet and capsule formulations of sulfanilamide, as well as many of its grandfathered products (which it offered before enactment of the Food, Drug, and Cosmetic Act of 1938). But the company was never really in the business of drug innovation, and Massengill provided a notice in 1939 saying that the firm would no longer prepare "new special formulas which were not prepared by our firm for a customer prior to the passage of this Act."[36] Despite a few bona fide attempts to develop novel drugs over the ensuing years, the company could not parlay these candidates into viable, marketable products, primarily because the firm 1) did not have the deep pockets or expertise for drug development and 2) could not successfully negotiate the evolving FDA standards for drug safety and efficacy. The number of prescription products offered by the Massengill company for human use declined from 1,317 in 1935 to 1,217 in 1939.[37] In 1946, the year of Massengill's death (due to coronary thrombosis at the age of 75), the company catalog offered 939 products for human consumption. This number declined by more than one-half 10 years later, and only 71 prescription products were listed in the firm's 1971 catalog. It seems fair to conclude that, while The S. E. Massengill Company survived the Elixir Sulfanilamide debacle, it became a victim of its aftermath—that is, increasing government regulation of the pharmaceutical industry.

From 1944 to 1951, the company was cited 12 times by the FDA for adulteration or misbranding.[38] In 10 cases, the counts against various remedies seemed to be part and parcel of the FDA's day-to-day surveillance at the time, and the products were destroyed by default decree, "no claimant having appeared." A gestalt reading of government records suggests that Massengill's products were no more likely to be targeted by the agency than others. Among notable citations, however, was the fact that the company was fined $3,000 in 1947 after pleading guilty to three counts of adulteration of an injectable B vitamin (mold was found in the solution).[39] In 1951, the company's popular Massengill powder, a consumer product to be mixed in water and used as a gargle or vaginal douche, was cited for misbranding. The powder—essentially a combination of boric acid, alum, and carbolic acid—was advertised to have a number of therapeutic effects, which, the FDA charged, were not supportable. Among the company's objectionable claims[40]:

Many medical authorities agree that such cleansing, two or three times a week, serves a useful purpose.

For maintaining normal acidity of the genital tract.

Most of the disease-producing organisms which may affect the vagina cannot survive when the medium in which they live becomes sufficiently acid. Nature attempts to keep the vagina acid in reaction. Massengill Powder assists Nature in this respect, and by helping maintain an acid reaction tends to suppress the growth of undesirable microorganisms.

The use of a bland, warm, slight acid douche is recommended two or three times a week as a cleansing wash for hygienic purposes.

The S. E. Massengill Company remained an overwhelmingly insular, family enterprise for 25 years after Dr. Massengill's death. Chief Counsel DeFriece became president, and many of the leading positions within the company were held by relatives of Massengill, either directly or by marriage. On DeFriece's retirement in 1959, his son succeeded him, and the junior DeFriece remained with the company when it was sold to the London-based drug company Beecham in 1971. At the time, 88% of Massengill company stock, which was first publicly offered in 1965, was owned by family members. Beecham paid out $27.25 per share and subsequently acquired two million shares for a grand total of $54.5 million.[41] The attraction of the Massengill company in the late 1960s and early 1970s was based almost exclusively on its over-the-counter feminine-hygiene products, which the firm had developed into a highly successful, multimillion-dollar business—in contradistinction to its prescription-drug business. Small, aromatic packets of Massengill Powder became stock items in drugstores and supermarkets across the country during the mid-20th century. At the time, sales of Massengill's feminine products consumed about one half of the country's vaginal-douche business (and yes, it was a business), according to company records. In 1970, the Massengill firm spent more than $1 million to market its feminine-hygiene products, which by then included liquid versions of its popular douche line.[42] The year's net intake exceeded $2.3 million, with sales surpassing $24 million. Beecham was evidently willing to capitalize on the brand equity in "Massengill," at least when the name was applied to feminine hygiene. To the good fortune of Massengill's heirs, America was either unaware of or had forgotten the surname's connection to mass death. In 1989, Beecham merged with the Philadelphia-based SmithKline Beckman to become SmithKline Beecham.[43] In 1994, King Pharmaceuticals, a contract-drug house, launched its business with the purchase of Massengill's Bristol campus.[44] Two years later, King began purchasing the rights to several branded pharmaceuticals from larger companies. At this time, Massengill's original plant was severed from any of Massengill's formulas or brands that had been acquired by Beecham in 1971.[45]

The maze of mergers and acquisitions continued. In 2000, the UK-based pharmaceuticals giant Glaxo united with SmithKline Beecham to become the world's largest drug company at the time, GlaxoSmithKline.[46] The Massengill feminine-hygiene product line survived the merger and was added to GSK's expansive consumer products division. The endurance of the Massengill brand was no doubt ensured through aggressive marketing by its various owners over the years, most notably in the form of the painfully memorable television advertisements that began airing during the 1970s and later (and which endure on YouTube).[47] The on-air campaign consistently emphasized the sentiment, "Massengill's a name you can trust." By 2009, however, the Massengill brand had slipped considerably from its monopolizing position. In the $32.8-million US market for vaginal douches in 2008, the brand held a distant number-two spot (behind Summer's Eve), with $4.1 million in annual sales.[48] In December of 2011, Prestige Brands Holdings of Irvington, New York, agreed to purchase 17 of GSK's consumer products, including the Massengill brands. In the SEC filing of January 18, 2012, noted declines in 2009 revenue from Massengill products were attributed to "general market declines in the category."

During the existence of The S. E. Massengill Company, it was a pervasive and enduring belief among executives that Elixir Sulfanilamide was never as deadly as charged by the FDA and the AMA, or that the product's erratic toxicity was due to the antibiotic and not the solvent. At their most gracious, Massengill executives would only admit that toxicologists might never agree on the true nature of the product. Company leaders generally viewed the firm as a hapless victim of circumstance and an exploited target of the FDA, which saw the "sulfanilamide problem" as "a gift from on high."[49] In an account of the company's history, Dr. Massengill's "determination" was described as "indomitable."[50] His denial of his role in the deaths of scores of Americans appears equally impregnable. When the fatalities from his elixir began to accumulate, his daughter reportedly asked what he would do if "this results in financial ruin for you and the company." The family account: He replied "with a twinkle in his eye" that he would start over. But Massengill's ultimate legacy is a harsh irony. For a man who conspicuously valued family heritage and civic reputation, he left his namesakes the embarrassment of a vaginal douche and the horror of mass death.

* * * * * *

There is little, if any, evidence to suggest that physicians who prescribed Elixir Sulfanilamide suffered tangible consequences, either because they innocently recommended the treatment or because they attempted to cover up their actions. Specifically there is no indication that dissembling physicians were charged with obstructing a federal investigation. Families of elixir victims, if they filed civil complaints, typically did so against the Massengill company and, perhaps, the dispensing pharmacy. Mississippi doctor Archie Calhoun was ultimately praised for his public candor about the unwitting role he played in his patients' deaths. According to a 2003 documentary of the event, the History Channel's "Elixir of Death," the doctor was initially the object of the kind of small-town gossip that might be expected in his home of Mt. Olive. His daughter recalled the whispered aspersions of her classmates and her father's distress at the fatal results of the medicine. "One night I can remember so clear hearing him crying, just sobbing. That really upset me [...]" she recollected, and "He was a very strong person, but it was just more than he could stand. I don't think he ever recovered from it. We could tell it was still on his mind." For the trouble and extra work he incurred while following up on his elixir-treated patients, Calhoun requested from the Massengill company and received $125 in compensation.[51] Twenty-four years later, the doctor was praised by the Mt. Olive community for half a century of medical service. He was honored with "Dr. Calhoun Day" and the "mighty nice gift" of a black-and-white television. Calhoun continued to serve the community as a physician for another 10 years, to the day of his death in 1971.

One of the largest prescribers of Massengill's elixir, Dr. Henri H. Weathers of East St. Louis served his community with venerable distinction for 13 more years, until his unexpected death at the age of 47. Practicing in the era of customary racial discrimination, Weathers nevertheless cultivated a vast and varied practice and broke through persistent racial barriers in medicine. In St. Louis, he became chief of surgery at St. Mary's Infirmary, a Catholic "hospital for colored people," and the associate director of surgery at the Homer G. Phillips Hospital, the city's only public inpatient facility for blacks in a time when segregated health care was the norm.[52] Weathers was also "one of the few Negroes ever admitted" to the American College of Surgeons and the International College of Surgeons. In 1943, he "startled the medical world" by sewing up the left ventricle of a stabbing victim; the patient survived the daring and lifesaving open-heart surgery.[53] Six years later, Weathers became one of three "negroes" appointed to the instructional staff of the Jesuit-based St. Louis University School of Medicine. The event was described by school officials as the "first appointment of its kind in the Midwest."[54] He was also the first African American admitted to his county medical society, at a time when the AMA provided equivocal leadership on the racially based exclusion of physicians from its member societies. On the night of August 2, 1950, Weathers collapsed at his home in East St. Louis and was rushed four miles, across the Mississippi River, to St. Mary's Infirmary, where he had provided years of medical service. He died there of a ruptured cerebral aneurysm. "Thousands" attended his funeral, and he was buried in a desegregated Catholic cemetery in St. Louis.

Logan Spann, the doctor who crumpled up and tossed Joan Marlar's prescription record, appears to have sustained no punishment for his attempted deception. In fact, Spann rose to a level of civic and medical leadership in Tulsa. According to a 1996 obituary, Spann practiced medicine for 48 years in the city, specializing in abdominal surgery and family practice. He delivered "thousands of babies, including two of his own grandchildren" and was a member of the AMA.[55] During World War II, he served as a navy flight surgeon for the 3rd Marine Division in the South Pacific and was discharged, after four years of service, as a lieutenant commander. Spann was elected vice-president of the Tulsa County Medical Society in 1953, was a cofounder of the city's Doctors' Hospital, and chaired the board of directors of the Tulsa Boys' Home.

* * * * * *

During their remaining careers, these doctors undoubtedly witnessed the ongoing revolution of chemical antibiosis. For the next decade, sulfanilamide, in tablet and capsule forms, remained an essential part of medical practice. But the groundbreaking drug had considerable limitations. In August of 1938, Wat Campbell advised caution in a letter to "distributors of sulfanilamide and related drugs." The compound was a "valuable aid in the treatment of several serious disease conditions when the dosage is properly adjusted," he admitted, but it could also be a "dangerous drug, capable of causing serious injury and even death."[56] The FDA chief attempted to rein in the injudicious use of sulfanilamide by using the agency's newly legislated power. He warned,

> Sulfanilamide and drug preparations containing sulfanilamide or related compounds for indiscriminate use by the general public, in a manner which constitutes a serious danger to health, are, when found in interstate commerce, actionable, in the opinion of the Food and Drug Administration, under section 502 (j) of the Federal Food, Drug, and Cosmetic Act [of 1938], which section of the law is now in effect.

A search for chemically related compounds that might be more efficacious, safer, or more soluble in traditionally potable liquids was immediate and active. It was a highly competitive race to create a better sulfanilamide among established drug makers—as well as producers of fine chemicals, which were making the transition to the pharmaceutical industry. The result was an explosion of newly designed compounds with therapeutic potential. By the mid-1940s, some 5,000 derivatives of sulfanilamide—known by the umbrella term sulfonamides (or more commonly, "sulfa drugs")—had been created. Only a handful of these compounds, however, ever made it to market. An early second-generation success was sulfapyridine, a drug originally manufactured by a British chemical firm. Sulfapyridine is notable for being the first, significant new drug to be judged and approved by the FDA under the Food, Drug, and Cosmetic Act.[57] The agency's five-month assessment of the required toxicology studies for sulfapyridine and its back-and-forth discussions with outside advisors, like the AMA's Council on Pharmacy and Chemistry, set the standard for the FDA's subsequent reviews of new drug applications.

Sulfa drugs were essential for reducing the infectious risks of injury in World War II, on both sides of the conflict, and sulfanilamide in particular was used widely and to great success in the immediate aftermath of the Japanese attack on Pearl Harbor in 1941. Millions of pounds of sulfa drugs were produced in the United States for the ensuing war effort, and sterile packets of sulfanilamide were famously contained in the first-aid kits of GIs, who were instructed to sprinkle the antibiotic into open wounds on the battlefield.[58] In addition to the attempted antibiosis of traumatic war injuries, sulfa drugs were instrumental in the prevention and treatment of other infections among enlisted men, including gonorrhea. No doubt, Tulsa physician Logan Spann used sulfa drugs extensively and preferentially during his military medical service, until the compounds were superseded by penicillin at the end of the war. Although penicillin had been discovered in 1928, before the infection-fighting properties of sulfanilamide were even realized, widespread use of the antibiotic was stymied by problems with mass production. However, once these manufacturing kinks were unraveled, growing supplies of penicillin in 1944 and 1945 eroded the use of sulfa drugs. The preferred treatment of various infections with penicillin—notably pneumonia, streptococcal sore throat, and venereal diseases—was due to the antibiotic's greater efficacy in these conditions and the emergence of sulfa resistance.[59]

With the progression of the 20th century, the use of sulfa drugs waned in the highly prolific and competitive field of antibiotic chemotherapy, but their importance and influence in pharmaceutical innovation remains. In the mid-1940s, the mode of sulfanilamide's action was correctly hypothesized. As it had been originally posited by Drs. Long and Bliss in 1937, sulfanilamide was confirmed to be bacteriostatic (not bactericidal). The drug competed with an essential bacterial compound (para-aminobenzoic acid) for the bacterial enzyme (dihydropteroate synthase) that produces folic acid. Without folic acid, bacteria like streptococcus cannot replicate. Consequently sulfanilamide was labeled an antimetabolite, and the discovery of its mode of action launched investigations into other compounds that might interfere with the essential functions of bacteria and, by extension, cancerous cells. As a result, "chemotherapy," as the term was originally applied by Paul Ehrlich in the late 19th and early 20th centuries to the treatment of infections, was transferred to the management of cancers in the mid-20th century and beyond.[60] Therefore sulfanilamide not only launched the age of antibiosis; the drug critically informed the focus of modern oncologic care.

17
NOTHING TO PREVENT INCIDENTS LIKE THIS OCCURRING IN THE FUTURE

In November of 1939, the FDA's Chief Medical Officer, Theodore Klumpp, and Chief Laboratory Scientist, Herbert Calvery, PhD, published their report on the deaths linked to Elixir Sulfanilamide.[1] The report ("The toxicity for human beings of diethylene glycol with sulfanilamide"), printed in the *Southern Medical Journal*, included information from 353 persons who had consumed the product in the fall of 1937. In the authors' estimation, data were "sufficient" to conclude that Massengill's elixir was the primary cause of 105 deaths; although they acknowledged that, in "several" cases, concomitant illness may have contributed to mortality. Among the dead, the drug was most often prescribed for the treatment of gonorrhea (39%) or sore throat (23%). The average length of survival, from the time of the first elixir dose to death, was 9.4 days (range, 2-22 days).

Klumpp and Calvery reported that the most common, initial symptoms of elixir poisoning were nausea and vomiting—symptoms which may have been lifesaving for some by prompting discontinuation of the toxic solution. Headache was also frequently experienced. These symptoms were followed in unpredictable fashion by a transient rise in urine output and then anuria. Signs of renal failure were often accompanied by considerable back, flank, or abdominal pain. As the toxicity advanced, dysfunction of the neurologic system, manifest by waning consciousness and then coma, preceded death. (Klumpp and Calvery did not comment on the possible direct neurotoxicity of diethylene glycol.) In only a minority of cases were laboratory studies performed during life to assess kidney function (for instance, in Charleston, South Carolina). The average elixir dose taken by the deceased was somewhat higher than that consumed by the assessed 248 survivors; although there was considerable overlap in the range of doses taken by the two groups (Table 17.1 and Figure 17.1).[2]

Table 17.1 and Figure 17.1. Mean Cumulative Doses of Elixir Sulfanilamide Among Deceased Victims and Survivors.

Group	Mean Dose, mL, ± SD (ounces)	Dose Range, mL, ± SD (ounces)
Adults		
Deceased (17-78 years; n = 71)	98.6 ± 39.7 (3.3 ± 1.3)	20-240 (0.7-8.1)
Surviving (≥15 years; n = 200)	83.7 ± 57.5 (2.8 ± 1.9)	1-240 (0.03-8.1)
Children		
Deceased (7 months-16 years; n = 34)	52.7 ± 32.8 (1.8 ± 1.1)	5-120 (0.2-4.1)
Surviving (1-14 years; n = 48)	44.2 ± 30.2 (1.5 ± 1.0)	3-105 (0.1-3.6)

SD = standard deviation.

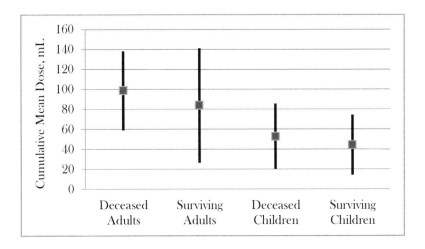

Given that Elixir Sulfanilamide was 72% diethylene glycol and assuming that all consumers sufficiently mixed the product before drinking it, the mean cumulative doses of diethylene glycol taken by the deceased and surviving adults were 71 and 60 mL, respectively (or 2.4 and 2.0 ounces).[3] The mean difference between life and death therefore appeared to be a little more than two teaspoons of diethylene glycol.[4] These data suggest that some individuals are peculiarly susceptible to the toxicity of diethylene glycol, although Klumpp and Calvery were more circumspect in their interpretation. They wrote,

> This is consistent with the well-recognized biological principle that under ordinary conditions the individual tolerance of noxious agents is not a fixed function of dosage. An accurate expression of the fatal dose of any drug can be made only in terms of a range of values. The information available in this study fails to throw light on the factors which influenced the varying tolerance to diethylene glycol.

A comprehensive, independent review of government records by this author reveals that at least 399 persons consumed some portion of Elixir Sulfanilamide (either from prescriptions, over-the-counter purchases, or samples), and that the elixir was the definite, probable, or possible cause of 105 deaths (see Appendix A). Consequently the crude fatality rate associated with Elixir Sulfanilamide was roughly 26%. Among the 276 consumers for whom a clinical reaction (positive, neutral, or negative) was documented in NARA records, 142 (51%) reportedly experienced no ill effects whatsoever (and many of these persons reportedly drank substantial portions, if not all, of their prescriptions). Among consumers who experienced adverse effects but did not die, the overwhelming majority of symptoms were limited to nausea and vomiting; very few patients who developed more severe problems, particularly a drop in urine output, survived.

In 1950, an FDA official claimed that if the entire 240 gallons of Massengill's antibiotic solution had been dispensed and consumed, more than 4,000 people would have died.[5] However, some practical assumptions and a few easy calculations project a substantially smaller, although still shocking, death tally. The entire volume of the elixir, 30,720 ounces, would have allowed for a total of 7,680 four-ounce prescriptions or 10,240 three-ounce prescriptions (the two most common prescription volumes). At a death rate of 26%, this volume, if either partly or wholly consumed (as was the case in 1937), would have caused between 2,000 and 2,700 deaths. In their 1938 toxicology report in *JAMA*, University of Chicago scientists Geiling and Cannon surmised a much less dramatic tally, while crediting the "intelligent, energetic and cooperative manner" of the AMA, the FDA, and several academic centers for their "speedy solution" to the disaster.[6] "Had it not been for their splendid service," they concluded, "the toll of human life would probably have amounted to several hundreds."

* * * * * *

The Food, Drug, and Cosmetic Act of 1938 and subsequent milestone federal legislation (the subject of which is beyond the scope of this book) can be credited for enabling the prevention of similar episodes of mass death in the United States. However, some parts of the world—particularly developing nations—do not have the same government protection or oversight to prevent such disasters. Consequently there have been at least 15 episodes of fatal mass poisoning due to diethylene glycol–contaminated drugs or other consumer goods. The most recent episode occurred in 2009. In many cases, diethylene glycol served as a cheap substitute for potable, but more expensive, solvents like glycerin or propylene glycol (both of which are FDA approved for use in drugs, cosmetics, and food).[7]

However, the FDA is not an absolute failsafe for Americans in the expanding global market. Long and complicated chains of international commercial suppliers for ingredients in medicines and other goods, including those consumed by US citizens, have allowed some nefarious dealers to operate anonymously and without repercussion. Mass poisoning has also been facilitated by interim brokers of bulk solvents, who often rely on the original, falsified certificates of analysis, while slapping their company logos on shipping records.

1. 1969: South Africa

In the summer of 1969, physicians in Cape Town recognized that seven deaths in young children (aged six to 31 months) were due to the consumption of liquid sedatives, branded as Pronap and Plaxim.[8] It was discovered that these sedatives were tainted with diethylene glycol. The children presented with rapidly progressive liver and kidney dysfunction (with BUN levels ranging from 132 to 240 mg/dL). Signs of profound metabolic acidosis, a condition in which the bloodstream harbors excess acid, were also seen. The recognized metabolic derangement was due to the kidney's inability to properly excrete acid. Attempted, but unsuccessful, therapies included hydration, correction of the metabolic acidosis, dialysis (in two cases), and assisted ventilation. Nevertheless "inexorable" death occurred within several days of hospitalization. All victims came to autopsy. The most striking and consistent finding was "extensive" necrosis of the microscopic, convoluted tubules of the kidney, specifically the proximal portion. Epidemiologic inquiries identified the common treatments, and chemical tests identified the presence of diethylene glycol in the liquid medications. The poisonous solvent was a substitute for propylene glycol. The write-up of the case series, published in 1972, revealed that both Pronap and Plaxim "were made under licence by the same manufacturing pharmaceutical firm, which immediately withdrew them from the market." Like in the case of Elixir Sulfanilamide, the South African public was warned through newspapers and radio broadcasts to avoid the products. The authors of the medical report, however, did not identify the manufacturer and did not reveal whether surviving children had also consumed the tainted drugs. They only cryptically wrote, "It then remained to establish how diethylene glycol could have been substituted for propylene glycol in the mixtures, and *this was subsequently done* [emphasis added]." A search of available, digitized newspapers of the era failed to return coverage of the event.

2. 1985: Spain

In 1985, five burn victims at a Barcelona hospital died of acute renal failure with metabolic acidosis.[9] The deaths prompted an investigation of prescribed treatments, and the inquiry ultimately led to the detection of diethylene glycol in an antibiotic ointment, silver sulfadiazine, a routine salve for burns.[10] It was concluded that the toxic solvent had been absorbed through the damaged skin of the five inpatients. The inquiry revealed that the hospital's pharmacy had recently purchased a new formulation of the ointment. The official medical report, published as a letter to the editor in a 1987 issue of the *Annals of Internal Medicine*, did not disclose the source of the toxin or how it ended up in the ointment. It is notable that application of the product was discontinued in "some patients" after they had developed allergic skin reactions. The authors concluded that the deceased victims were more vulnerable to the deadly effects of the tainted ointment because they tolerated it (from an allergic standpoint), thereby allowing for repeated applications. In addition, broad sections of skin were treated in these burn victims, allowing for absorption of the toxin through wide surface areas.

3. 1985: Austria

From an international investigation that began in the spring of 1985 and extended well into 1986, it was determined that diethylene glycol was an intended ingredient in millions of gallons of Austrian wine.[11] In a disturbingly widespread form of industrial corruption, the solvent was systematically added to compensate for the limitations of Austrian grape crops and to boost the sweetness and body of wines from more than 135 Austrian winemakers. At least 1,000 labels were implicated, with vintage years ranging from 1978 to 1984. The US Bureau of Alcohol, Tobacco, and Firearms, which had purview over the domestic investigation of imported wines (as opposed to the FDA), found through widespread testing of more than 12,000 imported bottles that nearly 100 Austrian, German, or Italian labels harbored tainted wine.[12] Reported concentrations of diethylene glycol in the contaminated wine, however, were typically very low, ranging from three to 45 parts per million (ppm); although high-end outliers reached 720 and 2,400 ppm.[13] (The FDA advised that a diethylene-glycol level of 160 ppm was potentially harmful, although no level was deemed safe.) Despite the contamination, there were no reported episodes of death due to the consumption of the tainted wine.[14] The scandal led to the arrest of at least 70 wine growers, importers, or wholesalers in Austria and the conviction of at least 11 individuals on charges of fraud. The Austrian government quickly passed legislation to tighten regulatory control over the country's winemaking industry and its extensive export business.

4. 1986: India

In January and February of 1986, 14 patients in a Bombay (Mumbai) hospital died of acute renal failure after receiving intravenous glycerin therapy for a variety of neurologic conditions.[15] The glycerin, which was later found to be 18.5% diethylene glycol, was purchased by the hospital through intermediate brokers, who had bought the product on the cheap from an industrial (not medical) supplier in India. Treatment of the poisoned patients with various diuretics, sodium bicarbonate (to counteract the ensuing metabolic acidosis), and dialysis (in 12 cases) was unsuccessful. A lengthy public inquiry slammed the hospital executives, charging that there was rampant corruption within India's drug agency. Even as the presiding judge of the inquiry submitted his extensive report to the government in 1987, it was learned that a similar incident had led to the deaths of seven people in northeast India, more than 1,800 miles away.

5. 1990: Nigeria

Between June and September of 1990, at least 111 Nigerian children (aged six months to six years) died of acute renal failure after being given an acetaminophen syrup that was tainted with diethylene glycol.[16] The syrup had been prepared by two hospital pharmacies with what was believed to be propylene glycol. However, it was learned that the pharmacies had actually purchased intentionally mislabeled diethylene glycol by nefarious traders, who had "diverted" the toxic solvent "from oil drilling sites, run by multi-national companies." Nigeria's Food and Drug Administration and Control, through its Task Force on Fake and Counterfeit Drugs, managed the crisis by banning the use of acetaminophen syrups and seizing nearly 350 gallons of the toxin (which could have been used in future lots of pharmaceutical syrups). The alleged traders were also arrested. The official report of the incident, in the *Nigeria Bulletin of Epidemiology*, concluded that sales of chemicals in Nigeria were not adequately monitored; the preparation of pharmaceuticals was not properly supervised; and "oil companies apparently do not have adequate security on their premises to ensure dangerous chemicals do not get into the wrong hands." "In fact," the terribly prescient report continued, "there is presently nothing to prevent incidents like this occurring in the future."

6. 1990-1992: Bangladesh

In the wake of the Nigerian deaths, a dramatic rise in cases of unexplained renal failure was observed in children at the major pediatric hospital in Dhaka, Bangladesh.[17] With assistance from the Massachusetts Department of Public Health and the World Health Organization, local investigators ultimately determined that many of the affected children had consumed one of several brands of acetaminophen elixir that contained diethylene glycol.[18] Laboratory testing revealed that the poisonous solvent had been used as a complete substitute for propylene glycol or glycerin. In an epidemiologic assessment extending to December 1, 1992, consumption of the tainted elixir was documented in at least 67 hospitalized children and suspected in another 272 pediatric inpatients. The poison was implicated in 51 fatalities and suspected in another 185 pediatric deaths. After the Bangladeshi government banned the sale of acetaminophen elixirs in December of 1992, pediatric hospitalizations for unexplained renal failure dropped precipitously, by 84%. In a 1995 report of the incident in the *British Medical Journal*, the authors were unable to state the source of the diethylene glycol, although they surmised that it was likely introduced unknowingly by the drug manufacturers, who had purchased mislabeled solvents from any number of foreign sources or importers.[19]

7. 1992: Argentina

In 1992, 29 people in Argentina (mostly residents of Buenos Aires or nearby La Plata) died of acute renal failure after consuming a popular "natural" over-the-counter syrup containing propolis, a structural resin of beehives.[20] The syrup, "Propoleo Huilen," taken for its supposed antimicrobial effects, was found to contain up to 66% diethylene glycol.[21] According to contemporaneous news reports, Argentinian health officials closed Huilen Laboratories and began searching for the approximately 4,000 at-large bottles of the distributed syrup. The general manager and technical director of Huilen Laboratories were jailed on charges of "crimes against public health" but were freed shortly thereafter on a $200,000 bond each. A brief follow-up by the *New York Times* in 2007, citing an Argentinian court official, revealed that no one had ever been prosecuted for the incident.[22]

8. 1994: Venezuela

In 1994, the ingestion of acetaminophen syrup contaminated with diethylene glycol resulted in the "intoxication and death" of an unknown (or merely unreported) number of children in and around Maracaibo, Venezuela.[23] A chemical analysis of several suspect liquid drugs (including two vitamin syrups) was published in 2000 by pharmacologists from the Universidad Central de Venezuela and the Instituto Nacional de Higiene. Concentrations of diethylene glycol in the syrups reached 29% (in a weight-to-volume ratio). The published report, however, did not provide any clinical information on the casualties, the manufacturer of the syrups, or how diethylene glycol might have ended up in them. A search of several online catalogs of English-language newspapers (eg, Proquest NewsStand, LexisNexis, NewspaperARCHIVE.com, and Google News Archives) failed to return any coverage of the incident. Inquiring emails (written in English) to the Venezuelan authors of the 2000 report went unanswered.

9. 1995-1996: Haiti

An acetaminophen syrup tainted with diethylene glycol was again implicated in at least 109 cases of unexplained multisystem failure, including renal failure, this time in Haitian children (aged one month to 13 years).[24] From October 1995 to mid-July of the following year, at least 85 died, although the numbers of cases and deaths were possibly much higher. An international medical investigation, which included the Centers for Disease Control and Prevention (CDC), had to rely almost exclusively on the recall of Haitian physicians, given that local medical records and any systematic access to them were limited. The tainted brands of liquid acetaminophen, Afebril and Valodon, which were made locally by the drug company Pharval, were found to contain anywhere from 1.2% to 19.6% diethylene glycol (the median volume-to-volume concentration was 14.4%).[25] Survival was significantly more likely among the 11 children who were lucky enough to be transported to the United States for intensive care. Although even with the most advanced treatments at American referral centers, the odds of recovery were slightly better than those of a random coin toss (54% versus 2% with Haitian care).

In a response that mirrored the reactions of Massengill, the AMA, and the FDA to Elixir Sulfanilamide, Pharval recalled its acetaminophen products, public warnings across Haiti were widely and repeatedly broadcasted (including by bullhorn), and police officers confiscated bottles of the implicated products. A "traceback investigation," led by invited agents of the CDC and the FDA, revealed that the glycerin used by Pharval was, in fact, 24% diethylene glycol. The contaminated glycerin had been imported into Haiti from China by way of European brokers, who had routinely concealed the origin of their goods, investigators learned. (The concealment, termed "neutralization," was an accepted business practice designed to ensure a broker's middleman status for future sales.) The FDA conducted a follow-up investigation in China and was able to trace the tainted glycerin to a chemical (not pharmaceutical) plant. But the agency's investigation was protracted and ultimately fruitless, thanks to the skillful stonewalling of Chinese drug officials, the state-sponsored exporter, and finally the plant manager. By the time an FDA agent found the bricks-and-mortar location of the implicated company (the Tianhong Fine Chemicals Factory in Dalian, a major northeastern seaport) at the end of 1997, the plant no longer made glycerin, and there were no records to examine.[26] According to the international authors of the official medical report, published in a 1998 issue of *JAMA*, "It is unknown how and at which point the contamination occurred or if other countries received [diethylene glycol]-contaminated glycerin."

10. 1998: India

During the spring and summer of 1998, 36 Indian children (aged two months to six years) with unexplained acute renal failure were admitted to one of two New Delhi hospitals.[27] An extensive and expansive epidemiologic investigation, including searches for potential infectious causes, ultimately led to the detection of diethylene glycol in a prescribed cough syrup, "Enchest expectorant." The syrup, which had been produced by a company in nearby Gurgaon, an industrial and financial center, was found to contain 17.5% diethylene glycol (on a volume-to-volume basis). The breakthrough in the case came after investigators read the published case series of diethylene-glycol poisonings in Haiti, which was printed in *JAMA* in April of 1998. In the article's comments section, prior episodes of similar poisonings were described, including the 1986 incident in Mumbai. This knowledge alerted investigators to the possibility of another episode of mass poisoning in India. At least 33 of the affected children died despite undergoing dialysis. Most were younger than two years of age. How and when diethylene glycol entered the syrup was unknown at the time of the medical report, which was published in the *Bulletin of the World Health Organization* in 2001.

11. 1998: India

Also in the spring of 1998, a "sudden rise" in cases of acute renal failure and encephalopathy in children (aged seven to 42 months) was observed at a separate New Delhi hospital.[28] At least 11 cases were identified, and eight of these children died despite undergoing dialysis and receiving other intensive supportive care. The consumption of an acetaminophen syrup contaminated with diethylene glycol (2.3%-22.3%, on a weight-to-weight basis) was identified in six cases. The published medical report, contained in a 2006 issue of the *Journal of Tropical Pediatrics*, did not reveal the source of the tainted syrup or whether its manufacturer was connected to that of the tainted cough syrup, which was ingested nearly simultaneously by local children.

12. 2003: France

In 2003, the French government suspended the marketing of an herbal weight-loss remedy, Pilosuryl, after several consumers developed severe renal impairment and coma.[29] According to the French equivalent of the FDA (l'Agence francaise de sécurité sanitaire des produits de santé, or Afssaps), the cases were related to the "excessive" consumption of the product, which contained a chemical form (monoethyl ether) of diethylene glycol at a relatively low concentration (6%). Astonishingly the chemical toxin was an intended ingredient of the dubious product, produced by Pierre Fabre Laboratories. A report of six affected adults in 2004 indicated that all developed acute renal failure; most exhibited a profound metabolic acidosis.[30] Five patients experienced severe neurologic complications, including coma. Kidney biopsies demonstrated acute necrosis of the proximal tubules. Despite the prompt institution of dialysis, four patients required long-term therapy for chronic renal failure. Another patient died a few months after hospital admission. The manufacturer agreed to develop a new formulation of the product.

13. 2006: China

The appearance of acute renal failure among Chinese inpatients led to the discovery of an intravenous drug tainted with diethylene glycol.[31] In the spring of 2006, 64 inpatients with preexisting liver failure received the contaminated drug, but only 15 (23%) developed signs of poisoning. Fourteen of the symptomatic patients died, despite aggressive supportive treatment.[32] It was discovered that the administered drug, armillarisin-A, a compound designed to promote the secretion of bile, contained 30% diethylene glycol by volume. The toxin had been introduced by the Chinese drug manufacturer, Qiqihar No. 2 Pharmaceutical Company, which had purchased the solvent as intentionally mislabeled propylene glycol from a criminal Chinese supplier, Wang Guipang.[33]

Common symptoms of poisoning, when they occurred, were nausea and vomiting, and 10 patients showed signs of delayed neurologic injury, specifically dysfunction of various cranial nerves. Paralysis and other nervous system abnormalities were also seen in a few symptomatic recipients of diethylene glycol. Death, when it occurred, was usually within a week or two of exposure. Microscopic views of kidney biopsies, taken from two patients, revealed the hallmark of diethylene-glycol poisoning: necrosis of the proximal filtering tubules. Notably the patients' glomeruli, the blood-filtering structures of the organ, were intact—just as Tulsa pathologist Ivo Nelson had witnessed nearly 70 years earlier in victims of Elixir Sulfanilamide.

According to international and Chinese news coverage, five executives of the drug company received jail sentences of up to seven years in April of 2008 for the "crime of major responsibility in a fatal accident."[34] Weeks later, Wang Guipang was sentenced to life in prison, evidently escaping a possible death sentence. In behavior reminiscent of Harold Cole Watkins, Wang admitted to Chinese authorities that he had shipped the mislabeled diethylene glycol after swallowing a small amount of the toxin. When nothing happened, he figured the switched-out liquid was acceptable for mass consumption.[35] The drug company was also fined "millions of dollars," and Wang was ordered to pay 400,000 yuan ($57,670 USD). Another 290,000 yuan was confiscated from the rogue supplier. Contemporaneous news coverage indicated that the families of the deceased patients were suing the hospital for 20 million yuan (more than $3 million USD).

14. 2006: Panama

In September of 2006, a Panamanian physician reported an odd spike in cases of unexplained renal failure and acute neurologic abnormalities (eg, cranial nerve palsies, flaccid paralysis, and encephalopathy) in adults.[36] Despite the institution of dialysis, 12 of the initially reported 21 patients died. An ensuing investigation by Panama's Ministry of Health, with assistance from the CDC, identified the common use of a government-manufactured prescription cough syrup. The implicated syrup was promptly shipped to a CDC lab in Atlanta, Georgia, where it was found to contain approximately 8% diethylene glycol. An examination of the syrup's bulk solvent, labeled as nearly pure glycerin, was determined to be about 22% diethylene glycol. Like in the Haitian poisonings, a traceback investigation revealed that the tainted glycerin had been imported from China by way of European brokers. However, the official medical report of the crisis, published in the October 2008 issue of the *Bulletin of the World Health Organization*, provided no further details of the supply trail. Because the tainted glycerin had been used to manufacture other pharmaceutical products in Panama, more than 60,000 medications had to be recalled. At least 119 patients were believed to have been poisoned by the cough syrup. A total of 78 died despite hemodialysis and other supportive care (for a fatality rate of 65.5% among symptomatic consumers).[37]

In contradistinction to prior international episodes of mass poisoning with diethylene glycol–tainted drugs, the American press, specifically the *New York Times*, conducted a comparatively exhaustive investigation of the Panamanian incident. The findings were published in May of 2007.

The *Times* reporters, namely Walt Bogdanich and Jake Hooker, were able to trace 46 barrels of imported, mislabeled glycerin (the source of the diethylene glycol in the tainted cough syrup) from the Panamanian port of Colon back to two international brokers: the Barcelona-based Rasfer International and a Beijing exporter, CNSC Fortune Way, a state-owned chemical broker.[38] The reporters discovered that neither interim broker had tested the glycerin to ensure its stated purity of 99.5%. Likewise the Panamanian importer, Medicom Business Group, and the Panamanian government's pharmaceutical laboratory, which had created the tainted syrup, failed to ensure the quality of the ersatz glycerin (which sat in Panama for two years before being used). Like in previous cases of mass poisoning, the middlemen changed the labeling on the barrels of solvent to ensure their companies' role in future transactions while obscuring the origin of the merchandise. Regardless the *Times* was able to further trace the mislabeled glycerin from the Beijing broker to the Taixing Glycerine Factory, a chemical plant near the Yangtze delta (in an area colloquially known as "chemical country"). The factory, Chinese officials admitted to the *Times*, was not licensed to deal in pharmaceutical ingredients. The original producer of the diethylene glycol was not identified by the paper, although it was reported that both the Taixing Glycerine Factory and broker Wang Guipang (convicted in connection with the diethylene-glycol poisoning of Chinese inpatients) had obtained their toxin from the same source.[39]

15. 2007: Worldwide

On May 5, 2007, a 51-year-old Kuna Indian noticed a large display of toothpaste in a Panama City discount store.[40] The listed ingredients on the tubes were large enough for Eduardo Arias to read from a distance, and he immediately recognized one of the chemical names, diethylene glycol, thanks to the publicized local deaths caused by tainted cough syrup. This accidental discovery, in which the toxic solvent was blatantly printed on the label of a consumer item, triggered the worldwide seizure of millions of tubes of Chinese-made toothpaste, which were found to contain diethylene glycol at concentrations of up to 14%. The toothpaste, some of which had been smuggled internationally, first turned up in Latin America and Australia, with brand names like Mr. Cool and Mr. Cool Junior. But over the ensuing weeks, contaminated tubes were discovered on at least five continents and in dozens of countries, including the United States and Canada. In June, the FDA announced that it had detected, through random testing, diethylene glycol in various US-imported brands of Chinese toothpaste. The labels of these products did not divulge the toxin.

The suspect tubes had been distributed to discount stores, luxury hotels, prisons, public hospitals, juvenile detention centers, and state institutions for the mentally ill.[11] (It was also learned that the tainted toothpaste had been offered for sale in American discount stores under the pilfered brand names of Colgate and Sensodyne.) The original sources of the contaminated toothpaste were identified as two Chinese producers in the eastern coastal province of Jiangsu, a high-volume center for Chinese exports: Goldcredit International Trading and the Suzhou City Jinmao Daily Chemicals Company, which were (and are) manufacturers of oral care products. Chinese regulators initially defended the toothpaste, stating that small amounts of diethylene glycol had long been standard in personal-care products that were unlikely to be ingested. But the FDA differed, stating that no amount of the toxin was acceptable in toothpaste. The admonition was especially true for fruit- and bubblegum-flavored toothpaste marketed to children, who would be more likely to swallow the product while brushing. Although there were no confirmed reports of injury due to the toxin-containing toothpaste, the Chinese government said in July that it had banned the use of diethylene glycol in toothpaste, weeks after Mr. Arias's astute observation.

The international focus on China as a source of dubious and potentially dangerous goods, thanks mostly to the investigative work of the *New York Times*, prompted the now-publicly embarrassed Chinese government to conduct, with relative earnest, an internal investigation of its chemical pipelines; although the state investigation remained a limited and bizarre one. Chinese officials eventually acknowledged "some misconduct" on the part of two chemical suppliers of tainted glycerin, but the responsibility was only partial, they hedged.[12] In the case of the tainted cough syrup in Panama, Chinese regulators stressed that the Panamanian importer "bore most of the blame," because it had failed to test the purchased glycerin. Not to anyone's surprise, the Panamanian importer and the implicated wholesalers objected to the outlandish charge. Likewise the FDA countered (while urging site testing of bulk pharmaceutical supplies) that the Panamanian deaths would never have occurred if Chinese suppliers had not spiked the glycerin with diethylene glycol in the first place. A more in-depth investigation by Chinese officials appeared to be stalled by nonsensical bureaucracy. The Taixing Glycerine Factory, the source of the tainted glycerin in the Panamanian cough syrup, was not licensed to produce pharmaceutical chemicals. Therefore, Chinese regulators said, they did not have purview over the business and could do very little, if anything. Similarly the state-owned Chinese broker that had exported the tainted glycerin was not under the regulatory control of the Chinese food and drug administration, state officials argued.

However, a few weeks later, the Chinese government flip-flopped and reported that it had revoked the license of the Taixing Glycerine Factory.[43] More astonishing, Chinese officials informed the world that the government had executed the former head of its drug-regulatory agency, 62-year-old Zheng Xiaoyu, on July 10th.[44] Zheng had pleaded guilty to bribery, officials said. Nevertheless it was unclear if he or other drug regulators had anything to do with the exportation of diethylene glycol–tainted glycerin. Rather the execution appeared to be a troubling political act, its message being: China is serious about overhauling the regulation of its chemical and pharmaceutical exports and ensuring their safety. China's newly found introspection led to months of negotiations between the US FDA and Chinese regulators, the intent of which was to toughen China's oversight of its exported drugs and chemicals.[45] An accord was signed in December of 2007, but the agreement, said the *New York Times*, addressed "only a tiny fraction of the pharmaceutical ingredients being marketed worldwide by thousands of unlicensed chemical companies." Furthermore it remained dubious whether the Chinese government had the manpower to oversee the country's massive and fractured drug and chemical industries.

16. 2008: Nigeria

In November of 2008, a startling increase in cases of unexplained renal failure among Nigerian children was traced to the use of a liquid teething medication containing acetaminophen ("My Pikin").[46] During an international investigation conducted by Nigerian officials, the CDC, and the FDA, batches of the product made from August to October of 2008 were found to contain diethylene glycol at a concentration of 17%-21% by weight. Investigators, reporting their results in the December 2009 issue of *Morbidity and Mortality Weekly Report*, identified 57 children (aged one week to 27 months) who were affected by diethylene-glycol poisoning due to consumption of the product; 54 died.[47] The quick discovery of exposure to the toxin in cases of renal failure led to an immediate recall of the product (7,616 of approximately 15,000 bottles were recovered) and the shutting down of the manufacturer, Barewa Pharmaceuticals, in Lagos. Despite these efforts, more than a quarter (28%) of the 57 poisonings occurred after the recall was announced. The CDC reported, "Although the exact mechanism of contamination was not identified, facility inspection revealed multiple errors common to previous [diethylene glycol]-associated large-scale poisoning events." These included the use of unknown or unapproved suppliers of the intended solvent (in this case, propylene glycol); a lack of certificates of analysis from suppliers; and a failure to assay the purchased solvent for diethylene glycol. According to contemporaneous news coverage in the *New York Times*, Nigerian officials traced the intentionally mislabeled diethylene glycol to an unlicensed chemical supplier in Lagos, who had sold the toxic solvent to Barewa.[48] In February of 2009, Nigerian officials arrested five "operators" of Barewa and seven employees of the original bulk-chemical supplier. In May of 2013, a federal court in Nigeria dissolved the firm and convicted two Barewa employees for "conspiracy and selling of a dangerous drug."

17. 2009: Bangladesh

In the summer of 2009, at least 28 children in eastern Bangladesh died of acute renal failure after consuming an acetaminophen syrup that was tainted with diethylene glycol. The contaminated syrup was manufactured by Rid Pharma, a company located outside of the capital, Dhaka. The plant was reportedly not licensed to produce the drug. Official details of the incident are scarce and confined to local and regional newspapers, most notably the Bangladeshi *Daily Star*.[49] (There is apparently no official report in catalogued medical journals and no relevant coverage in American news sources.) In late July of 2009, the toxin was detected in the syrup by state drug officials, and the manufacturing plant was "sealed," reported the *Daily Star*. Shortly thereafter, court proceedings were initiated against Rid Pharma managers and pharmacists. However, the legal case has been protracted. Local police inexplicably delayed the necessary arrest warrants for the implicated parties, and some of the accused went into hiding. The prosecution has also been stalled by repeated requests from the defense to postpone hearings. A trial reportedly began in early 2012.[50]

* * * * * *

The answer to why diethylene glycol becomes an ingredient in liquid pharmaceuticals is relatively transparent. It is a cheap substitute for more expensive, potable solvents, like glycerin and propylene glycol. And there are criminal traders who are willing to capitalize on this fact, and others who are willing to ignore the possibility. It is particularly distressing that the most likely victims of contaminated solvents are children, because they are most likely to need and consume liquid medications. It is especially troubling that the children who are most vulnerable to mass poisoning with diethylene glycol are those in impoverished countries, where there is limited or no regulatory oversight of the manufacture and distribution of chemicals and pharmaceuticals.

Yet how diethylene glycol exerts its toxicity in consumers remains unclear, and this uncertainty continues to hamper the successful treatment of poisoning. Much of what we know about diethylene glycol and how it behaves in the human body has been extrapolated from studies in animals, specifically rats.[51] After diethylene glycol is taken by mouth, it is rapidly absorbed from the gut and widely distributed throughout the body, particularly the kidneys, brain, and liver. The metabolism of diethylene glycol occurs primarily in the liver, where a percentage of the chemical is sequentially broken down by two workhorse enzymes: alcohol dehydrogenase (ADH) and aldehyde dehydrogenase (ALDH), the same enzymes that break down ethyl alcohol (ethanol). Investigators of diethylene-glycol poisoning, specifically scientists at Louisiana State University (LSU) reported in 2011 that the chemical breakdown products of diethylene glycol (known by the merciful abbreviations 2-HEAA and DGA)[52] are probably the chief toxic offenders. Recent laboratory studies at LSU indicated that DGA, not the parent compound diethylene glycol or the initially produced metabolite HEAA, is the primary instigator of damage to cells of the proximal convoluted tubules of the human kidney.[53] Moreover blocking the metabolic enzyme ADH with the drug fomepizole (foe MEP eh zole) in rats has been shown to block the metabolism of diethylene glycol and prevent the development of both kidney and liver damage.[54] But to effectively prevent toxicity, the antidote most likely needs to be administered quickly—for instance, within 15 minutes of diethylene-glycol ingestion in rats.

Another animal study supports the benefit of preventing diethylene-glycol metabolism to reduce the solvent's toxicity. Chinese investigators examined rats with chemically induced liver damage, which stunts the activity of the enzymes ADH and ALDH.[55] When exposed to diethylene glycol, the experimental animals with liver disease were less likely to show signs of diethylene-glycol toxicity, including kidney toxicity, than the control animals—presumably because the animals with liver disease were less able to break down diethylene glycol to one or more toxic metabolites. These animals could therefore excrete the intact parent compound (diethylene glycol) more efficiently in their urine, before significant organ damage could occur. The rodent data may have a real-world human correlate. Among the 64 Chinese inpatients with preexisting liver disease who were exposed to intravenous diethylene glycol in 2006, only 15 developed clinical symptoms of poisoning. It is therefore conceivable that liver disease (and the relative inability to break down diethylene glycol) was protective in some of these human cases.

Use of fomepizole for preventing or delaying injury from diethylene glycol is theoretically sound, particularly if the antidote is given quickly;

however, practical experience remains limited. According to the CDC, only two Nigerian children who were exposed to diethylene glycol in 2008 received fomepizole. The treatment (along with dialysis) did not improve the chances of survival in these patients, however.[56] Otherwise there is at least one case report of the successful treatment of diethylene-glycol poisoning in a 17-month-old child, who received fomepizole and hemodialysis within hours of ingesting the toxin.[57]

Data recorded by the FDA indicate that not everyone who was exposed to Elixir Sulfanilamide, even a considerable volume, showed signs of toxicity. These accounts were the basis of Massengill's defense, which rested on the observation that not everyone who drank the toxic elixir became ill. In fact, some patients actually improved, presumably because of the antibiotic's beneficial effects. A review of NARA records shows that roughly half of consumers (for whom reactions to the product were recorded) tolerated the elixir without any ill effects. This phenomenon of an asymptomatic ingestion of diethylene glycol is supported by the 1939 article of Drs. Klumpp and Calvery. They reported a minimal difference (and tremendous overlap) between the amounts of elixir that were consumed by survivors and victims. The observation is reinforced by data from Chinese inpatients with liver disease who were exposed to diethylene glycol in 2006. There was no statistically significant difference between the median cumulative dose of diethylene glycol among symptomatic patients and that among asymptomatic patients (24 and 36 mL, respectively).[58] Yet the examination of relatively asymptomatic consumers of diethylene glycol has otherwise been limited.

Recently published studies of mass diethylene-glycol poisoning rely on case-control methods, an approach used by epidemiologists to identify the likely causes of an observed disease or injury. In case-control studies of renal failure, for example, subjects whose condition is unexplained are compared with subjects whose renal failure has a known cause or causes. A statistical association is then examined between the exposure to possible instigators of renal dysfunction—for instance, exposure to a suspect medication—in the two patient populations. If exposure to a suspect medication is significantly greater in the patients with unexplained renal failure, it may be concluded that the unexplained renal failure is, in fact, due to the suspect medication. However, a case-control study is limited in that it neglects the assessment of potentially asymptomatic consumers of diethylene glycol–tainted products (a population that may be, admittedly, hard to quantify in developing countries).

In the Panamanian poisoning of 2006, the CDC identified at least 28 individuals who consumed the tainted cough syrup but did not develop symptoms of poisoning.[59] Among the conjectures for the absence of symptoms in these patients was the possibility that they did not consume a sufficiently toxic dose of syrup, or they were not compromised by coexisting illnesses. The investigators acknowledged that the minimum toxic dose of diethylene glycol is not well documented. The official report concluded that "there may be thousands of people who were exposed to the contaminated syrup but who displayed only minor symptoms and did not develop acute renal failure or even seek medical care." Obviously the possibility is not without precedent.

* * * * * *

The activity of the liver enzymes that break down diethylene glycol, ADH and ALDH, are known to vary on the basis of a number of factors, including how they are genetically expressed.[60] Some variations in the genes (known as alleles) encoding for ADH and ALDH are more efficient at breaking down ethyl alcohol (and by extension, diethylene glycol) than others. It is therefore possible that certain individuals may be relatively resistant to diethylene-glycol poisoning, because their ADH or ALDH enzymes are not particularly efficient at creating the toxic metabolites of the solvent. Yet a follow-up examination of selected alleles for ADH and ALDH among 34 of the 64 Chinese inpatients who were exposed to intravenous diethylene glycol in 2006 did not show significantly different patterns of allelic expression.[61] Patients who developed acute renal failure after receiving the tainted drug (n = 10) showed a similar allelic pattern for the metabolic enzymes as those who did not (n = 24). However, the sample size may have been too small to show significant statistical variations.

Yet if the metabolism of diethylene glycol does vary on the basis of the genetically programmed activity of ADH and ALDH, then identifying the toxic or lethal dose of diethylene glycol among the general population may be difficult (as it has been) or even irrelevant. The lethal dose may only have meaning as it applies to certain subpopulations who have similar genetic profiles for the metabolic enzymes that break down diethylene glycol. Regardless the matter may be of scientific interest only. As the FDA has repeatedly advised: Diethylene glycol at any level does not belong in consumer products. The fact that diethylene glycol appears to have no or minimal effects on a substantial portion of the population does not negate its fatal effects on susceptible individuals.

* * * * * *

Only within the last decade or so has it been fully appreciated that diethylene glycol (or its metabolites) is directly toxic to the nervous system.

In laboratory animals, diethylene glycol rapidly crosses the blood-brain barrier, a membranous fence between the brain capillaries and the central nervous system.[62] Diethylene glycol's ease of transmission into the brain may account for the direct neurotoxic effects of the solvent or its metabolites (although other unknown mechanisms may be at work). In 2002, physicians at the University of Colorado reported a case of diethylene-glycol poisoning in a suicide who drank Sterno fluid (pure diethylene glycol).[63] Prolonged survival, which may have been promoted by the suicide's immediate consumption of a large volume of ethyl alcohol[64] and the later administration of fomepizole, was associated with a delayed, but rapidly progressive, paralysis of the limbs and the respiratory muscles. Function of the cranial nerves, nerves emerging directly from the brain and the brainstem (as opposed to nerves from the spinal cord), was also disrupted. These cranial-nerve abnormalities manifested as paralysis of the eye muscles and loss of the pupils' constricting reaction to light. Nerve tests performed during life indicated that the neurologic injury was primarily confined to the myelin, the fatty insulation of nerve fibers; these findings were confirmed at autopsy. (The patient died about two weeks after the toxic ingestion.) In some areas of the nerve fibers, the myelin had been completely destroyed, leaving the underling extension of the nerve cell, the impulse-transmitting axon, vulnerable to injury.

In 2005, physicians at the University of Pennsylvania described the subacute development of complete paralysis, dysfunction of the cranial nerves, and coma in a 24-year-old man who had ingested vodka and a "fog solution," which was found to be 28% diethylene glycol.[65] The neurologic signs and symptoms followed the well-recognized effects of diethylene-glycol poisoning—namely, renal failure with metabolic acidosis. In contradistinction to the case report from Colorado, nerve testing in this case suggested a primary insult to the axons with later damage to the surrounding myelin. The process by which diethylene glycol injured the nerves remained unclear and could only be guessed at (on the basis of nerve damage known to be caused by other chemical toxins). The patient survived the poisoning and, after months, recovered much of his neurologic function; although his kidney injury was permanent, and he remained dependent on dialysis. The authors concluded that an "animal model would be helpful to determine the mechanisms underpinning the damaging effects of [diethylene glycol] on peripheral nerves." However, there are apparently no published reports to this end.

In another recent case of diethylene-glycol poisoning, due to the intentional ingestion of wallpaper stripper by a man with a psychiatric disease, studies performed several days after exposure to the poison suggested mild damage to the sensory and motor axons in the arms and legs.[66] The neurologic injury progressed rapidly to quadriparesis and profound dysfunction of the cranial nerves. About two months later, nerve studies indicated severe damage to the surrounding myelin of the axons. At three months, the man recovered to the point of being able to "walk a few steps with assistance." At six months, "his neurologic function continued to improve," although he remained dependent on dialysis.

Delayed neurotoxic effects of diethylene glycol were observed in three of seven Australian inmates who intentionally consumed a diluted cleaning solution, which contained the toxin.[67] Neurologic signs and symptoms, which emerged during the second week after ingestion, included blindness, deafness, and a profound, generalized weakness. In one case, electrical studies of the legs suggested damage to the sensory and motor axons. In another case, an MRI study of the brain showed multiple small areas of either edema or infarction (ie, stroke). This patient died on the 19th day after ingestion. A limited autopsy showed no evidence of myelin damage in the brain (eg, central demyelination). Of the two patients who survived, neurologic deficits were evident two years later. Both patients remained dependent on dialysis, because of the toxin-induced kidney failure.

Paralysis was a prominent feature of the Panamanians who were poisoned with the diethylene glycol–tainted cough syrup in 2006, and the neurologic manifestations of the poisonings (including encephalopathy and cranial-nerve dysfunction) were believed to be due to the direct neurotoxicity of diethylene glycol.[68] Because the effects of diethylene glycol on the nervous system appear to be a relatively delayed effect of the toxin, these manifestations may be more likely in people who initially survive or endure the early toxicity of diethylene-glycol poisoning—specifically renal failure—for longer periods of time. End-of-life signs and symptoms for many victims of Elixir Sulfanilamide included descriptions of weakness, delirium, encephalitis, blindness, difficulty talking, throat paralysis, respiratory paralysis, deafness, convulsions, or coma, which may have been due to the direct neurotoxicity of diethylene glycol. Although many of the deceased victims of Massengill's elixir underwent autopsy, detailed examinations of nervous tissue in these cases were apparently not performed or not reported.

* * * * * *

Of course, the prevention of diethylene-glycol poisoning is ideal. The toxin has multiple legitimate uses: as an ingredient in antifreeze solutions,[69] brake fluids, industrial lubricants, wallpaper strippers, artificial fog solutions, and heating and cooking fuels (like Sterno)—to name several.[70] However, protective packaging and warnings to deter the intentional or accidental ingestion of these liquid products are variable and often insufficient.[71] Prompted by the mass diethylene-glycol poisoning in Panama in 2006, the FDA issued a warning to "pharmaceutical manufacturers, suppliers, drug repackers, and health professionals who compound medications."[72] They were urged "to be especially vigilant in assuring that glycerin, a sweetener commonly used worldwide in liquid over-the-counter and prescription drug products, is not contaminated with diethylene glycol"; although the FDA believed that there was little threat to US consumers. The agency's guidance stipulated that "certain analytical testing procedures must be performed on all lots of glycerin," specifically an identity test for diethylene glycol.[73] The FDA's safety limit for the toxin in bulk glycerin was 0.1%, as recommended by the US Pharmacopeia.

The most reliable and accurate test for detecting diethylene glycol in solvents is a two-part method known as gas-liquid chromatography (GC) and mass spectrometry (MS).[74] But this bipartite test necessitates resources—specifically money for the purchase of expensive equipment and technical training for proper use of the equipment—which are characteristically limited in developing nations. Relatively simpler and less costly techniques exist for the detection of diethylene glycol in commercial solvents, but these methods—namely infrared spectrometry and thin-layer chromatography (TLC)—have failed to identify diethylene glycol in some instances of mass poisonings. In the FDA's investigation of the tainted acetaminophen syrup in Haiti during the mid-1990s, infrared spectrometry—which was recommended by the US Pharmacopeia to identify diethylene glycol—did not reveal the substance.[75] Only GC and MS signaled the poison. And in India in 1998, TLC missed the toxin in the contaminated cough syrup. The authors of the Indian medical report concluded,

> [T]hin layer chromatography alone may not identify contamination with diethylene glycol. On the other hand, gas-liquid chromatography or other appropriate methods are not available in all the laboratories that may be asked to test medicines. Appropriate tests must be available in laboratories that test medicines for contaminants.
>
> The failure to detect the contamination using thin layer chromatography had an important bearing on these cases.[76]

Despite the apparent limitations of TLC in the detection of diethylene glycol, the FDA recommended an inexpensive, simple, and quickly performed version of the assay in 2007 for use in the field.

Created by FDA scientists after the mass poisoning in Haiti, the revised, but less sensitive, technique employs TLC, a method that separates components of a liquid solution for their identification.[77] This on-site version of TLC can be used to identify diethylene glycol (as well as ethylene glycol) to a concentration as low as 6% in glycerin and 2% in elixirs, according to FDA scientists.[78] The method requires a technician to visually inspect a thin "plate" or sheet of specialized testing paper that has been exposed to the solvent in question. No other testing equipment is necessary. (Chemical spraying of the testing sheets in a laboratory is required to identify diethylene glycol at lower concentrations, below 0.1%.) Although the assay is relatively insensitive when compared with the reference standard of GC and MS, its use would certainly have increased the odds of identifying diethylene glycol in most cases of mass poisoning to date. Unfortunately this basic method and more sophisticated tests for diethylene glycol in bulk pharmaceutical ingredients have not been proactively used on a routine basis. Consequently repeated episodes of mass poisoning due to diethylene glycol–tainted drugs are expected.

APPENDIX A: ELIXIR DEATHS BY STATE

Further details of deaths due to Elixir Sulfanilamide, including specific FDA sources, can be found at http://bmartinmd.com/elixir-sulfanilamide-deaths.html. The race or ethnicity of victims who were other than Caucasian or white is indicated by quoted descriptors used in contemporaneous FDA or other public records.

Alabama (nine confirmed, two possible)

Alabama's history with Massengill's Elixir Sulfanilamide is distinctive in that the first documented prescriptions for the product, specifically three written on September 16, 1937, were dispensed there. In addition, America's first known elixir-related death, on September 24th, occurred in Alabama.

During the FDA's investigation in the state, which continued into December, the agency discovered 11 elixir-related casualties (two of which were only possibly related to Massengill's product). However, the outcomes of two nameless prescriptions and two over-the-counter purchases were apparently never determined, despite local radio broadcasts that warned of the elixir's dangers and urged the return of the product.

John (Johnay) C. Holloway, 22, a married "colored" farmhand from Clayton, died on September 24th. (See Chapter 10 for a description of this case.)

Syble Gwendolyn Singleton, a 10-month-old girl from Georgetown, Georgia, died on September 25th at the Salter Hospital in Eufaula. (See Chapter 10 for a description of this case.)

Anderson Crews (or Cruce), 63, a married "colored" or "mulatto" farmer from Headland, died on September 25th. (See Chapter 10 for a description of this case.)

(Berry) Edward Walker, a single 26-year-old man from Chancellor, died on October 3rd in a Dothan hospital after consuming about three ounces of Elixir Sulfanilamide, which was prescribed as treatment for gonorrhea.

Ethel (or Ether or Ester) Colston, 49, a widowed black laborer from Ariton, died in Dothan on October 4th after drinking about eight tablespoons of elixir for an unknown ailment.

Mary Frances "Fannie" Zeanah , 68, a widowed housekeeper from Eufaula, died on October 13th at the Salter Hospital after consuming an unknown quantity of Elixir Sulfanilamide.

Ed (or Edd) Scott, a five-year-old "colored" boy from the Demopolis area, died on October 14th after consuming two ounces of Elixir Sulfanilamide, which was prescribed for an unknown ailment.

Nettie Joe (or Betty Jo) Story, a two-year-old girl from Guntersville, died on October 16th after drinking one-and-a-half ounces of a six-ounce prescription for Elixir Sulfanilamide. The medication was intended as treatment for acute streptococcal pharyngitis. (See Chapter 10 for a description of this case.)

Alfred "Alf" McDade (or McDay), 47, a married "colored" plasterer from Eufaula, died on October 17th after consuming about two ounces of Elixir Sulfanilamide. The product was prescribed for an unspecified ailment.

Possible

Rita Glendyne (or Glendine) Mallon, a six-month old girl from Dauphin Island, died on October 10th in the Mobile Infirmary. She consumed "three or four doses" of Elixir Sulfanilamide, which was prescribed for symptoms of fever, inability to digest, and urinary pus.

Martin Smith, 42, a man from Pisgah, died on October 17th after consuming three ounces of Elixir Sulfanilamide for an unknown ailment.

Arkansas (one confirmed)

For a description of the FDA's confiscation of Elixir Sulfanilamide in Arkansas and the agency's discovery of a related death—that of seven-year-old *Ruth Jeanell Long*—see Chapter 10.

California (one confirmed)

FDA Chemical Analyst Morris Yakowitz, 26, was charged with tracing and impounding Elixir Sulfanilamide in the Fresno area, where 19 pints had been shipped. During his investigation in late October, Yakowitz discovered four prescriptions in the area, one of which was associated with a death.

Orvin Charles Kutz, Jr., a five-year-old boy from Fresno, died on October 24th after consuming one ounce of Elixir Sulfanilamide in divided doses as treatment for a streptococcal sore throat and high fever.

Florida (two confirmed, one possible)

In its investigation in Florida, which extended into November, the FDA learned of three deaths among six prescriptions (including two for one individual) that were dispensed in the state.

Fred L. (possibly Leroy) Williams, 35, a "colored" merchant tailor from Jacksonville, died on October 12th after consuming an unknown quantity (but probably six ounces) of Elixir Sulfanilamide, which was prescribed for gonorrhea.

Emanuel Cauley, 37, a "colored" laborer with the Atlantic Coast Line Railroad, died on October 16th in Jacksonville. He consumed more than four ounces of Elixir Sulfanilamide, which was prescribed for probable gonorrhea. (For a description of the related civil case against Massengill and its outcome, see Chapter 16.)

Possible

J. C. Donalson (or Donaldson), a four-year-old "colored" boy from Seaboard, died on October 16th at Quincy. He consumed probably two ounces of Elixir Sulfanilamide, which was prescribed for an unclear illness.

Georgia (11 confirmed, two possible)

The FDA's investigative efforts in Georgia, which were hampered by repeated stonewalling and deception on the part of several pharmacists and physicians, extended well into November (see Chapter 11). A total of 25 prescriptions (including one for two individuals) and three over-the-counter purchases of Elixir Sulfanilamide were discovered. Thirteen known elixir-related deaths occurred in the state.

Ewell Daughtrey (or Daughtry), 32, a railroad foreman from Dillard, Alabama, died on September 26th at the Atlantic Coast Line Railroad Hospital in Waycross, Georgia. Daughtrey received two ounces of Elixir Sulfanilamide on September 16th, as treatment for gonorrhea.

Jewell Fitts, a 36-year-old man from Dahlonega, died on October 5th at the Downey Hospital in Gainesville. (For details of this case, see Chapter 11.)

Betty Louise Satterfield, a three-year-old girl from Greensboro, died on October 7th. She received a four-ounce prescription for Elixir Sulfanilamide, which was intended as treatment for erysipelas.

Luther N. (or O.) Gillham, a 29-year-old man from Porterdale, died on October 8th at a Covington hospital. Gillham received a four-ounce prescription for Elixir Sulfanilamide as treatment for gonorrhea.

Herman Bolton, a 34-year-old taxi driver from Millen, died on October 16th at a local hospital. After a lengthy investigation, the FDA determined that Bolton had received six ounces of Elixir Sulfanilamide, without a prescription from a local pharmacy. The elixir was intended as a remedy for gonorrheal symptoms.

Robert Lee Fields, a 68-year-old farmer, and **Lillie Lyons,** a 45-year-old widow and farm laborer, both from Aaron, died on October 17th and 19th, respectively. The couple shared an eight-ounce prescription of Elixir Sulfanilamide as treatment for gonorrhea.

Leonard J. Dees, a 22-year-old "colored" man from Griffin, died on October 18th in Lamar County. (See Chapter 11 for a description of this case.)

Robert L(ee) Parks, a 19-year-old man from Dahlonega, died on October 19th at the Downey Hospital in Gainesville. (See Chapter 11 for details of this case and its investigation.)

Seth L(awton) Durden, a 28-year-old single, "colored" farmer from Wadley, died on October 21st in a Millen hospital. (See Chapter 11 for details of this case and its investigation.)

Will (William Leon) Portwood, a 34-year-old farmer from Swainsboro, died on October 26th at the town's Franklin Hospital. (See Chapter 11 for details of this case and its investigation.)

Possible

Arnette (or Anett) Lewis, a one-year-old "colored" girl from McDonough died on October 6th at home. She consumed one ounce of a two-ounce prescription for Elixir Sulfanilamide, which was given as treatment for streptococcal pharyngitis.

Mrs. Mark (Morning Catherine) Reynolds (née Bracewell), a 77-year-old farmer's wife from Dublin, died on October 12th. She consumed between one and two ounces of Massengill's elixir as treatment for pyelitis, or kidney inflammation.

Illinois and Missouri (eight confirmed, one possible)

Among the 71 elixir prescriptions ultimately identified by the FDA in Illinois and Missouri (with 67 known exposures), nine deaths were discovered. All but one of these prescriptions were dispensed in Illinois, and most of these (about 70%) were dispensed by two East St. Louis pharmacies (the Walter J. Daut Pharmacy and the Lincoln Pharmacy).

Hazel Mildred Fea, a 23-year-old manicurist from Potosi, Missouri, died on October 10th at the Barnes Hospital in St. Louis. (For details of this case, see chapter 8.)

J. D. Kimbrough (or Jee D. Kimbrew), a 26-year-old married black laborer from East St. Louis, Illinois, died on October 15th at the city's St. Mary's Hospital after consuming three or four tablespoons of a compounded prescription containing Elixir Sulfanilamide. The treatment was intended as a remedy for a "sore throat."

Edwin Maurice Slaughter, a four-year-old boy from East St. Louis, died on October 16th at the city's St. Mary's Hospital. The child probably drank "all but two doses" of a four-ounce compounded formula containing Elixir Sulfanilamide. The treatment was prescribed for gonococcal urethritis and inguinal adenitis (inflammation of the lymph nodes in the groin).

George W. Nixon, a five-year-old boy from Pine Bluff, Arkansas, died on October 18th at St. Mary's Infirmary in St. Louis. The child drank less than one ounce of a four-ounce compounded mixture containing Elixir Sulfanilamide, which was prescribed as a remedy for strep throat.

Joseph L. Henry, a 60-year-old switchman from East St. Louis, Illinois, died on October 18th at St. Mary's Hospital in St. Louis, Missouri. Henry drank all but three or four doses of a four-ounce compounded treatment containing Elixir Sulfanilamide, which was prescribed for a bladder infection.

Alexander A. Brooks, 70, a "colored" widowed electrician from East St. Louis, died on October 21st at the city's St. Mary's Hospital. Brooks consumed about three ounces of a compounded mixture containing Elixir Sulfanilamide, which was prescribed for epididymitis.

Gertrude Lee (Mrs. Ellis Z.) Black, a 38-year-old housewife, from East St. Louis, died on October 24th at the Homer G. Phillips Hospital in St. Louis, Missouri. Black drank about two ounces of a compounded solution containing Elixir Sulfanilamide, which was prescribed for a streptococcal sore throat.

William L. Schroeder, a 50-year-old brewery employee from St. Louis, died on October 24th at the city's Barnes Hospital. (For details of Schroeder's death, see chapter 8.)

Possible

Bessie Lee Bosley, a 53-year-old "Negro" woman from East St. Louis, died on October 8th at the city's St. Mary's Hospital. She consumed an unknown quantity of a four-ounce compounded prescription containing Elixir Sulfanilamide. The treatment was intended, presumably, for a streptococcal infection of the neck and jaw, which was the official cause of death (along with septicemia).

Mississippi (23 confirmed, two possible, one unlikely)

Mississippi's history with Elixir Sulfanilamide is notable for the fact that the confirmed death toll in the state (as determined by the FDA's extended investigation) was almost twice that in any other state. The high elixir-related death tally in Mississippi, however, was not due to a disproportionately large volume of elixir shipped to the state. Rather the large number of fatalities among Mississippians appeared to be the result of the individual and chance willingness of certain physicians—like the unsuspecting Archie Calhoun of Mt. Olive, Joe Green of Laurel, and John

V. James of Bentonia—to write relatively large numbers of prescriptions for the untested product.

Working out of the agency's New Orleans station, Inspector Roland Sherman was instrumental in not only investigating the first publicized deaths, but in uncovering fatalities by reviewing state death records—which he continued to do into December of 1937. It was ultimately determined that 71 prescriptions for Elixir Sulfanilamide were written and dispensed in Mississippi to 70 individuals (two of whom died in Tennessee (*Columbus Bryant* and *James E. Byrd*). In addition, there was at least one over-the-counter purchase of the product (which caused the death of *William Corneel Howell*).

Henry G. Taylor, a 28-year-old "colored" man from Bentonia, died on September 25th at the Afro-American Hospital in Yazoo City after consuming four and three-quarter ounces of Elixir Sulfanilamide. The product was prescribed as treatment for gonorrhea.

"Little" Martin Shelby, a 24-year-old "colored" man from Bentonia, died on September 29th at the Charity Hospital in Vicksburg. He consumed about two and three-quarter ounces of Elixir Sulfanilamide, which was prescribed as treatment for gonorrhea and epididymitis.

Franklin Jones, a 28-year-old "colored" man from Bentonia, died on the night of October 2nd after consuming less than three ounces of Elixir Sulfanilamide, which was prescribed for a "[p]eritonsillar abscess."

Joe Hewitt, a 32-year-old "colored" cotton farmer from Deasonville, died on October 4th (presumably at home) after consuming an unknown quantity of Massengill's elixir, which was prescribed for "a severe attack of tonsillitis."

Claiborne L(evell) Anderson, a 37-year-old Masonite employee from Laurel, died on October 4th at the Laurel General Hospital. Anderson consumed about three and one-half ounces of Elixir Sulfanilamide, which was prescribed for a "sore throat and headache."

Albert Cole, a 19-year-old "negro" laborer from Laurel, died on October 5th, presumably at his mother's home. He consumed about three ounces of Elixir Sulfanilamide, which was intended as treatment for gonorrhea.

Hettie (or Ettie) Young, an 18-year-old "colored" girl from Sanatorium, died on October 5th at the nearby Magee General Hospital.

She consumed an unknown quantity of Elixir Sulfanilamide, which was prescribed for gonorrheal cystitis and vaginitis.

Essie Davis, a 48-year-old "colored" man from Bentonia, died on October 8th at the Charity Hospital in Vicksburg. He consumed an unknown amount of Elixir Sulfanilamide, which was prescribed as treatment for gonorrhea.

Leffie Easterling, a 25-year-old "Negro" from Collins, died on October 9th at the Magee General Hospital. (For details of this case, see Chapter 9.)

Robert A. Boutwell, a 27-year-old Masonite employee from Ellisville, died on October 10th at the Laurel General Hospital after taking several doses of Massengill's elixir, which was prescribed as treatment for protracted gonorrhea.

Walter Bell, an 11-year-old "colored" boy from Benton, died on October 11th (presumably at his home) after taking nearly two ounces of Elixir Sulfanilamide. The treatment was prescribed for an "abscessed throat."

William Corneel Howell, a 38-year-old "colored" man from New Albany, died at the town's Mayes Hospital on October 14th. He consumed probably three ounces of Elixir Sulfanilamide, which was sold over the counter as a remedy for gonorrhea.

Mrs. Henry (Katie or Katy) Stuckey (née Meadows), a 39-year-old farmer's wife and mother from Collins, died on October 14th at the Magee General Hospital. (For details of this case, see Chapter 9.)

Steve Demus, a 25-year-old married "colored" man from Bentonia, died on October 15th at Vicksburg's Charity Hospital. He drank nearly four ounces of Elixir Sulfanilamide, which was prescribed as treatment for gonorrhea.

Mrs. Gussie Mae (or Jessie May) Grubbs, a 22-year-old "colored" woman from Mt. Olive, died on October 15th at the Magee General Hospital. She took three ounces of Elixir Sulfanilamide, which was intended as treatment for "severe pyelitis and cystitis."

Edie (or Eddie) Sullivan, a 49-year-old farmer from Mize, died on October 17th at the Magee General Hospital. He drank about two and one-half ounces of Elixir Sulfanilamide, which was prescribed as treatment for a "large carbuncle" on the back of his neck.

Otis Coulter, a 36-year-old farmer from Mt. Olive, died on October 19th at the Magee General Hospital. He consumed a little more than four ounces of Elixir Sulfanilamide, which was prescribed as treatment for gonorrhea.

James Monroe Vick, a 53-year-old Masonite employee from Ellisville, died on October 20th in hospital. He drank an unknown quantity of Elixir Sulfanilamide, which was prescribed as treatment for a chronic prostate infection.

Mrs. J(ulius) E(dmond) (Nola) Penn (née Derrick), a 62-year-old farmer's wife, died on October 20th at the Magee General Hospital. The woman drank two and one-half ounces of Elixir Sulfanilamide, which was prescribed as treatment for pyelitis (a kidney infection).

Lorene (or Lorece) Lewis, a seven-year-old "colored" girl from a "plantation" about 14 miles from Philadelphia, died on October 20th at home. She consumed an unknown quantity of a four-ounce prescription for Elixir Sulfanilamide, which was intended as treatment for an incised and drained inguinal abscess.

Emmett (or Eva or Era) Pickens, a 21-year-old "colored" man from Laurel, died on or about October 21st at an undescribed location. He consumed about one ounce of Elixir Sulfanilamide, which was prescribed as treatment for gonorrhea.

Jerry Gordon Strickland, a 33-month-old boy from Burnsville, died on October 22nd at Corinth Hospital after drinking less than two ounces of Elixir Sulfanilamide. The drug was prescribed as treatment for suspected streptococcal pharyngitis.

Sallie Louise Brown, a seven-year-old "colored" girl from Benton, died on October 24th, presumably at home, after taking two-thirds of an ounce of Massengill's elixir. The liquid antibiotic was prescribed as treatment for a streptococcal sore throat and "acute tonsillitis."

Possible

Elnora (Mrs. Robert) Perkins, a 46-year-old farmer and farmer's wife from Itta Bena, died on October 1st at the Colored King's Daughters

Hospital in Greenville. She consumed three ounces of Elixir Sulfanilamide, which was prescribed as treatment for a "pelvic infection."

Julia Brown, a 67-year-old woman from Weathersby, died on October 12th. She consumed four doses of Elixir Sulfanilamide, which was prescribed as a remedy for pyelitis (a kidney infection).

Unlikely

John W. Gibbons, a 71-year-old farmer from Mt. Olive, died on October 9th at the Baptist Hospital in Jackson. (For details of this case, see Chapters 9 and 16.)

North Carolina (two confirmed, one probable)

From the FDA's initial canvass in North Carolina, beginning on October 21st, the agency learned that more than four gallons of elixir remained at large, much of it concentrated within the Rocky Mount area. After persistent investigation, which extended into December of 1937, the FDA discovered at least three elixir-related deaths in the state.

Charles "Charlie" Richardson, a 24-year-old "negro" farmer from Nashville, died on October 17th at the Rocky Mount Sanitarium. He took approximately four ounces of Elixir Sulfanilamide, which was prescribed as a treatment for gonorrhea.

John Thomas Tanner, a 59-year-old logger from Rocky Mount, died on October 31st at the town's Park View Hospital. He consumed four ounces of Elixir Sulfanilamide, which was prescribed as treatment for "chronic gonorrhea."

Probable

Master Billy Lee Lindsey, a three-year-old boy from Nashville, died on October 23rd at the Park View Hospital in Rocky Mount. The child consumed an unknown quantity of Elixir Sulfanilamide, which was prescribed as treatment for streptococcal pharyngitis.

Ohio (one confirmed)

For a description of Ohio's lone death due to Elixir Sulfanilamide-- that of six-year-old *Jo Anne Cramer*—see Chapter 10.

Oklahoma (11 confirmed)

Although the first deaths due to Elixir Sulfanilamide did not occur in Oklahoma, elixir-related fatalities there were the first to be recognized on a national scale—thanks to the early-warning efforts of Tulsa physicians. The FDA ultimately determined that Elixir Sulfanilamide caused the deaths of 11 Oklahomans, including eight children.

Robert "Bobbie" Sumner (or Summer), a two-year-old boy from Leonard, died on September 30th at his aunt's home in Tulsa. (See Chapter 1 for a description of this case.)

Mary Earline Watters, an 11-month-old girl from Tulsa, died on October 1st at the city's St. John's Hospital. (See Chapter 1 for a description of this case.)

John "Jack" King, Jr., an eight-year-old boy from Tulsa, died on October 1st at the city's St. John's Hospital. (See Chapter 1 for a description of this case.)

Millard Wesley "Sonny" Wakeford, a five-year-old boy from Tulsa, died on October 4th at Tulsa's St. John's Hospital. (See Chapter 1 for a description of this case.)

Joan Marlar, a six-year-old girl from Tulsa, died on October 5th at the city's Morningside Hospital. (See Chapter 1 for a description of this case, and Chapter 7 for an account of the FDA's investigation of it.)

Michael S. Sheehan, a six-year-old boy from Tulsa, died on October 6th at the city's St. John's Hospital. (See Chapter 1 for a description of this case.)

Kathleen Estelle Hobson, an eight-year-old girl from Red Fork, died on October 9th at Tulsa's Morningside Hospital. (See Chapter 1 for a description of this case.)

Glen(n) F(rederick) Entler, 19, of Tuscola, Illinois, died on October 9th in Tulsa while visiting his aunt and uncle. (See Chapter 3 for a description of this case.)

Charlene Mardell Canady, a four-year-old girl from Tulsa, died on October 12th at the city's St. John's Hospital. She consumed two ounces of Elixir Sulfanilamide, which was prescribed for presumptive streptococcal pharyngitis.

Earl Lee Beard, a 25-year-old air-conditioning engineer from Tulsa, died on October 16th at an unnamed city hospital. He consumed five ounces of Elixir Sulfanilamide, which was prescribed as treatment for gonorrhea. (For a description of the related civil case against Massengill and its outcome, see Chapter 16.)

Wilmer L. Morris, a 22-year-old man from Osage, died on October 27th at St. John's Hospital in Tulsa. Morris drank about two and one-half ounces of Elixir Sulfanilamide, which was prescribed as treatment for gonorrhea.

South Carolina (nine confirmed)

In South Carolina, the FDA quickly learned that most of the distributed commercial packages of Elixir Sulfanilamide, eight-and-a-half of 11 gallons, had not been returned intact to Massengill headquarters in Bristol, Tennessee. A total of 19 prescriptions were ultimately discovered in the state, nine of which resulted in death.

Oscar Chisolm, a 26-month-old "colored" boy, died on September 30th at the Roper Hospital in Charleston after consuming an unknown quantity of a two-ounce prescription for Elixir Sulfanilamide. The elixir was intended as a remedy for a sore throat.

Ella Blanche Washington, a three-year-old "colored" girl, also died on September 30th at the Roper Hospital in Charleston. The amount of Elixir Sulfanilamide consumed by the toddler (from a three-ounce prescription) was never determined, and the reason for treatment was not described by the FDA.

Pearl Locklair (née Miles), a wife, mother, and 37-year-old "colored" domestic worker for a private family, died on October 4th at the Roper Hospital in Charleston after consuming an unknown quantity of a six-ounce prescription for Elixir Sulfanilamide. The antibiotic solution was intended to treat a "retropharyngeal abscess or tumor." (For a description of the related civil case against Massengill and its outcome, see Chapter 16.)

Susie Mae DeLoach, a 16-year-old farmer's daughter from Brunson, died on October 7th. She consumed about two ounces of Elixir Sulfanilamide, which was prescribed for a posttraumatic skin infection on her leg.

James Stewart, a 10-year-old "colored" boy from Union Heights, died on October 12th at the Roper Hospital in Charleston. He received a four-ounce prescription for Elixir Sulfanilamide as treatment for a sore throat.

Ward St. John O'Brien, a 38-year-old married "negro" cook from Charleston, died on October 13th at the city's Hospital and Training School. He consumed four ounces of Elixir Sulfanilamide, which was prescribed for an undescribed ailment.

Harry M. Terry, a 34-year-old laborer from Estill, died on October 14th. He drank a total of three ounces of Elixir Sulfanilamide, which was intended as a remedy for gonorrhea.

John McDaniel (or J. J. McDanil), a 35-year-old "colored" lumber mill worker from Luray or Ellenton, died on October 14th at the Cohen's Bluff Camp of the Hendrix Lumber Mill in Estill. (For details of this case and its investigation, see Chapter 11.)

Willie Badger, a 25-year-old laborer from Scotia, died on October 18th. (For details of the FDA's investigation of this death, see Chapter 11.)

Tennessee (six confirmed, one unlikely)

The government's investigation of elixir shipments throughout Tennessee, Massengill's home state, was coordinated out of the FDA's station in Cincinnati, Ohio. The inspector assigned to the job, Ohio native Carl Stone McKellogg, 43, was sent to determine the whereabouts of more than 16 gallons of Elixir Sulfanilamide, which had been shipped directly from Massengill's headquarters in Bristol throughout The Volunteer State. Although these shipments were not interstate and therefore not strictly a federal matter, the FDA nevertheless assumed the authority and responsibility to pick up outstanding bottles of the deadly product.

Among these elixir shipments, the FDA discovered that less than one-third had been returned intact to Bristol (presumably as a result of Massengill's recall telegrams). This left more than 11 gallons at large within Tennessee. The confirmed death count due to Elixir Sulfanilamide in the state, from 21 prescriptions or over-the-counter purchases, came to six and included the deaths of two individuals who had received their elixir treatments in Mississippi.

Horace N. Williams, a 25-year-old road construction worker from Sevierville, died on October 12th at St. Mary's Hospital in Knoxville. He drank most of a two-ounce supply of Massengill's elixir, which was prescribed for symptoms of gonorrhea.

William E. Kyte, a 38-year-old married "colored" butcher from the Bearden neighborhood of Knoxville, died on October 17th at Knoxville General Hospital. Kyte drank four ounces of Elixir Sulfanilamide, which was prescribed as treatment for chronic gonorrhea.

Columbus Bryant, a 34-year-old "colored" road worker (or "concrete finisher") from Memphis, died on October 17th at the city's John Gaston Hospital, an inpatient facility for African Americans. Bryant drank four ounces of Elixir Sulfanilamide, which was prescribed in Mississippi as a remedy for gonorrhea.

C(harles) W(illiam) Miller, a 25-year-old filling-station attendant from Memphis, died on October 20th at the city's Methodist Hospital. Miller consumed about four ounces of Elixir Sulfanilamide, which was purchased over the counter and intended as self-treatment for gonorrhea.

Reverend James Edward Byrd, a 65-year-old Baptist preacher from Mt. Olive, Mississippi, died in the early morning hours of October 21st at St. Mary's Hospital in Knoxville. (For details of this death, see Chapters 8 and 9.)

Charles "Charlie" Alexander Meredith, Jr., a 17-year-old "colored" student from Cleveland, died on October 24th at the Physicians and Surgeons Hospital in the piedmont community. The teenager consumed less than two ounces of Elixir Sulfanilamide, which was prescribed for a suspected streptococcal infection.

Unlikely

"Baby" Thompson, an infant of about one year of age from Jacksboro, died on October 9th. The child probably consumed about one teaspoon of a two-ounce prescription for Elixir Sulfanilamide, which was intended as treatment for "an advanced stage of erysipelas."

Texas (seven confirmed, two possible, one unlikely)

The FDA's search for outstanding lots of Elixir Sulfanilamide and related deaths in Texas extended well into 1938. Among 34 known prescriptions, 10 deaths were identified; although at least one of these deaths was not convincingly linked to the elixir.

Johnnie (or Johnie) Fay Kay, a 12-year-old girl from Hemphill, died on October 4th after taking about three ounces of Elixir Sulfanilamide, which was prescribed for an unspecified illness.

William Taft Parker, a 27-year-old married "tool dresser" for an oil company, died on October 10th at the Bethania Hospital in Wichita Falls. He consumed about three and one-half ounces of Elixir Sulfanilamide, which was prescribed as treatment for gonorrhea.

Robert Montgomery Goode, a 29-year-old married fishing pier operator from Texas City, died on October 9th at the John Sealy Hospital in Galveston. (For details of this case, see Chapter 10.)

Levi (or Levy) Kelly, a 19-year-old married "colored" farmer from Highbank, died on October 12th. Kelly probably drank his entire four-ounce supply of Elixir Sulfanilamide, which was prescribed as treatment for gonorrhea.

Alberta Yvonne Howell, a two-year-old girl from Hatchel, died on October 13th at the Halley-Love Sanitarium in nearby Ballinger. She probably drank one ounce of a two-ounce prescription for Elixir Sulfanilamide, which was intended to cure an "infected throat."

Lois Jean Wilkins (or Wilkinson), a four-year-old girl from Centerville, died on October 18th. She consumed about two ounces of Elixir Sulfanilamide, which was prescribed for an "inflamed" throat.

Mollie May Schmittou, an 18-year-old student at the East Texas State Teachers College in Commerce, died on October 20th. She took about three ounces of Elixir Sulfanilamide, which was dispensed on prescription as a treatment for "boils."

Possible

Lillie Maurye Howard, a five-year-old girl from Goree, died on October 6th after drinking about two ounces of Elixir Sulfanilamide, which was prescribed for a streptococcal infection of the throat.

Margrita Rosas, a seven-month-old girl living near Tahoka, died at the Mercy Hospital in Slaton on October 7th. The infant received a one-ounce prescription for Elixir Sulfanilamide for "apparent meningitis symptoms with slight middle ear disturbance and respiratory embarrassment." The FDA estimated that the baby consumed about one-half ounce of Massengill's elixir.

Unlikely

Mrs. C(larence) D. Hammock (probably Eleanor, née Gates), a 23-year-old housewife and mother from Hemphill, died on October 14th at the Memorial Hospital in Nacogdoches. The woman consumed an unknown quantity of Elixir Sulfanilamide, which was likely prescribed as treatment for a postpartum infection.

Virginia and West Virginia (two confirmed, two probable)

The government's investigation of Massengill's elixir in Virginia and West Virginia was coordinated out of the FDA's Baltimore Station. From this hub, FDA veteran Frank Wollard assigned three inspectors, McKay McKinnon, Jr., Louis Leahy Judge, and James C. Pearson, to retrieve outstanding lots within the combined territory of 67,000 square miles. The FDA's efforts were complemented by several Virginia state health officials and, in West Virginia, by 24-year-old Joseph E. Settle, Jr., from the state health department. Their search, including the retrieval of any bottles secreted within the coal-rich Allegheny Mountains along the states' common border, prompted an investigation of 10 prescriptions in Virginia and eight in West Virginia.

During the government's extended investigation of Dr. Dibrel Crowder Mayes, of Church Road, Virginia, who had received seven pints of Elixir Sulfanilamide, Inspector Pearson learned of two deaths that were deliberately concealed by the doctor. Likewise in West Virginia, persistent efforts by the FDA led to the discovery of two deaths among the patients of an African-American physician in Beckley, Dr. Robert J. Howard, who initially refused to name his vulnerable clients.

Martha "Bettie" Agnes Cairns (née Green), a 24-year-old farmer's wife and mother, died at the Petersburg Hospital in Petersburg, Virginia, on October 7th. She took about four ounces of Massengill's elixir, which was prescribed as a remedy for gonorrhea.

Robert Harrison Mayes, a seven-year-old boy from Church Road, Virginia, died on October 17th at the Petersburg Hospital. He drank three ounces of Elixir Sulfanilamide, which was prescribed as treatment for a "typical streptococcus sore throat."

William Irvin (or Irvine), a 17-year-old "colored" student from Beckley, West Virginia, died at the Beckley Hospital on October 11th. The teenager consumed about one ounce of a three-ounce prescription for Elixir Sulfanilamide, which was possibly intended as treatment for gonorrhea.

Jonathan Walter Lyons, a 35-year-old married coal miner from Beckley, West Virginia, died at the Beckley Hospital on October 18th. Lyons drank an unknown quantity of Elixir Sulfanilamide, which was prescribed as treatment for presumptive gonorrhea.

APPENDIX B:
ELIXIR DISTRIBUTION BY STATE

The Confiscation Roundup and Final Assessment

Distribution of Commercial Packages

Nearly 160 gallons of Elixir Sulfanilamide—the majority of which were shipped in pint bottles—were distributed by The S. E. Massengill Company to 620 commercial recipients in 31 states and Puerto Rico.[1] The elixir was shipped as far north as Harvey, North Dakota, and as far south as San Juan, Puerto Rico, and from coast to coast (see the FDA's historical map [p 141]). However, shipments were disproportionately high in Texas and the Southeast (specifically Georgia, Alabama, and Mississippi), and the number of direct commercial recipients in a state correlated roughly with the total amount of elixir received in that state. For instance, Georgia received more than 21 gallons of the antibiotic solution, which was directly shipped in individual packages to at least 83 sites, and Alabama received nearly 16 gallons, which were distributed among 78 sites. The number of prescriptions in each state was also roughly proportional to the number of commercial recipients and the volume distributed; however, elixir prescriptions were also dependent on the peculiar readiness of some enthusiastic and trusting physicians—like Dr. Archie Calhoun of Mt. Olive, Mississippi, and Dr. Henri H. Weathers of East St. Louis, Illinois—to write large numbers of prescriptions for the untested product.

Table. Elixir Sulfanilamide Distribution, Consumption, and Death Tally by State

State	Direct Recipients of Commercial Packages	Total Amount (Gallons) Shipped Directly Into State	Known Exposures Through Prescriptions, OTC Sales, or Samples	Deaths (Confirmed, Probable, or Possible)
Mississippi	42	13	70	24[a]
Georgia	83	21.375	29	13
Alabama	78	15.75	46	11[b]
Oklahoma	18	6.625	40	11
Texas	100	17	35	9
Illinois/Missouri	47	11.125	67	9
South Carolina	12	11	19	9
Tennessee	43	16.25	21	6
North Carolina	24	14.25	19	3
Florida	18	2.375	5	3
Virginia	12	5.125	11	2
West Virginia	13	1.75	7	2
California	16	3.875	5	1
Ohio	15	2.125	3	1
Arkansas	3	0.375	3	1
Indiana	25	4.5	8	0
Michigan	17	3.25	1	0

Kentucky	14	2.375	2	0
Louisiana	13	1.75	6	0
Pennsylvania	7	1.5	–	0
Maryland	3	0.75	1	0
Puerto Rico	1	0.75	0	0
Minnesota	3	0.375	0	0
North Dakota	2	0.375	1	0
Colorado	1	0.25	–	0
Iowa	2	0.25	0	0
Kansas	2	0.25	0	0
New York	2	0.25	–	0
Oregon	1	0.25	–	0
Wisconsin	2	0.25	0	0
Connecticut	1	0.125	–	0
	620	159.25	399	105

OTC = over the counter.
a. Excludes two deaths that occurred in Tennessee (Bryant and Byrd).
b. Excludes one death that occurred in Georgia (Daughtrey).
N.B.—Commercial recipients were drug wholesalers, retail pharmacies, doctors' offices, and hospitals. The amount of elixir directly shipped (column 3) does not account for distributed sample vials. Among the 399 recorded exposures, eight (2.0%) were OTC purchases (one in Alabama, three in Georgia, one in Mississippi, and three in Tennessee); five OTC purchases resulted in death (Bolton, Durden, and Portwood in Georgia; Howell in Mississippi; and Miller in Tennessee). At least nine samples were dispensed; two resulted in death (Singleton in Alabama and Cramer in Ohio). Prescription data for New York, Pennsylvania, Connecticut, Colorado, and Oregon were not available in acquired FDA records; but no prescriptions were likely written in these states, given the relatively small volume of elixir distributed and the absence of state-specific prescription data in FDA accounts.

FDA's Seizure of Commercial Packages and Samples

In the end, FDA officials calculated that 11 gallons and six pints of Massengill's elixir had been dispensed as prescriptions or sold over the counter, and that about one half of this volume had been consumed.[2] (Massengill claimed that only five gallons and one pint had been dispensed as prescriptions or otherwise sold to individuals.)[3] The remainder was taken, in some cases literally, out of the hands of consumers by FDA agents. During the last months of 1937, the FDA managed to pick up, destroy, or otherwise account for 228 gallons and 2 pints of elixir from the 240 gallons that had been produced.[4] (According to the Massengill company, 1,879 pints [nearly 235 gallons] were "found" and returned.) But clearly some elixir recipients or their legal representatives were allowed to retain partially filled bottles, ostensibly for use in civil litigation against Massengill.

APPENDIX C: RACIAL BREAKDOWN OF ELIXIR SULFANILAMIDE VICTIMS

Were African Americans Targeted for Use of Elixir Sulfanilamide?

In his comprehensive book on the history of the FDA, *Reputation and Power*, Daniel Carpenter writes that use of Massengill's elixir "appears to have been disproportionately common among African Americans,"[1] implying that elixir prescriptions to African Americans were disproportionately high and/or that African Americans were particularly susceptible to the toxicity of diethylene glycol. Among the adult victims, Carpenter calculates that 54% were African American; among pediatric victims, 56% were African American. Carpenter's calculations rely on the incomplete recording of race in FDA records, of which he claims, "[O]f the records from 72 cases that remain in FDA archives, 57 can be identified by race. Of these 57, 31 (54 percent) were identified as African Americans."[2]

These calculations are presented within Carpenter's discussion of a longstanding misconception, specifically among white Americans in the early 20th century, that venereal disease (for which Elixir Sulfanilamide was often prescribed) is a peculiar ailment of black males. Carpenter writes, "The link between Elixir Sulfanilamide, syphilis, and blackness was one established in myth," and "[T]his subtle link greatly empowered the rumors and reduced the vitality and visibility of the sufferers."[3] Carpenter's point about the nexus between African Americans, venereal disease, and Elixir Sulfanilamide is otherwise murky, but his loaded implication—particularly when he alludes to the Tuskegee Syphilis Study in a footnote—is this: Physicians in 1937, meaning predominantly white physicians, consciously or unconsciously used African Americans as real-world test subjects for Elixir Sulfanilamide. Such a potentially explosive implication (or perhaps merely a loaded inference on my part) demands further examination and merits defusing.

A more in-depth and detailed assessment of the Elixir Sulfanilamide victims here, drawing on FDA, NARA, census, and death records, enables the determination of the race or ethnicity of all 105 confirmed, probable, or possible victims with reasonable certainty. These calculations, based on the complete data, provide somewhat lower percentages for African Americans among the Elixir Sulfanilamide victims: 46 (44%) of the 105 were African American (African American being noted typically in contemporaneous records as "colored," "Negro," or "black"). Fourteen (30%) of these African Americans were 18 years of age or younger, thereby accounting for 36% of the 39 confirmed, probable, or possible pediatric victims of Elixir Sulfanilamide (Figure).

Figure. Racial Breakdown of Elixir Sulfanilamide Victims

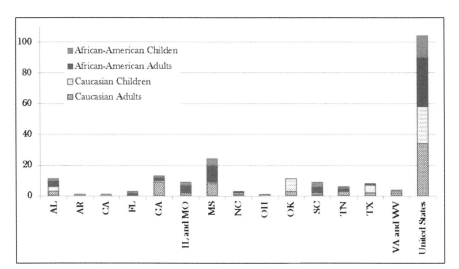

N.B.—One possible infant victim in Texas, not included graphically here, was Hispanic (Mexican), and an Oklahoma pediatric victim (included here as "Caucasian") was probably of mixed Native American heritage.

According to data from the US Census Bureau for 1930 and 1940, "blacks" made up 9.7% and 9.8%, respectively, of the US population. These national percentages were substantially lower than the percentage of African Americans (44%) among those who fell victim to Elixir Sulfanilamide. However, it cannot be determined with any certainty whether a disproportionate percentage of African Americans died of Elixir Sulfanilamide poisoning, without knowing the racial makeup of the individual communities where elixir shipments were distributed or, more specifically and more accurately, the racial makeup of the prescribing doctors' patient populations. The closest we can probably come to estimating these subpopulations is by examining contemporaneous census data for states. (Although conclusions to be drawn from this exercise are diluted owing to the smaller numbers of elixir victims within these subpopulations.)

In the 1940 census, the percentage of blacks in the South Atlantic and East South Central divisions, areas where shipments of Elixir Sulfanilamide were especially concentrated, was considerably higher than the national average: approximately 26%. In Alabama and Georgia—states with high numbers of deaths due to Massengill's elixir—blacks made up approximately 35% of the population. Among the elixir victims for each of these respective states, 45% (5/11) and 23% (3/13) were African American, and the average percentage of black victims for these states combined is 33% (8/24), which closely approximates the African-American makeup of the two states. Most notably in Mississippi, the state with the highest death toll overall and that for blacks specifically, African Americans made up about 50% of the population in 1930 and 1940. Among the state's 24 elixir-related casualties, 15 (62%) were African American. Among the 19 adult victims, 11 (58%) were African American. Consequently an examination of the racial makeup of state populations suggests that the regional percentage of African Americans was either roughly equivalent to or somewhat lower (but not dramatically lower) than the state-specific percentage of African Americans who died of Elixir Sulfanilamide poisoning (insofar as these generalizations can be made when dealing with relatively small numbers).

It should also be emphasized that white physicians were not the only physicians who prescribed Elixir Sulfanilamide. Despite the heavily white, paternalistic view we may have of healthcare delivery during the early part of the 20th century, it is, at least to some extent, a condescending one. Black physicians in the 1930s undoubtedly sustained substantial hardship during their segregated medical education and training; however, many prevailed and were important providers of healthcare, specifically to black populations of the era, including those African Americans who had the misfortune to consume Elixir Sulfanilamide. Among the high prescribers of Massengill's product were Dr. Henri H. Weathers, a prominent African-American surgeon of East St. Louis, and Dr. J. A. C. Jackson, a black physician in Charleston, South Carolina. Of the 46 African-American victims of Massengill's elixir, at least 43 received their treatment by means of prescription, and the race or ethnicity of the named prescribing physician in all 43 cases can be determined through FDA or census records or both. It can therefore be concluded that more than one-third of African-American victims (specifically 18 or 42%) received their prescriptions from African-American physicians. (All white victims who received prescriptions for Elixir Sulfanilamide, except one patient in West Virginia, received them from white physicians.) The point being: There is no evidence that white physicians preferentially prescribed Elixir Sulfanilamide to black patients, at least when considering the fatalities. And black physicians who prescribed Elixir Sulfanilamide prescribed the product for black patients, because their patient population was uniformly (or nearly so) black.

There is also no evidence that The S. E. Massengill Company or its
sales force made any concerted effort to promote Elixir Sulfanilamide to
African-American physicians and, by extension, to promote the
prescription of the product to African Americans. Specifically and bluntly,
there is no indication that Massengill was interested in testing his elixir on
the African-American population. On the contrary, Massengill's primary
transgression was that he wantonly distributed his untested product to the
largest possible consumer base—which, given his established distribution
network, included large chunks of the southeast and south-central United
States, which were heavily populated by African Americans. Like just
about every drug company executive, Massengill was primarily interested
in expansive drug sales and wanted his product prescribed and sold widely,
regardless of the color (or age or sex) of the consumer.

Were African Americans Unusually Susceptible to Elixir Sulfanilamide (Diethylene Glycol)?

A related question is whether African Americans were (or are) more
susceptible to the toxicity of diethylene glycol than whites. To begin to
answer this question, the racial makeup of all consumers of Elixir
Sulfanilamide would have to be determined, and these data would have to
be compared with the racial makeup of the fatalities. However, in FDA
and NARA records, the race or ethnicity of *surviving* consumers is
infrequently recorded, and an attempt to determine the race of these
survivors through census records is hindered by a number of factors—
particularly the inability to positively identify elixir consumers in the
available census records of 1930 and 1940 to determine their recorded
race. Given the current state of the publicly available records, the question
cannot be answered confidently. No scientific data produced in the
interim, meaning during the last 77 years, indicate that blacks are
peculiarly (eg, genetically) susceptible to the toxicity of diethylene glycol;
however, the absence of evidence on this point is, as it is often said, not
necessarily evidence of absence.

ENDNOTES

Frequently Cited Sources

FDA historical records: Correspondence and other FDA documents pertaining to Elixir Sulfanilamide are contained within the collection of the FDA's historical records, AF1258, at Rockville, MD. Information for locating and viewing these records can be found at the FDA website ("Research Tools on FDA History").

Jackson: Jackson CO. *Food and Drug Legislation in the New Deal*. Princeton, NJ: Princeton University Press; 1970.

NARA: FDA correspondence (c1937-1938) and other documents (eg, newspaper clippings) pertaining to Elixir Sulfanilamide are housed at the National Archives and Records Administration, Record Group (RG) 88, College Park, MD.

Pully, DeFriece: Pully P, DeFriece FW. *Masengill Brothers and Company and The S. E. Massengill Company, 1897-1971*. Knoxville, TN; Tennessee Valley Publishing; 1996.

Wallace report: Report from the Secretary of Agriculture, Henry A. Wallace to Congress, submitted November 25, 1937. *Elixir Sulfanilamide: Letter From the Secretary of Agriculture Transmitting in Response to Senate Resolution No. 194— A Report on Elixir Sulfanilamide-Massengill*. Washington, DC: Government Printing Office; 1937. Document no. 124.

Preface and Acknowledgements

1. Prescription antibiotic therapy, however, is not necessarily appropriate in these cases. For instance, Linder et al reported that the throat swabs of only 37% of children presenting with sore throat test positive for Group A streptococcus, the infectious cause of strep throat. Yet physicians prescribe antibiotics in about one-half of an estimated 7.3 million annual visits in the United States for sore throat. Linder JA, Bates DW, Lee GM, Finkelstein JA. Antibiotic treatment of children with sore throat. *JAMA*. 2005;294(18):2315-2322.
2. Young JH. Sulfanilamide and diethylene glycol. In: Parascandola J, Whorton JC, eds. *Chemistry and Modern Society: Historical Essays in Honor of Aaron J. Ihde*. Washington, DC: American Chemical Society; 1983: 105-125.
3. Email communication with direct descendants of Dr. Massengill suggests that this book represents the bulk, if not the entirety, of publicly accessible company records.
4. FDA Oral History Transcripts. Interview of Morris Fishbein by Charles O. Jackson, May 12, 1968. Available at http://www.fda.gov/AboutFDA/WhatWeDo/History/OralHistories. Last accessed August 12, 2013.

5. However, I was surprised to learn that most relatives with whom I communicated were unaware of the details of the elixir-related death in their family. Moreover many were ignorant of the national scope of the Elixir Sulfanilamide tragedy. Nevertheless the publication of *Elixir* may prompt other victims' relatives to investigate and reveal their family stories and thus add to the ongoing patchwork record.

Chapter 1: At Least Six Deaths in Tulsa

1. The telegraph text, written by an unidentified physician or physicians from Tulsa's Springer Clinic, is contained in "Correspondence and Items" from the American Medical Association's Council on Pharmacy and Chemistry. October 13, 1937 (NARA, Box 931, Folder 510-.20S). It is uncertain who drafted and sent the alerting dispatch, although Dr. Homer Ruprecht—a member-physician of the Springer Clinic—is a likely candidate.
2. Leech received a PhD from the Department of Chemistry at the University of Chicago in 1913.
3. Details of the Tulsa deaths are contained in an FDA investigative report from Kansas City Station Chief William H. Hartigan to the agency's Central District Chief. November 3, 1927 (FDA historical records). This information is supported by data from the Oklahoma death certificates of the victims.
4. *Streptococcus pyogenes* or Group A (beta-hemolytic) *Streptococcus* and specifically its toxin were established as the cause of scarlet fever in the early 1920s by the husband-and-wife team of George and Gladys Dick (The etiology of scarlet fever. *J Am Med Assoc.* 1924;82:301-302). The Tulsa nephrologist, 48-year-old Garabed A. Z. Garabedian, may have been aware of a recently published pathologic review of acute nephritis by E. T. Bell (The pathology and pathogenesis of clinical acute nephritis. *Am J Pathol.* 1937;13:497-552). The review described the clinical and pathologic findings of streptococcal nephritis. Specifically the interval between the onset of scarlet fever and nephritis, when it occurred, was observed to be usually between two and three weeks. In an odd turn of events, Garabedian died seven months later, on April 26, 1938, of a coronary thrombosis, which was curiously ascribed to a streptococcal pharyngitis. (Anonymous. Southern medical news. *South Med J.* 1938;31[9]:36).
5. For an account of the first successful hemodialysis in the United States, see Peitzman SJ. *Dropsy, Dialysis, Transplant: A Short History of Failing Kidneys.* Baltimore, MD: Johns Hopkins University Press; 2007: 82-87.
6. According to FDA records, the girl's mother also consumed some portion of the elixir (at "twice the dose") during the same time period, but the mother also "took large quantities of fluids, water, lemon juice, etc. This [...] was probably responsible for her suffering no ill effects." On the basis of the prescription's directions, the girl may have taken as much as three ounces of elixir; however, given the fact that she shared the prescription with her mother, it is likely that she consumed substantially less than three ounces.

7. The victim's mother could not state accurately how much of the elixir was consumed, because a nurse was employed to take care of the child during his illness.

8. According to Wakeford family history (obtained from email and telephone correspondence in 2009 with Onslow Stevenson Wakeford III and Karyn Tunks), both children shared a hospital room, and Millard's younger sister survived because she was asleep when the nurse entered the room to administer the elixir (suggesting that Elixir Sulfanilamide was continued in hospital despite the children's deteriorating clinical status). Family history also indicates that Sonny suffered with "encephalitis," a term that may have been used to describe what was actually uremic encephalopathy, an end-stage coma-inducing manifestation of kidney failure. An alternative explanation is a direct neurotoxic effect of the elixir. The children's father, local hockey star Millard "Sonny Boy" Wakeford was reportedly urged by the hospital staff to read to his children to keep them awake (and presumably from lapsing into coma). A 2009 email request to interview the surviving younger sister of Sonny, then 75 years of age, was refused.

9. A description of Joan Marlar's symptoms is contained in a letter written on November 8, 1937, by the girl's mother, Maise Nidiffer, to President Franklin D. Roosevelt. See Wallace report (p 8).

10. See letter from Perrin H. Long to Mr. Wollard (US Department of Agriculture). October 15, 1937 (NARA, Box 934, Eastern District sulfanilamide correspondence).

11. Letter from C. E. Halstead (of E. R. Squibb and Sons) to Charles L. Greenlee. November 5, 1937 (NARA, Box 934, Eastern District sulfanilamide correspondence); and Part I, Elixir Sulfanilamide Investigation. January 17, 1938 (NARA, Box 935, Central District Sulfanilamide Report). The representative from E. R. Squibb and Sons was identified as J. D. Nance of Tulsa.

12. For a contemporaneous case study of mercury poisoning, see Hull E, Lonte LA. Bichloride of mercury poisoning. *South Med J.* 1934;27:918-924.

13. Biographical data on Drs. Ivo A. Nelson and Homer A. Ruprecht were obtained from telephone interviews with Kathryn Brownfield (June 8, 2009) and Dick Ruprecht (August 24, 2009), respectively. Biographical data were also found in the *American Medical Dictionary, 14th ed* (Chicago, IL: AMA; 1936); Everett MR. *Medical Education in Oklahoma* (Norman: University of Oklahoma Press; 1972); and Leitner J. Leaders in medicine: Homer A. Ruprecht, MD. *J Okla State Med Assoc.* 1982;75:137-143.

14. For a description of the clinical course of Jack Voorhees after his consumption of Elixir Sulfanilamide, see court records for *Voorhees v Massengill.* National Archives Southeast Region, Atlanta, GA.

15. Telephone interview with Charlotte Cox, June 16, 2009.

16. Another important medical-investigative government agency, the Centers for Disease Control and Prevention (CDC), first known as the Communicable Disease Center, did not come into existence until 1946. See the CDC web site: About CDC, our story. Available at

http://www.cdc.gov/about/history/ourstory.htm. Last accessed August 12, 2013.

17. Biographical details for Morris Fishbein are derived from the relevant entry in the *National Cyclopaedia of American Biography*. New York, NY: James T. White and Company; 1930: 466. See also, Fishbein M. What I have learned in life. *Int Rec Med*. 1957;170:259-261.

18. Anonymous. Medicine: nationalized doctors? *Time*. June 21, 1937; 29(25):26,28,30.

19. Cushny AR, Diehl CL, Hallberg CSN, et al. AMA Council on Pharmacy and Chemistry. *Cal State J Med*. 1905;3:103-104. See also, Smith A. The Council on Pharmacy and Chemistry and the Chemical Laboratory. In: Fishbein M. *A History of the American Medical Association, 1847 to 1947*. Philadelphia, PA: W. B. Saunders; 1947: 865-886.

20. In 1888, the American Pharmaceutical Association began separately publishing its *National Formulary* on an irregular basis. Later the US Pharmacopeia acquired the *National Formulary*, and the compendia were published together, beginning in 1980. Annual revisions were not provided until 2002.

21. Anonymous. Synthetic drugs. *New York Times*. July 10, 1913 (p 6).

22. Anonymous. Sulfanilamide: a warning. *J Am Med Assoc*. 1937;109:1128. Although sulfanilamide was largely dispensed by means of prescription in the United States, there were apparently no laws in 1937 that prevented pharmacists from selling the drug directly to consumers, on request.

23. Kohn SE. Acute hemolytic anemia during treatment with sulfanilamide. *J Am Med Assoc*. 1937;109:1005-1006; Bucy PC. Toxic optic neuritis resulting from sulfanilamide. *J Am Med Assoc*. 1937;109:1007-1008; Menville JG, Archinard JJ. Skin eruptions in patients receiving sulfanilamide: report of four cases. *J Am Med Assoc*. 1937;109:1008-1009; Goodman MH, Levy CS. The development of a cutaneous eruption (toxicodermatosis): during the administration of sulfanilamide; report of two cases. *J Am Med Assoc*. 1937;109:1009-1011; Frank IJ. Dermatitis from sulfanilamide. *J Am Med Assoc*. 1937;109:1011-1012; Schonberg IL. Purpuric and scarlatiniform eruption following sulfanilamide. *J Am Med Assoc*. 1937;109:1035; Newman BA, Sharlit H. Sulfanilamide: a photosensitizing agent of the skin. *J Am Med Assoc*. 1937;109:1036-1037; Salvin M. Hypersensitivity to sulfanilamide. *J Am Med Assoc*. 1937;109:1038-1039.

24. Council on Pharmacy and Chemistry. Sulfanilamide and related compounds. *J Am Med Assoc*. 1937;108:1888-1890; Chemical Laboratory. Examination of certain American brands of sulfanilamide. *J Am Med Assoc*. 1937;109:358; and Council on Pharmacy and Chemistry. New and non-official remedies: sulfanilamide. *J Am Med Assoc*. 1937;109:358-359.

Chapter 2: The Best Thing Ever Discovered for Gonorrhea

1. Although the antibacterial properties of penicillin were discovered by Scotsman Alexander Fleming in 1928, several years before the systematic clinical study of sulfanilamide, human trials of penicillin did not gain steam

until the late 1930s, and mass production of the drug was not worked out until the mid-1940s. See for example, Lax E. *The Mold in Doctor Florey's Coat: The Story of the Penicillin Miracle.* New York, NY: Henry Holt and Company; 2004. For a much more detailed and nuanced history of sulfanilamide, see Lesch JE. Chemistry and biomedicine in an industrial setting. In: Mausfopf SH, ed. *Chemical Sciences in the Modern World.* Philadelphia: University of Pennsylvania Press; 1993: 159-215; and Lesch's comprehensive book, *The First Miracle Drugs: How the Sulfa Drugs Transformed Medicine.* New York, NY: Oxford University Press; 2007. Briefer chronologies are also provided by Long PH, Bliss EA. *The Clinical and Experimental Use of Sulfanilamide, Sulfapyridine and Allied Compounds.* New York, NY: The MacMillan Company; 1939: 1-13; and Dowling HF. *Fighting Infection: Conquests of the Twentieth Century.* Cambridge, Mass: Harvard University Press; 1977: 108-124.

2. For a history of the synthetic-dye industry and how it gave birth to and revolutionized the chemical industry in Western Europe, see Wilcock CC, Ashworth JL. *Whittaker's Dyeing With Coal-Tar Dyestuffs.* Princeton, NJ: D. Van Nostrand Company, Inc.; 1964; and Travis AS. *The Rainbow Makers: The Origins of the Synthetic Dyestuffs Industry in Western Europe.* Bethlehem, PA: Lehigh University Press; 1993.

3. Short for *Interessen-Gemeinschaft Farbenindustrie* (literally community in the interests of the dye industry). I. G. Farben was formed in 1925 in a mass-merger of several established German dye and chemical companies—namely, BASF [Badische Anilin und Soda Fabrik (Baden Aniline and Soda Factory)], Bayer, Höchst, AGFA [Aktiengesellschaft für Anilin-fabrication (Corporation for Aniline Fabrication)], and two other firms.

4. See Lesch JE. Chemistry and biomedicine in an industrial setting (endnote 1). For a discussion of Bayer's early history, see also Mann CC, Plummer ML. *The Aspirin Wars: Money, Medicine, and 100 Years of Rampant Competition.* New York, NY: Alfred A. Knopf; 1991: 15-31.

5. Lister's first use of carbolic acid, as a solution on wound dressings, was reported in March 1867 (On a new method of treating compound fracture, abscess, etc. *Lancet.* 1867;89:326-329).

6. In fact English chemistry whiz William Perkin, while attempting to produce an artificial quinine from the coal-tar derivative benzene, created instead the seminal dye aniline purple, or mauve, in 1856.

7. Which was to become, like Bayer, another subsidiary of I. G. Farben.

8. See for instance, Morgan GT. Synthetical drugs. *Sci Prog Twent Century.* 1908;2:572-588.

9. Cahn A, Hepp P. Antifebrin, a new antipyretic. *Am J Pharm.* 1886;58:565-567.

10. American Chemical Society. *The Pharmaceutical Century: Ten Decades of Drug Discovery.* Washington, DC: American Chemical Society; 2000. Bayer's later synthetic pharmaceutical triumphs—although not coal-tar derivatives—were the blockbusters acetylsalicylic acid (c1897), diacetylmorphine (c1898), and phenobarbital (c1902). The first two

compounds are better known by their respective Bayer trade names of Aspirin and Heroin.

11. See for instance, Bosch F, Rosich L. The contributions of Paul Ehrlich to pharmacology: a tribute on the occasion of the centenary of his Nobel Prize. *Pharmacology.* 2008;82:171-179.

12. Hörlein H. The chemotherapy of infectious diseases caused by protozoa and bacteria. *Proc Roy Soc Med.* 1935;29:313-324.

13. See for instance, Wilson LG. The early recognition of streptococci as causes of disease. *Med Hist.* 1987;31:403-414. Because the cocci resemble beaded necklaces under the microscope, German surgeon Theodor Billroth applied the moniker streptococcus—from the Greek words *streptos* and *kokkos*, meaning twisted chain and berry, respectively.

14. In the late 1920s and early 1930s, innovative American microbiologist Rebecca Lancefield established the cellular technology to type various species of streptococcal bacteria on the basis of their major surface antigens. Her methods enabled the confirmation of *S. pyogenes* (Lancefield Group A) as the causative agent of a wide variety of infectious diseases in humans. See for example, McCarty M. *Rebecca Craighill Lancefield, 1895-1981.* Washington DC: National Academy of Sciences; 1987: 227-246.

15. The Bayer chemists who created these azo dyes were Fritz Meitzsch and Joseph Klarer.

16. When selecting azo dyes for therapeutic examination, Domagk did not exclude substances without antibacterial effects in the laboratory. He had often witnessed the promising in vitro effects of compounds, only to be disappointed by their activity in systemic infections. Although lacking clear explanation, some distinction between the two bacterial environments was evident to the prescient Domagk, who did not dismiss the reverse situation: the apparent inactivity of a substance in culture and its activity in vivo.

17. Domagk G. Ein beitrag sur chemotherapie der bakteriellen infektionen. *Deutsche Medizinische Wochenschraft.* 1935;61:250-253. An English translation is available in Brock TD. *Milestones in Microbiology.* Englewood Cliffs, NJ: Prentice-Hall; 1961: 195-199. For his work with Prontosil, Domagk was awarded the Nobel Prize in Physiology or Medicine in 1939; however, he was prevented from accepting the prize at the time by the Nazi government. The coinventors (and patent holders) of Prontosil, chemists Fritz Meitzsch and Joseph Klarer, were passed over by the Nobel committee.

18. The author's Google-aided translation of, "Es wirkt wie ein echtes Chemotherapeutikum nur im lebenden Organismus."

19. Presented at the Association of Düsseldorf Dermatologists on May 17, 1933. See Foerster R. Sepsis im Anschluß an ausgedehnte periporitis: heilung durch streptozon. *Zentralblatt für Haut-und Geschlechtskrankheiten.* 1933;45:549-550. It was acknowledged in the printed report of the presentation that I. G. Farben recommended the drug for the treatment of streptococcal infections; however, in this case, the documented cause of sepsis was staphylococcus.

20. Domagk G. Chemotherapie der streptokokkeninfektionen. *Klinische Wochenschrift.* 1936;15:1585-1590. Cited in Lesch, *The First Miracle Drugs* (pp 105-106).

21. Klee P, Römer H. Prontosil bei Streptokokkenerkrankungen. *Deutsche Medizinische Wochenschraft.* 1935;61:253-255; Schreus HT. Chemotherapie des Erysipelas und anderer Infektionen mit Prontosil. *Deutsche Medizinische Wochenschraft.* 1935;61:255-256; and Anselm E. Unsere Erfahrungen mit Prontosil bei Puerperalfieber. *Deutsche Medizinische Wochenschraft.* 1935;61:264. All cited in Lesch, *The First Miracle Drugs* (pp 86-87).

22. See Long and Bliss, *The Clinical and Experimental Use of Sulfanilamide, Sulfapyridine and Allied Compounds* (pp 4-5); and Dowling, *Fighting Infection* (p 20).

23. For a detailed description of these experiments and their quick publication, see Lesch, *The First Miracle Drugs* (pp 126-130).

24. Tréfouël J, Tréfouël J, Nitti F, Bovet D. Activité due p-aminophénylsulfamide sur les infections streptococciques expérimentales de la souris et du lapin. *Biologie Comptes Rendus.* 1935;120:756-760.

25. Although Prontosil was a commercial success, at least initially. Sales of the drug shot up from 175,000 Marks (approximately $70,000 USD) in 1935 to 5 million Marks (approximately $2 million USD) in 1937. See Lesch, *The First Miracle Drugs* (p 104).

26. Gelmo P. Über sulfamide der p-amidobenzolsulfonsäure. *J Praktische Chemie.* 1908;77:369-382. See p 372 in this citation for a description of "sulfanilsäureamid" (German for sulfanilamide).

27. Bayer had actually obtained a patent on sulfanilamide soon after its creation by the Austrian chemist, Gelmo; however, Bayer's chemists, presumably oblivious to the compound's therapeutic potential, had only used sulfanilamide as an intermediate for the creation of synthetic dyes. English bacteriologist Ronald Hare—mistrusting German pharmaceutical development—later argued that Bayer's management, in fact, knew in 1932 that the no-longer-patented sulfanilamide was the active ingredient of Prontosil. Hare further posited that the intervening time between Domagk's initial experiments and his 1935 publication was consumed by the creation and testing of a patentable analog of sulfanilamide (that is, Prontosil). See for instance, Dowling, *Fighting Infection* (p 108). However, medical historian John Lesch contests Hare's argument. See Lesch, *The First Miracle Drugs* (pp 89-90).

28. Colebrook L, Kenny M. Treatment of human puerperal infections, and of experimental infections in mice, with Prontosil. *Lancet.* 1936;227:1279-1286. For a description of these studies, see Lesch, *The First Miracle Drugs* (pp 141-144).

29. Buttle GAH, Gray WH. Protection of mice against streptococcal and other infections by *p*-aminobenzenesulphonamide and related substances. *Lancet.* 1936;227:1286-1290.

30. Colebrook L, Kenny M. Treatment with Prontosil of puerperal infections. *Lancet.* 1936;228:1319-1322.

31. Colebrook L, Buttle GAH, O'Meara RAQ. The mode of action of p-aminobenzenesulphonamide and Prontosil in hæmolytic streptococcal infections. *Lancet.* 1936;228:1323-1326.
32. Foulis MA, Barr JB, Prontosil album in puerperal sepsis. *Br Med J.* 1937;1:445-446; Colebrook L, Purdie AW. Treatment of 106 cases of puerperal fever by sulphanilamide (streptocide). *Lancet.* 1937;230:1237-1242.
33. See Dowling, *Fighting Infection* (p 107). I. G. Farben's subsequent version of sulfanilamide was dubbed Prontosil album to denote its colorless (ie, white) nature and to distinguish it from the original Prontosil (aka Prontosil rubrum).
34. Long PH, Bliss EA. Para-amino-benzene-sulfonamide and its derivatives. *J Am Med Assoc.* 1937;108:32-37.
35. In addition, a pharmacologist at Hopkins, E. K. Marshall, Jr., fastidiously dissected the pharmacokinetics of sulfanilamide and provided a method for assaying the substance in blood and urine. His work was instrumental for calculating the optimum dosages for human treatment. See Marshall EK, Emerson K, Cutting WC. Para-aminobenzenesulfonamide: absorption and excretion—method of determination in urine and blood. *J Am Med Assoc.* 1937;108:953-957.
36. Associated Press. F D Roosevelt Jr is in Boston hospital. *New York Times.* November 27, 1936 (p 2); Associated Press. Sinus attack calls mother to bedside. *New York Times.* November 27, 1936 (p 2); Associated Press. Young Roosevelt better. *New York Times.* November 28, 1936 (p 5); Associated Press. Mrs Roosevelt visits ill son. *New York Times.* December 11, 1936 (p 29); Associated Press. Roosevelt operation delayed till Monday. *New York Times.* December 12, 1936 (p 12); Anonymous. Young Roosevelt better. *New York Times.* December 13, 1936 (p 24); Associated Press. President's son still ill. *New York Times.* December 14, 1936 (p 17); Anonymous. Franklin D Jr improving. *New York Times.* December 15, 1936 (p 27); Anonymous. Young Roosevelt saved by new drug. *New York Times.* December 17, 1936 (p 1). According to news reports, FDR, Jr., received Prontylin, Winthrop Chemical's brand-name version of sulfanilamide.
37. Anonymous. Medicine: Prontosil. *Time.* December 28, 1936;28(26):21.
38. Anonymous. Medicine: Prontylin for gonorrhea. *Time.* May 17, 1937; 29(20):63-64.
39. See for example, Squire PW. *Squire's Companion to the Latest Edition of the British Pharmacopoeia, 18th ed.* London, England: J. A. Churchill; 1908: 462; Hoffman E. The routine treatment of gonorrhoea and syphilis. *Br J Vener Dis.* 1926;2:231-234; and Harrison LW. The routine management of syphilis and gonorrhœa employed in the St. Thomas's Hospital Venereal Diseases Department. *Br J Vener Dis.* 1926;2:19-35.
40. Osler W, McCrae T. *The Principles and Practice of Medicine, 9th ed.* New York, NY: D. Appleton and Company; 1921: 125-128.
41. Dees JE, Colston JAC. The use of sulfanilamide in gonococcic infections. *J Am Med Assoc.* 1937:108:1854-1858. In a footnote, the authors noted that

they had treated an additional 28 cases, for a total of 47 cases. In 36 of these cases (77%), "the gonococci and the urethral discharge disappeared in less than five days."

42. Anonymous. The limitations of sulfanilamide. *Drug Cosmet Ind.* 1937;41:37. The notice also warned of "trouble" as use of the antibiotic exploded, including use of over-the-counter treatments.

43. Advertisement for Prontylin and Prontosil by the Winthrop Chemical Company. *S Med J.* 1937;30:33. Winthrop was the US subsidiary of I. G. Farben.

44. Prontosil 2.5% aqueous solution for intramuscular injection was sold in the United States by Winthrop Chemical. The compound, disodium 4-sulphamido-phenyl-2-azo-7-acetyl-amino-1-hydroxynaphthalene 3,6-disulphonate, was soluble in water to a solution of about 4%. Sulfanilamide was known to be less soluble in water, to a solution of only about 1%. See Long PH, Bliss EA. The use of para amino benzene sulphonamide (sulfanilamide) or its derivatives in the treatment of infections due to beta hemolytic streptococci, pneumococci, and meningococci. *S Med J.* 1937;30:479-487.

45. Council on Pharmacy and Chemistry. Sulfanilamide and related compounds. *J Am Med Assoc.* 1937:108:1888-1890.

Chapter 3: Something Is Wrong With the Elixir

1. Council on Pharmacy and Chemistry. Correspondence and items. October 13, 1937 (NARA, Box 931, Folder 510-.20S). The separate dispatches of Drs. Ruprecht and Childs were dated October 11, 1937.

2. Root T. Frantic fight on death is heart-breaking job. *Kansas City Journal-Post.* October 31, 1937 (NARA, Box 933, sulfanilamide clippings); Tulsa County Medical Society. Meeting notes. October 11, 1937. Dr. Underwood prescribed the elixir on September 24th (for Bobbie Sumner), September 25th (for Mary Earline Watters), September 26th (for the Wakeford children), and October 4th (for Charlene Canady). Two other elixir-prescribing doctors were also present at the society meeting: Dr. Childs and Dr. William Turnbow, who prescribed the elixir for Kathleen Hobson.

3. Nelson described the non-protein nitrogen, or NPN, level as an indicator of uremia and renal insufficiency. This terminology was supplanted by the blood urea nitrogen (BUN) level in the mid-20th century. See Dunea G, Freedman P. The nonprotein nitrogen level of the blood in renal disease. *JAMA.* 1968;203:1125-1126.

4. See for instance, Bell ET. Nephritis and nephrosis. *Cal West Med.* 1931;34:393-395.

5. Anonymous. Probe started in deaths of Tulsa children. *Tulsa Tribune.* October 15, 1937 (p 1, col 6).

6. von Oettingen WF, Jirouch EA. The pharmacology of ethylene glycol and some of its derivatives in relation to their chemical constitution and physical chemical properties. *J Pharmacol Exper Ther.* 1931;42:355-372.

7. Hansen K. Äthylenglykol vergiftung. *Samml Vergiftungsf.* 1930;1:A175; Anonymous. Possible death from drinking ethylene glycol ("Prestone"). *J Am Med Assoc.* 1930;94:1940. Both are cited and described in von Oettingen and Jirouch (p 356).
8. Ruprecht HA, Nelson IA. Clinical and pathologic observations. *J Am Med Assoc.* 1937;109:1537.
9. Anonymous. New deaths spur inquiry: four die in Illinois; Tulsa boy recovering. *Tulsa Tribune.* October 19, 1937 (p 1, col 2; p 4, col 7).
10. de Navasquez S. Experimental tubular necrosis of the kidneys accompanied by liver changes due to dioxan poisoning. *J Hyg (Lond).* 1935;35:540-548.

Chapter 4: Return Our Expense

1. Deaths due to Elixir of Sulfanilamide-Massengill: report of Secretary of Agriculture submitted in response to House Resolution 352 of Nov 18, 1937, and Senate Resolution 194 of Nov 16, 1937. *J Am Med Assoc.* 1937;109:1985-1988. In a footnote to the notice, on p 1985, it was revealed that the AMA had also telegraphed the FDA on October 14, 1937, about the presence of diethylene glycol in Massengill's product.
2. Letter from Perrin H. Long to Mr. Wollard (US Department of Agriculture). October 15, 1937 (NARA, Box 934, Eastern District sulfanilamide correspondence). On the basis of Dr. Long's letter and correspondence from E. R. Squibb and Sons to the FDA (dated November 5, 1937), Long's friend was most likely J. D. Nance, Squibb's representative in Tulsa.
3. Associated Press. Drug preparation blamed in deaths. *New York Times.* October 19, 1937 (p 27, col 2). See also, Anonymous. Deaths following Elixir of Sulfanilamide-Massengill. *J Am Med Assoc.* 1937;109:1367.
4. In 1933, a *JAMA* editorial praised dinitrophenol, stating that the weight-loss drug possessed the "remarkable power of stimulating metabolism enormously, producing pyrexia [fever], and without such deleterious symptoms as would result from equivalent doses of thyroid gland." But the commentary also advised, "A drug with the potency and effects of dinitrophenol is a two-edged sword with appalling possibilities for harm as well as for good" (Anonymous. Dinitrophenol, a metabolic stimulant. *J Am Med Assoc.1933;*101:213-214). By July of 1937, Fishbein was alerting his newspaper readers, "So much harm was done to people who endeavored to reduce their weight with dinitrophenol," and that the drug was "exceedingly dangerous" (Fishbein M. Choose diets on advice of your doctor. *Pittsburgh Press.* July 6, 1937 [p 22, col 8]).
5. Associated Press. Drug preparation blamed in deaths. *New York Times.* October 19, 1937 (p 27, col 2).
6. AMA Chemical Laboratory. Elixir Sulfanilamide-Massengill: Part I—Introduction. *J Am Med Assoc.* 1937;109:1531; Anonymous. Deaths due to Elixir of Sulfanilamide-Massengill. *J Am Med Assoc.* 1937;109:1367; and Schoeffel EW, Kreider HR, Peterson JB. Part II: chemical examination of Elixir of Sulfanilamide-Massengill. *J Am Med Assoc.* 1937;109:1532.

7. Root T. Frantic fight on death is heart-breaking job. *Kansas City Journal-Post.* October 31, 1937 (NARA, Box 933, sulfanilamide clippings).

8. Telegram from J. O. Clarke to FDA, Washington, DC. October 16, 1937 (NARA, Box 935, Central District sulfanilamide correspondence).

9. Anonymous. Probe started in death of Tulsa children. *Tulsa Tribune.* October 15, 1937 (p 1, col 6).

10. Anonymous. Death answer may be late: Tulsa investigators are to be thorough. *Tulsa Tribune.* October 16, 1937 (p 1, col 5).

11. For a brief history of jake-related paralysis in the United States, see Parascandola J. The Public Health Service and Jamaica ginger paralysis of the 1930s. *Public Health Rep.* 1995;110:361-363.

12. Associated Press. Drug preparation blamed in deaths. *New York Times.* October 19, 1937 (p 27, col 2). For variable wording of the statement, see Anonymous. Deaths following Elixir of Sulfanilamide-Massengill. *J Am Med Assoc.* 1937;109:1367.

13. Geiling EMK, Coon JM, Schoeffel EW. Preliminary report of toxicity studies on rats, rabbits, and dogs. *J Am Med Assoc.* 1937;109:1532-1536. These data were consistent with roughly concurrent experiments performed by the FDA's chief pharmacologist, Herbert Calvery. See also a final, follow-up report from the Chicago investigators: Geiling EMK, Cannon PR. Pathologic effects of Elixir of Sulfanilamide (diethylene glycol) poisoning: a clinical and experimental correlation—final report. *J Am Med Assoc.* 1938;111:919-926.

14. Associated Press. Drug preparation blamed in deaths. *New York Times.* October 19, 1937 (p 27, col 2). See also, Anonymous. Deaths following Elixir of Sulfanilamide-Massengill. *J Am Med Assoc.* 1937;109:1367.

15. Anonymous. Finality of AMA report resented: doctors here continue laboratory work with drug. *Tulsa Daily World.* October 19, 1937; Associated Press. Tulsa medical group acts. *New York Times.* October 19, 1937 (p 27).

16. Associated Press. Shipments of fatal drug are seized by federal food body. *Daily Capital News (Jefferson, Missouri).* October 20, 1937 (p 10, col 6).

17. Letter from W. G. Campbell to Chiefs of Districts. October 18, 1937 (NARA, Box 931, Folder 510.20S).

18. Circulating reports suggested that an identical product was being marketed by the William S. Merrell Company of Cincinnati, Ohio. See dispatch from W. G. Campbell to FDA, San Francisco. October 20, 1937; letter from John L. Harvey to Western District Stations. October 20, 1937 (both in NARA, Box 934, miscellaneous correspondence on sulfanilamide). However, these reports were apparently false.

19. Wallace report (p 4). Excerpts of the report were printed in *JAMA* (1937;109:1985-1987).

Chapter 5: Much Prejudice Against Tablets

1. Information about Samuel Evans Massengill and The S. E. Massengill Company is largely derived from Pully, DeFriece. Biographical information on the Massengill family can also be found in Massengill SE. *The*

Massengills, the Massengales and Variants, 1472-1931. Bristol, TN: King Printing Company; 1931.

2. Pully, DeFriece (p 31).
3. Ibid (p 32).
4. Ibid (p 32).
5. Ibid (p 137). Massengill's entire medical education, for which he was given a medical doctorate (MD), consisted of three years of lectures, each lasting from three to six months in duration. The lectures were attended, consecutively, at the Tennessee Medical College in Knoxville; in St. Louis, Missouri; and at the University of Nashville (which was later absorbed by the Vanderbilt University School of Medicine).
6. Ibid (p 36).
7. Adams SH. *The Great American Fraud.* P. F. Collier's and Son; 1905. A discussion of Adams's articles can be found in Young JH. *The Toadstool Millionaires.* Princeton, NJ: Princeton University Press; 1961: 205-225.
8. For a brief, early history of Charles Pfizer and Company, see Swift TP. $2500 Started chemical concern in 1849; business now $10,000,000. *New York Times.* June 14, 1942 (p F1).
9. For a contemporaneous commentary on the nature of drug manufacturing near the turn of the century, see Anonymous. Adulteration of drugs: what Dr. Edward Squibb, Jr., has to say on the subject. *New York Times.* December 3, 1895 (p 9).
10. For a discussion of Wiley's influence on the passage of the Food and Drugs Act of 1906, see Young, *The Toadstool Millionaires* (pp 226-244).
11. The law is also known as the Pure Food and Drug Act of 1906. For the contents of the Act, see FDA. Federal Food and Drugs Act of 1906. Available at http://www.fda.gov/regulatoryinformation/legislation/ucm148690.htm. Last accessed August 12, 2013. For background on the Act, see Bakran ID. Industry invites regulation: the passage of the Pure Food and Drug Act of 1906. *Am J Public Health.* 1985;74:18-26. Shortcomings of the Act are discussed in Jackson (pp 4-8).
12. Pully, DeFriece (p 38). The guaranty provision of the Food and Drugs Act of 1906 was designed to protect dealers from charges of adulteration or misbranding, providing that they could show a guaranty from a supplying wholesaler, jobber, or manufacturer. The guaranty was intended to be used between commercial parties (for example, on bills of sale) and not as a public endorsement of the drug. Drug labels advertising slogans like, "Guaranteed under the Food and Drugs Act," were considered misleading and prohibited after May 1, 1915. See for instance, Anonymous. Abolish guaranty number and serial number on food and drugs. *South Pharmaceut J.* 1914;6(10):441-442.
13. Pully, DeFriece (pp 38-39).
14. See hiring notice for H. L. Troxel, PhD. Mostly personal. *Pharm Era.* 1910;43:906.
15. *Complete Catalog of the Products of the Laboratories of The S. E. Massengill Company.* Bristol, TN: King Printing Co; 1936.

16. Pully, DeFriece (p 18).
17. Ibid (p 170). Samuel Massengill became sole owner of the company in 1917, after the departure of his older brother, Norman, from the business, reportedly for health reasons. (Norman died, according to his Tennessee death certificate, in 1926 at the age of 56 of "acute uremia following chronic Bright's disease.") The expansion of the company at Bristol was largely accomplished by purchasing the "entire" property of King College (now King University), which moved its campus to a new location in the city.
18. See entry for Massengill, Samuel Evans. In: *National Cyclopaedia of American Biography*. New York, NY: James T. White and Company; 1948: 504-505.
19. *Complete Catalog of the Products of the Laboratories of The S. E. Massengill Company* (p 8).
20. A company assessment was reported by Dun & Bradstreet, Inc., on November 8, 1937 (NARA, Box 934, miscellaneous correspondence on sulfanilamide).
21. Letter from P. B. Dunbar to Drug Division. July 23, 1938 (NARA, Box 47, sulfanilamide correspondence, March-December 1938).
22. Pully, DeFriece (p 194).
23. Stone G. *Bristol*. Mount Pleasant, SC: Arcadia Publishing; 2008: 65.
24. Pully, DeFriece (p 79).
25. In 1931, Massengill published a 908-page book of his genealogic research (see endnote 1). Massengill also erected a 24-foot monument to his pioneer ancestors in 1937. The monument was located in north Johnson City, Tennessee, at a highway intersection, until 1990, when it was moved to nearby Winged Deer Park.
26. Pully, DeFriece (p 106).
27. Ibid (p 111).
28. Ibid (pp 176-184).
29. Ibid (p 177).
30. Wallace report. See also FDA Notices of Judgment collection at http://archive.nlm.nih.gov/fdanj/community-list (*US v Samuel Evans Massengill, MD*. Adulteration and misbranding of fluidextract of colchicum [23228]; *US v Samuel Evans Massengill, MD*. Adulteration and misbranding of Tablets Tinct. Aconite [27136]; and *US v Five 1-Pint Bottles et al*. Adulteration and misbranding of elixir terpin hydrate and codeine [24030]).
31. Pully, DeFriece (pp 169-170).
32. Ibid (p 169).

Chapter 6: At Least 2 Sheets in the Wind

1. Pully, DeFriece (p 18).
2. Wallace report (p 3).
3. According to *Time* magazine (Anonymous. Medicine: fatal remedy. November 1, 1937;30[18]:61), Massengill knew "that his Southern customers prefer their medicines in bottles," and that "New Englanders prefer pills." This geographic bias was otherwise unexplained. In his 1978 interview for the

FDA Oral History project, Inspector Roland Sherman, who operated out the agency's New Orleans Station in 1937, bluntly reminisced, "Sulfanilamide was a powder—and down south, if you can't give colored people or children a red liquid medicine, you aren't any kind of a doctor at all." FDA Oral History Transcripts. Interview of Roland D. Sherman by Robert G. Porter, July 4, 1978.

4. See Wallace report (p 9): "Some [drug manufacturers] are known to have considered making a solution of sulfanilamide in diethylene glycol before the 'elixir' was put on the market but abandoned the idea on investigating the toxicity of the solvent."

5. Klumpp TG, Ford WT. Report of factory inspection. October 18, 1937 (FDA historical records).

6. Wallace report (p 3).

7. Amaranth, a synthetic bright-red azo dye, was presumably added so that the color of Elixir Sulfanilamide would resemble Bayer/I. G. Farben's patented Prontosil. Amaranth, later known as Red Dye No. 2, was banned in the United States in 1976, after reports that the dye caused cancer in laboratory animals. See for instance, Franks L. Red Dye No. 2: the 20-year battle. *New York Times*. February 28, 1976 (p 45).

8. von Oettingen WF, Jirouch EA. The pharmacology of ethylene glycol and some of its derivatives in relation to their chemical constitution and physical chemical properties. *J Pharmacol Exper Ther*. 1931;42:355-372; Haag DB, Ambrose AM. Studies on the physiological effect of diethylene glycol. *J Pharmacol Exp Ther*. 1937;59:93-100. The 1931 report was cited by the AMA's Paul Leech on October 12, 1937, in his telegram to Dr. Ruprecht of Tulsa.

9. Letter from W. G. Campbell to Chief, Central District. November 12, 1937 (NARA, Box 931, Folder 501-.20S). See also, Wallace report (p 3).

10. Report from Leo J. Cramer to Chief, Baltimore Station. October 20, 1937 (NARA, Box 934, Easter District sulfanilamide correspondence).

11. Letter from Frank L. Wollard to Chief, Eastern District. November 3, 1937 (FDA historical files). On October 22nd, a representative of the Union Carbide and Carbon Corporation reported to the FDA that, in 1936, the company had shipped 2,500 pounds of diethylene glycol to The S. E. Massengill Company in Bristol and another 1,000 pounds to its Kansas City, Missouri, branch. In 1937, 2,500 and 1,000 pounds of diethylene glycol were shipped to the Bristol and Kansas City hubs, respectively. Memorandum of telephone conversation between J. J. Durrett and I. M. Stewart. October 22, 1937 (NARA, Box 934, miscellaneous correspondence on sulfanilamide).

12. In addition, Massengill's Bristol plant sent approximately five-and-a-half gallons in the form of commercial packages (37 pints) and 58, two-ounce samples to its Kansas City branch. Part IV, Elixir Sulphanilamide Investigation (NARA, Box 935, Central District Sulfanilamide Report).

13. The cited costs of pint and gallon bottles of Elixir Sulfanilamide are based on invoice exhibits included with the court records for *Gibbons et al v Massengill et al*. National Archives Southeast Region, Atlanta, GA.

14. S. E. Massengill Co. Briefs. No. 1. October 1937 (FDA historical records). Cited by Young JH. Sulfanilamide and diethylene glycol. In: Parascandola J, Whorton JC, eds. *Chemistry and Modern Society: Historical Essays in Honor of Aaron J. Ihde*. Washington, DC: American Chemical Society; 1983: 105. For confirmation of the salesman's talking point ("the elixir would appeal especially to children and those who objected to taking capsules and tablets"), see letter from J. F. Earnshaw to Chief, Baltimore Station. October 21, 1937 (NARA, Box 934, Eastern District sulfanilamide correspondence).

15. Letter from Theodore G. Klumpp to Perrin H. Long. November 1, 1937 (NARA, Box 931, Folder 510-.20S).

16. Klumpp TG, Ford WT. Report of factory inspection. October 18, 1937 (FDA historical records). For Massengill's quotations, see also Young JH (pp 111-112), which cites Klummp's April 1938 report of his visit to the Massengill firm on October 18, 1937.

17. Letter from Theodore G. Klumpp to Perrin H. Long. November 1, 1937 (NARA, Box 931, Folder 510-.20S). According to a follow-up investigation by the FDA, fatalities due to Massengill's colloidal sulfur preparation could not be substantiated. Although Watkins said that there were complaints from Massengill's New York branch, the FDA's direct inquiries to the branch, the New York Medical Examiner's Office, and the New York Department of Health failed to reveal any possible associated deaths. Likewise a search of the recent medical literature did not return reports of suspect cases. See telegram from W. T. Ford to Larrick. November 19, 1937; and memorandum of Charles Hyak and L. L. Lusby. November 25, 1937 (FDA historical records).

18. Cinchophen preparations were frequently used in the early 20th century to alleviate joint- or nerve-associated pain. A 1931 medical review cited 34 published deaths caused by cinchophen or its derivatives as a result of liver toxicity (Parsons L, Kimball T. Fatalities due to cinchophen. *Cal West Med.* 1931;35:307-308). Massengill's 1936 catalog offered a cinchophen-salicylate-iodide compound for intravenous administration.

19. Klumpp TG, Ford WT. Report of factory inspection. October 18, 1937 (FDA historical records).

20. Letter from Theodore G. Klumpp to Perrin H. Long. November 1, 1937 (NARA, Box 931, Folder 510-.20S).

21. According to historian James Harvey Young, Watkins claimed later that there was no point in testing the product, because the properties of the ingredients were "well understood," and that the glycols were "well known not to be toxic." Young JH. Sulfanilamide and diethylene glycol. In: Parascandola J, Whorton JC, eds. *Chemistry and Modern Society: Historical Essays in Honor of Aaron J. Inde*. Washington, DC: American Chemical Society; 1983: 105-125. (Young cited Klummp's April 1938 report of his visit to the Massengill firm on October 18, 1937 [FDA historical records].)

22. Harold C. Watkins appears in the general registers of the University of Michigan for the academic years of 1899-1900, 1900-1901, and 1901-1902. He was enrolled as an undergraduate in the school of pharmacy, where he was pursuing the degree of either pharmaceutical chemist (PhC) or bachelor

of science (BS), which required two and four years of study, respectively. He does not appear in the 1902-1903 general register. His name (but not his photograph) also appears in the *Michiganensian* (the University of Michigan yearbook) for the years 1900, 1901, and 1902. Alumni directories indicate that Watkins left the University of Michigan in 1902, after approximately three years of study and with a PhC.

23. At the University of Michigan, Watkins shared the F. Stearns & Co. Fellowship, totaling $350, with another pharmacy student, Charles Eckler. The 1902 Ebert Prize was bestowed for contributions to the chemistry of *Stylophorum diphyllum* (aka poppywort), and the 1906 prize was given for contributions to the chemistry of "chelidone" (probably *Chelidonium majus* or greater celandine). See Funkhouser JA. Prize winners in chemistry. *Chem Eng News.* 1936;14(7):123. The Ebert Prize is still given out annually.

24. *State of California v Harold C. Watkins.* Criminal court records were obtained from the Center for Sacramento History. Watkins also admitted to stealing another small platinum dish, 13.5 ounces of mercury, three ounces of morphine (valued at $13 per ounce), and "a few other small medicinal articles."

25. Although it is possible that Watkins received written permission to move out of California to gain employment in New York.

26. Evidently the 1917 pregnancy did not reach term, or the child died an early death.

27. For a company description, see Pennsylvania Department of Internal Affairs, Woodward JF. *Fourth Industrial Directory of the Commonwealth of Pennsylvania.* Harrisburg, PA: J. L. L. Kuhn; 1922; 926.

28. Anonymous. Revenue agents seize stock of Scranton firm. *Reading Eagle.* March 16, 1921 (p 7, col 3). According to a brief mention in the March 28, 1921, issue of the *Oil, Paint and Drug Reporter,* Watkins also worked for the Scranton Dental and Supply Company.

29. See Wallace report (pp 8-9). This fact was presumably discovered after Klumpp and Ford interviewed Watkins on October 18th. In response to the author's direct query, a representative from NARA responded that she found no relevant Post Office records about or judgments against Harold Cole Watkins or Watkins Laboratories circa 1929. A search of the FDA Notices of Judgment database failed to return any citations against Harold Cole Watkins, Watkins Laboratories, Watkins Products, or Nature's Products of Scranton.

30. According to the *Official Gazette of the United States Patent Office* (June 25, 1929; p 862), Watkins (as Nature's Products, Inc., of Scranton) registered a "print" for "Takoff," a reducing compound. An entry in the *Official Gazette* for 1923 (vol 306, p vi) indicates that "Watkins, Harold C. doing business as Watkins Chemical Company, Scranton, Pa." applied for a trademark on a cathartic. In a 1927 issue of the *Official Gazette* (January 11, 1927 [p 309]), Nature's Products of Los Angeles is listed as having registered a label for Takoff (published November 4, 1926). In 1928, the Nature's Product's Company of Los Angeles applied for a trademark on "EXIT" laxative pills, with claims used since 1926 (*Official Gazette.* May 29, 1928; p 1030). It is

therefore possible that Watkins's Takoff product was merely a laxative or cathartic. The composite information also suggests that Watkins may have relocated from Scranton to Los Angeles between 1925 and 1929.

31. Notice in *American Druggist*. 1928;77-78:41. Given the ad's references to the Pacific Coast and Denver, Watkins may have relocated to these areas between 1926 and 1928, before returning to the Scranton area. A 1926 newspaper advertisement for Takoff from Nature's Products, Inc., indicates that the company was located in Hollywood, California (*Salt Lake Tribune*. May 9, 1926 [p 10, cols 6-8]).

32. Advertisement ("EAT WHAT YOU LIKE"). *Ireton Ledger*. February 7, 1929 (p 3, col 7); *Sioux County Index*. February 8, 1929 (p 3, col 6).

33. Advertisement for Takoff. *Motion Picture*. March 1929 (p 110).

34. Klumpp TG, Ford WT. Report of factory inspection. October 18, 1937 (FDA historical records).

35. Pully, DeFriece (p 170).

36. In addition to publicly available primary and secondary sources, information about the early life of Harold Cole Watkins is importantly informed by David C. Larsen, the chemist's great-nephew. Biographical sketches of George Watkins, Harold's father, can be found in Lapham WB, Maxim SP. *The History of Paris, Maine: From its Settlement in 1800* (Paris, ME: Wm. B. Lapham and Silas P. Maxim; 1884) and in the *Oxford Democrat* (March 11, 1890 [p 2, col 1]). The Bethel Historical Society of Bethel, Maine, provided genealogic information on the Watkins family and transcribed relevant newspaper reports.

37. County probate records indicate that the care, board, and clothing of Harold and Edith Watkins from 1887 to 1889 were provided by Dr. A. E. Bessey, Mrs. Wyman (Harold's caretaker), and "others."

38. Anonymous. Death of Geo. H. Watkins. *Oxford Democrat*. March 11, 1890 (p 2, col 2).

39. Anonymous. In the schoolroom. *Daily Kennebec Journal*. February 9, 1901 (p 9, col 4).

40. Letter from Paul B. Dunbar to Chiefs of District. October 22, 1937 (NARA, Box 934, miscellaneous correspondence on sulfanilamide).

41. Wallace report (p 5).

42. Telegram (text in written script) from W. T. Ford to Mr. Clarke. October 23, 1937 (NARA. Box 935, Central District sulfanilamide correspondence). A wire of the same date was directed to Massengill's salesmen: "IMPERATIVE YOU TAKE UP IMMEDIATELY ANY CASE OF PHYSICIANS SAMPLES YOU MAY HAVE GIVEN TO PHYSICIANS OR ANYONE ELSE AND RETURN TO US (Part II, Report on Elixir Sulfanilamide manufactured by S. E. Massengill Company [NARA, Box 935, Central District Sulfanilamide Report]).

43. Letter from W. T. Ford to Central District Chief. October 31, 1937 (FDA historical records). Massengill's other suspect products included Phe-Mer-Nite, a solution of 25% diethylene glycol and nearly 50% alcohol; the product was intended as a skin antiseptic, a vaginal or nasal douche, and a gargle. Other concerning products included ear drops composed of 87.5% ethylene glycol, and a local, intramuscular anesthetic containing "about" 100%

ethylene glycol. It is unclear if any of these products caused any harm during their use (or if they were, in fact, ever used).

44. Letter from W. G. Campbell to Dr. George A. Denison. November 6, 1937 (NARA, Box 931, Folder 501-.20S).

Chapter 7: A Technical and Trivial Charge of Misbranding

1. Associated Press. Drug fatality cause is traced to 'elixir.' *New York Times.* October 20, 1937 (p 18).
2. FDA Notices of Judgment Under the Food and Drugs Act. *US v 1 Gallon of Elixir Sulfanilamide.* Adulteration and misbranding of elixir sulfanilamide (30776). Default decree by condemnation and destruction. January 1939.
3. See for instance, Sollman TH. *A Manual of Pharmacology and Its Applications to Therapeutics and Toxicology, 2nd ed.* Philadelphia, PA: W. B. Saunders; 1922: 32.
4. Fuller HC. *The Story of Drugs.* New York, NY: The Century Company; 1922.
5. American Pharmaceutical Association. *The National Formulary, 6th ed.* Washington, DC: American Pharmaceutical Association; 1935: 98-131.
6. Anonymous. Deaths following Elixir of Sulfanilamide-Massengill: III. *J Am Med Assoc.* 1937;109:1544-1545.
7. Information about Campbell and specifically his political views on legislative reform are derived from Dunbar PB. Memories of early days of Federal Food and Drug law enforcement. *Food Drug Cosmet Law J.* 1959;14:87-138; Jackson; and contemporaneous coverage in *Time* magazine (eg, Anonymous. Fatal remedy. *Time.* November 1, 1937;30[18]:61) and the *New York Times.* Information on Campbell's tenure at the FDA can also be found at the FDA web site: http://www.fda.gov/AboutFDA/CommissionersPage/ucm113609.htm. Last accessed August 13, 2013.
8. This law was praised by *JAMA* editors in 1908 as "being, perhaps, the best general pure food and drug law as yet adopted" (Anonymous. The Kentucky pure food law. *J Am Med Assoc.* 1908;52:968). However, given the year of the law's enactment, 1908, it's unlikely that Campbell had much actual experience enforcing the law.
9. *US v Johnson,* 221 US 488 (1911). For background on this case, see Propaganda Department of the Journal of the American Medical Association. *Cancer "Cures" and "Treatments."* Chicago, IL: American Medical Association; 1922: 30-34; Munch JC. A half-century of drug control. *Food Drug Cosmet Law J.* 1956;11(6):305-334.
10. For text of the Sherley Amendment (37 Stat. 416 [1912]), see FDA. Food and Drugs Act of 1906. Available at http://www.fda.gov/regulatoryinformation/legislation/ucm148690.htm. Last accessed August 13, 2013.
11. *FTC v Raladam Co.,* 283 US 643 (1931). For a discussion of this case, see Jackson (pp 5-7).

12. For a brief discussion of Harvey Wiley's tenure at the Bureau of Chemistry, a colorful topic that is most certainly beyond the scope of this book, see Linton FB. Federal food and drug laws: leaders who achieved their enactment and enforcement. *Food Drug Cosmet Law Quart*. 1949;4:451-470.

13. Carl Alsberg, a physician, succeeded Wiley as Chief in 1912. Chemist Charles A. Browne was named Chief of the Bureau in 1924.

14. Anonymous. Our medicinal drugs undergo severe tests. *New York Times*. August 3, 1930 (p 112).

15. See Jackson (pp 24-28).

16. Jackson (pp 6-7). Ruth DeForest Lamb, the FDA's information officer, wrote descriptions of these and other offending products in her *American Chamber of Horrors* (New York, NY: Farrar and Rinehart; 1936). Lamb published her work as a private citizen, although she received permission to do so from the agency.

17. For a more in-depth narrative of follow-up drug legislation, see Chapter 14.

18. Letter from Leo J. Cramer to Chief, Central District. October 18, 1937 (NARA, Box 935, Central District sulfanilamide correspondence). See also Part IV, Elixir Sulphanilamide Investigation (NARA, Box 935, Central District Sulfanilamide Report).

19. At the Kansas City branch, 384 one-ounce samples (24 pints) were produced. In addition, 58 two-ounce samples (7.25 pints) were shipped from Bristol to Kansas City for distribution. Among these samples (totaling 500 ounces or 31.25 pints), 24.5 pints (about 80%) were shipped out to salesmen. Part II, Report on Elixir Sulfanilamide manufactured by S. E. Massengill Company, Bristol, Tenn.; Part IV, Elixir Sulphanilamide Investigation (NARA, Box 935, Central District Sulfanilamide Report).

20. Telegram from W. G. Campbell to FDA, San Francisco. October 20, 1937 (NARA, Box 934, miscellaneous correspondence on sulfanilamide); letter from R. B. Bork to Chief, San Francisco Station. October 19, 1937 (NARA, Box 934, Western District sulfanilamide correspondence); and Part IV, Elixir Sulphanilamide Investigation (NARA, Box 935, Central District Sulfanilamide Report).

21. Memorandum from Charles Hyak. October 21, 1937 (NARA, Box 934, Eastern District sulfanilamide correspondence). Notably a one-pint shipment to the Ira J. Shapiro Company, a wholesaler in New York City, was traced to the Winthrop Chemical Company, the maker of Prontylin tablets (a branded version of sulfanilamide). The pint bottle was then traced to Winthrop's Albany, New York, laboratories, where it was sent for analysis.

22. Wallace report (p 3); Part IV, Elixir Sulphanilamide Investigation (NARA, Box 935, Central District Sulfanilamide Report). At the time, newspapers grossly underreported the distribution of Massengill's elixir, claiming a total of "375 shipments to drugstores throughout the country." See for example, Anonymous. Finality of AMA report resented. *Tulsa Daily World*. October 19, 1937.

23. Among this volume, only 24 ounces were on hand at Bristol (either 24 one-ounce or 12 two-ounce samples [or some combination thereof]). A total of 326 ounces had been shipped directly from Bristol to salesmen or physicians.

Among the 187 two-ounce samples produced at Bristol, 58 were shipped to Kansas City, 40 went to San Francisco, and New York received 30.

24. Anonymous. Earl Beard dies in Tulsa hospital. *Tulsa Daily World.* October 17, 1937; Anonymous. Tulsa newcomer ninth victim of mysterious, fatal malady. *Tulsa Tribune.* October 17, 1937 (p 1, cols 2, 3). Local news coverage misreported Beard as the ninth elixir victim in Tulsa.

25. Joint Committee on Radio Research. Estimated number of families owning radio sets: urban and rural. *Broadcasting.* 1938;14(10):20. For a more recent examination of radio ownership in the early 20th century, see Craig S. How America adopted radio: demographic differences in set ownership reported in the 1930-1950 US censuses. *J Broadcast Elect Media.* 2004;48:179-195.

26. Associated Press. Drug preparation named in deaths. *New York Times.* October 19, 1937 (p 27, col 2); Associated Press. Venereal disease 'cure' kills 8 of 10 patients in Oklahoma. *Washington Post.* October 19, 1937 (p 3); and Anonymous. Chicagoans warned against drug fatal to eight in Tulsa. *Chicago Daily Tribune.* October 19, 1937 (p 8).

27. United Press. Think medicine causes deaths. *Billings Gazette.* October 19, 1937 (p 7, col 3).

28. United Press. Says druggists warned. *Billings Gazette.* October 19, 1937 (p 7, col 3).

29. Associated Press. Strong drug is recalled. *Bristol New Bulletin.* October 19, 1937 (p 1, col 8).

30. Anonymous. Mrs. F. L. Harkrader, 83, dies in Virginia. *New York Times.* March 1, 1937 (p 19).

31. The Wallace report (p 5) indicated that Massengill had approximately 200 salesmen, although Massengill's own sources indicated that the company had 160 salesmen.

32. Part I, Elixir Sulphanilamide Investigation (NARA, Box 935, Central District Sulfanilamide Report).

33. Root T. Frantic fight on death is heart-breaking job. *Kansas City Journal-Post.* October 31, 1937 (NARA, Box 933, sulfanilamide clippings).

34. Report from W. H. Hartigan to Chief, Central District. November 3, 1937 (FDA historical files).

35. Spann, who graduated in 1931 from medical school at the University of Oklahoma in Norman, first admitted to Hartigan that he had written two prescriptions for Joan Marlar: one for Elixir Phenobarbital (two ounces) and one for Elixir Lactated Pepsin (three ounces). Both were filled at the Crown Drug Store on September 28th and were indicated to "control restlessness." Notably Crown had not received any shipment of Massengill's elixir.

36. Although Dr. Spann was not recorded as being present at the October 11th meeting of the Tulsa County Medical Society, it is reasonable to conclude that information from the meeting quickly circulated among Tulsa's physicians.

37. Associated Press. Pigs used in new drug quiz: doctors perform autopsy, find clues in strange death investigation. *Ada News Weekly.* October 21, 1937 (p 6, col 6).

38. Anonymous. New deaths spur inquiry; four die in Illinois; Tulsa boy recovering. *Tulsa Tribune*. October 19, 1937 (p 1, col 2; p 4, col 7).

Chapter 8: The Prescription Was a Legitimate One

1. Hagebusch OE. Necropsies of four patients following administration of Elixir of Sulfanilamide-Massengill. *J Am Med Assoc*. 1937;109:1537-1539.
2. For details of these deaths and those of Dr. Weathers's other patients, see Appendix A and http://bmartinmd.com/elixir-sulfanilamide-deaths.html. Sources: Letter from S. W. Ahlmann to Chief, Central District. October 18, 1937 (NARA, Box 935, Central District sulfanilamide correspondence); General Report from A. E. Lowe to Chief, Central District. October 27, 1937 (FDA historical records); correspondence from A. E. Lowe to Chief, Central District (with statement from Dr. Weathers). November 26, 1937 (FDA historical records); Geiling EMK, Cannon PR. Pathologic effects of Elixir of Sulfanilamide (diethylene glycol) poisoning: a clinical and experimental correlation—final report. *J Am Med Assoc*. 1938;111:919-926; and Anonymous. Four deaths here among 13 laid to use of new drug. *St. Louis Post-Dispatch*. October 19, 1937 (p 3A).
3. Consequently the amount of Elixir Sulfanilamide consumed by Dr. Weathers's patients is difficult to quantify accurately.
4. According to FDA historical records, Weathers prescribed Elixir Sulfanilamide to 50 patients, producing an ultimate fatality rate of 12%.
5. See for instance, Rollins YD, Filley CM, McNutt JT, et al. Fulminant ascending paralysis as a delayed sequela of diethylene glycol (Sterno) ingestion. *Neurology*. 2002;59:1460-1463; Hasbani MJ, Sansing LH, Perrone J, et al. Encephalopathy and peripheral neuropathy following diethylene glycol ingestion. *Neurology*. 2005;64:1273-1275; and Reddy NJ, Sudini M, Lewis LD, et al. Delayed neurological sequelae from ethylene glycol, diethylene glycol and methanol poisonings. *Clin Toxicol (Phila)*. 2010;48:967-973.
6. Another elixir-consuming patient of Dr. Weathers, a 53-year-old woman, died on October 8th. However, FDA inspectors attributed her death to her underlying illness: infection of the teeth and jaw. Part I, Elixir Sulphanilamide Investigation (NARA, Box 935, Central District Sulfanilamide Report). See also, Appendix A and http://bmartinmd.com/elixir-sulfanilamide-deaths.html.
7. Biographical information on Dr. Henri H. Weathers was obtained from documents supplied by and a telephone interview with (June 19, 2009) his son, William Weathers, MD. The first name of the senior Dr. Weathers is spelled variably in published notices as either "Henri" or "Henry." His Missouri death certificate, biographical data for which were supplied by his widow, gives the first name of Henri.
8. For a brief history of the Flexner Report, see Beck AH. The Flexner Report and the standardization of American medical education. *JAMA*. 2004;291:2139-2140. The report itself, *Medical Education in the United States and Canada: A Report to the Carnegie Foundation for the Advancement of Teaching*, can be found at

http://www.carnegiefoundation.org/sites/default/files/elibrary/Carnegie_Flexn
er_Report.pdf. Last accessed August 13, 2013.

9. See Everett MR. *Medical Education in Oklahoma*. Norman, OK: University
   of Oklahoma Press; 1972; University of Oklahoma. *General Catalog, 1918-
   1919*. Norman, OK: University of Oklahoma Press; 1919:323-352; *Western
   Reserve University in the City of Cleveland Annual Catalogue, 1925* (from a
   manuscript in the Case Western Reserve University archives); Tulsa County
   Medical Society. Ivo Amazon Nelson, MD [obituary]. *Bull Tulsa County
   Med Soc.* 1946;12:13; and Leitner J. Leaders in medicine: Homer A.
   Ruprecht, MD. *J Okla State Med Assoc.* 1982;75:137-143.

10. For a discussion of how the medical-education reform movement affected
    black medical education, see Savitt TL. Abraham Flexner and the black
    medical schools. In: Savitt TL. *Race and Medicine in Nineteenth- and Early-
    Twentieth-Century America.* Kent, OH: Kent State University Press; 1992:
    252.

11. For a discussion of Meharry's development under the controversial
    leadership of President John J. Mullowney, see Summerville J. *Educating
    Black Doctors: A History of Meharry Medical College.* Birmingham, AL:
    University of Alabama Press; 1983: 60-80.

12. Advertisement for Meharry Medical College in *The Crisis Advertiser.*
    1926;31(5):253.

13. At the time, only 12 states required participation in a medical internship as a
    prerequisite for licensure. See Bousfield MO. Internships, residencies and
    post graduate training. *J Natl Med Assoc.* 1940;32:24-30.

14. The contemporaneous bed capacity of the hospital is provided by Barrett
    WHA. The Missouri hospital situation. *J Natl Med Assoc.* 1930;22:140-141.

15. For a relevant timeline of racial discrimination in the AMA (which persisted
    well into the 1960s), see Race and the AMA: a chronology. Available at
    http://www.ama-assn.org/ama/pub/about-ama/our-history/timelines-ama-
    history/race-ama-a-chronology.page. Last accessed August 13, 2013.

16. Anonymous. Four deaths here among 13 laid to use of new drug. *St. Louis
    Post-Dispatch.* October 19, 1937 (p 3A). In addition to naming the four
    deceased patients of Dr. Weathers at the time of publication, the newspaper
    revealed that three of his patients were ill at the time (after taking Elixir
    Sulfanilamide). However, the FDA later determined that one of these
    patients had never taken the product. See General Report from A. E. Lowe
    to Chief, Central District. October 27, 1937 (FDA historical records).

17. General Report from A. E. Lowe to Chief, Central District. October 27,
    1937; bulletin from A. E. Lowe to Chief, Central District. October 20, 1937
    (FDA historical records).

18. Preliminary report from A. E. Lowe to Chief, Central District. October 18,
    1937 (NARA, Box 935, Central District sulfanilamide correspondence). See
    also, Part I, Elixir Sulphanilamide Investigation (NARA, Box 935, Central
    District Sulfanilamide Report).

19. General Report from A. E. Lowe to Chief, Central District. October 27,
    1937 (FDA historical records). See also, Part I, Elixir Sulphanilamide
    Investigation (NARA, Box 935, Central District Sulfanilamide Report).

20. The agents were ultimately aided in their search by Meyers Brothers' clerks, after Lowe advised the president of the firm of the seriousness of the matter.

21. In Lovejoy, Illinois, four ounces were dispensed on prescription to a "negro woman suffering from cancer." The elixir was consumed in its entirety "without apparent ill effects."

22. General report from A. E. Lowe to Chief, Central District. October 27, 1937 (FDA historical records).

23. Ibid. A check of these numbers against Part I, Elixir Sulphanilamide Investigation (NARA, Box 935, Central District Sulfanilamide Report) shows that five druggists in East St. Louis sold the drug, in variable amounts, to 10 pharmacies in Illinois. Lowe recorded "69 prescriptions" in his October 27th report. Part I indicates that 70 prescriptions for 68 individuals were dispensed in Illinois (from 14 druggists and two doctors' offices), and that one prescription was dispensed in St. Louis (from a doctor's office).

24. Details of this case are provided by the following: Part I, Elixir Sulphanilamide Investigation (NARA, Box 935, Central District Sulfanilamide Report); letter from A. E. Lowe to J. O. Clarke. November 12, 1937 (FDA historical records); and Anonymous. Two more deaths here from Elixir of Sulfanilamide. *St. Louis Post-Dispatch*. October 25, 1937 (p 3A, col 1). During a postmortem inquest, Dr. Murray admitted to prescribing sulfanilamide tablets to Schroeder as treatment for urethritis before prescribing Massengill's elixir; the tablets caused no ill effects. Schroeder's widow ultimately turned over the remaining elixir to a local attorney, Everett Hulverson, for use in a damage suit.

25. Bulletin from A. E. Lowe to Chief, Central District. October 20, 1937 (FDA historical files); letter from S. W. Ahlmann to Chief, Central District. October 18, 1937 (NARA, Box 935, Central District sulfanilamide correspondence). The Massengill rep for St. Louis was Kenneth Lusher.

26. Anonymous. 6th East Side death from sulfanilamide. *St. Louis Post-Dispatch*. October 21, 1937 (p 4A, cols 3, 4).

27. Associated Press. Drug fatality cause is traced to 'elixir.' *New York Times*. October 20, 1937 (p 18, col 6).

28. Anonymous. Alleged fatal drug is widely in use here. *Lima News*. October 21, 1937 (p 4, col 5).

29. Associated Press. Drug stores warned. *Kingsport Times*. October 21, 1937 (p 14, col 1).

30. Anonymous. 6th East Side death from sulfanilamide. *St. Louis Post-Dispatch*. October 21, 1937 (p 4A, cols 3, 4); General Report from A. E. Lowe to Chief, Central District. October 27, 1937 (FDA historical records). See also, Anonymous. Death in elixir case to be probed: Granite City woman may have succumbed to poison drug dose. *Globe-Democrat*. October 21, 1937 (NARA, Box 931, sulfanilamide clippings). For further details of the case of Hazel Fea, see Appendix A and http://bmartinmd.com/elixir-sulfanilamide-deaths.html.

31. Anonymous. 6th East Side death from sulfanilamide. *St. Louis Post-Dispatch*. October 21, 1937 (p 4A, cols 3, 4).

32. Anonymous. Poison 'elixir' kills Memphian who had druggist prescribe; medical society gives warning. *Commercial Appeal.* October 21, 1937 (p 1) (NARA, Box 931, sulfanilamide clippings). For further details of this case, see Appendix A and http://bmartinmd.com/elixir-sulfanilamide-deaths.html.
33. Associated Press. "Over the counter" drug prescriptions will be warred on. *Daily Democrat-Times* (Greenville, MS). October 21, 1937 (p 20, col 7); Associated Press. New drug fatal to pastor and gas station operator. *Kingsport Times.* October 21, 1937 (p 1, cols 7, 8; p 14, col 1).

Chapter 9: Nobody but Almighty God and I

1. Toler K. Dr. A. S. Calhoun commended by Mt Olive for candidness about lethal drug cases. *News-Commercial.* October 29, 1937 (pp 1, 2).
2. Newspaper accounts and official records disagree on the number of patients to whom Calhoun prescribed Elixir Sulfanilamide. FDA records indicate that Calhoun prescribed the drug to 13 or 14 patients. Calhoun himself reported to news sources on October 22nd that he had prescribed the elixir to 12 individuals.
3. For a description of the case of John W. Gibbons (and other deaths in Mississippi associated with Elixir Sulfanilamide), see New Orleans Report (Elixir Sulphanilamide [Fatalities]) to Chief, Central District. October 25, 1937; letter from R. D. Sherman to Chief, New Orleans Station. October 31, 1937 (both in FDA historical records). Other details of Gibbons's death can be found in the court records of *Gibbons v Massengill.* National Archives Southeast Region. Atlanta, GA.
4. Easterling was mistakenly identified as a "negress" in newspaper reports, but census records indicate that this elixir victim was the son of Louis Easterling of Mt. Olive. (The patient is recorded as "Lefey" in the 1930 census record.)
5. For details of these deaths, see Appendix A and http://bmartinmd.com/elixir-sulfanilamide-deaths.html. Gussie Mae Grubbs may be alternately known as Jessie May Grubbs. Edie, or Eddie, Sullivan was listed in contemporaneous newspaper reports as being a patient of Dr. Calhoun, but FDA records indicate that Sullivan was a patient of Dr. Wright W. Diamond of the Magee General Hospital. Calhoun himself publicly acknowledged that he prescribed Elixir Sulfanilamide for Sullivan. It seems reasonable to conclude that Calhoun prescribed the elixir to Sullivan, and that Diamond was Sullivan's physician in the hospital (although FDA records also indicate that Sullivan obtained his elixir prescription at the Magee hospital, not from the pharmacy of Calhoun's brother).
6. Associated Press. Sulfanilamide elixir kills 6 in Mississippi. *St. Louis Post-Dispatch.* October 22, 1937 (p 3A); Toler K. Dr. A. S. Calhoun commended by Mt. Olive for candidness about lethal drug cases. *News Commercial.* October 29, 1937 (pp 1-2).
7. For other details of this death, see Appendix A and http://bmartinmd.com/elixir-sulfanilamide-deaths.html.
8. Letter from C. S. McKellogg to Chief, Cincinnati Station. October 31, 1937 (FDA historical records). The letter indicates that Calhoun wired the

Knoxville hospital and "simply stated that [Byrd] had been taking the Elixir." A date for Calhoun's wire is not provided, but it is presumed that he sent it on October 19th or shortly thereafter.

9. Associated Press. Noted Pastor is victim of medical drug. *Laurel Leader-Call.* October 21, 1937 (p 1); Associated Press. Third death from drug. *Laurel Leader-Call.* October 21, 1937 (p 1).

10. Associated Press. Six of 12 die after doses of poison elixir. *Chicago Daily Tribune.* October 23, 1937 (p 11). The identified dead were Rev. Byrd, Mrs. J. E. Penn, Ed Sullivan, Otis Coulter, and "two negroes" (ie, Mrs. Gussie Mae Grubbs and Leffie Easterling).

11. AMA Chemical Laboratory. Special article from the American Medical Association Chemical Laboratory: Elixir of Sulfanilamide-Massengill. *J Am Med Assoc.* 1937;109:1539.

12. The experts were Johns Hopkins pharmacologist Eli Kennerly Marshall, Jr.; toxicologist W. F. von Oettingen, first author of the 1931 article on the toxicity of diethylene glycol; and Stanford pharmacologist P. J. Hanzlik.

13. Calhoun AS. Mississippi doctor tells own story of how 6 patients died. *New Orleans States.* October 22, 1937 (pp 1, 19) (NARA, Box 931, sulfanilamide clippings).

14. FDA records indicate that seven or eight of Calhoun's patients died. Missing from Calhoun's self-reported death tally, for unclear reasons, were John W. Gibbons and Katie Stuckey.

15. Calhoun's surviving patients were identified in news reports as Mrs. Frank Hamilton (29); Velma Lucas (21); Mrs. H. D. [or N. E.] Booth (60); Mrs. Baxter Pittman (38); Lula Herring (30); and his office nurse, Evelyn Sharbrough (29). See Breazeale J. Elixir victim is laid to rest. *Sunday Item-Tribune* (New Orleans). October 24, 1937 (NARA, Box 931, sulfanilamide clippings).

16. Anonymous. Styx elixir. *Delta Weekly.* October 25, 1937 (p 10, col 3).

17. United Press. Nurse works on though death threatens her as elixir victim. *Brooklyn Daily Eagle.* October 23, 1937 (p 1, cols 6, 7); United Press. Physician's nurse 13th of his patients to take "death drug." *Lima News.* October 24, 1937 (p 15, cols 2, 3).

18. United Press. She took "elixir" but lives. *Wisconsin State Journal.* October 25, 1937 (p 16, col 4).

19. See endnote 16.

20. Schoenberger P. Westwego child given elixir has no bad effects. *Times-Picayune–New Orleans States.* October 24, 1937 (pp 1, 2) (NARA, Box 931, sulfanilamide clippings).

21. Anonymous. Boy survives use of elixir. *Chattanooga Times.* October 26, 1937 (NARA, Box 933, sulfanilamide clippings).

22. Letter from R. B. Born to Chief, San Francisco Station. October 26, 1937 (NARA, Box 934, Western District sulfanilamide correspondence).

23. Fishbein M. Ailing tonsils scatter germs through body. *Spokane Daily Chronicle.* December 31, 1936 (p 4, col 3).

24. Extended follow-up of the victim, William Ellsworth Judson, Jr., is not found in official government records, but his obituary in the *Contra Costa Times,*

dated November 28, 2007, reveals that he finished his schooling at Berkeley, and studied medicine at Temple University.

25. Anonymous. Deaths following Elixir of Sulfanilamide-Massengill. *J Am Med Assoc.* 1937;109:1367.

26. Associated Press. Elixir Sulfanilamide manufacturer disclaims responsibility. *St. Louis Post-Dispatch.* October 24, 1937 (p 9A).

27. Anonymous. Reports not confirmed. *Laurel Leader-Call.* October 22, 1937 (pp 1, 10).

28. Anonymous. Confirmation lacking. *Laurel Leader-Call.* October 23, 1937 (p 1); Anonymous. Elixir of Sulfanilamide may have played part in death of five, states local doctor. *Laurel Leader-Call.* October 25, 1937 (p 1).

29. FDA records indicate that Green prescribed Elixir Sulfanilamide to probably 10 patients, five of whom died. See letter from R. D. Sherman to Chief, New Orleans Station (Dr. Green's memo). October 21, 1937; New Orleans Report (Elixir Sulphanilamide [Fatalities]) to Chief, Central District. October 25, 1937; and report of R. D. Sherman. Elixir Sulfanilamide: additional data on deaths at Laurel, Miss. November 2, 1937 (all in FDA historical records).

30. For details of these deaths (Claiborne L. Anderson, Robert A. Boutwell, James Monroe Vick, Emmett Pickens, and Albert Cole), see Appendix A and http://bmartinmd.com/elixir-sulfanilamide-deaths.html.

31. Anonymous. Elixir of Sulfanilamide may have played part in death of five, states local doctor. *Laurel Leader-Call.* October 25, 1937 (p 1).

Chapter 10: Nationwide Race With Death

1. Associated Press. Near end of chase for deadly elixir. *New York Times.* October 25, 1937 (p 21).

2. Anonymous. Lad questions safety of mother's elixir. *Food Drug Rev.* 1937;21:269.

3. See for instance, Cutting WC. *Actions and Uses of Drugs: A Textbook for Nurses.* Stanford, CA: Stanford University Press; 1946: 52-53, 130.

4. Associated Press. Sale deadly drug is under control. *Kingsport Times.* October 25, 1937 (p 3, col 8).

5. United Press. Federal and state agents search for bottles of elixir. *Oshkosh Northwestern.* October 25, 1937 (p 3, col 4).

6. United Press. Alabama counts victims. *Anniston Star.* October 25, 1937 (p 1).

7. Anonymous. Four persons died from drug over Alabama. *Alabama Journal.* October 23, 1937; Anonymous. Fatal elixir kills its 5th in this state. *Montgomery Advertiser.* October 24, 1937 (both in NARA, Box 931, sulfanilamide clippings).

8. Report from New Orleans Station to Chief, Central District (Elixir Sulphanilamide [Fatalities]). October 25, 1937 (FDA historical records).

9. W. C. White of Dothan.

10. See Appendix A and http://bmartinmd.com/elixir-sulfanilamide-deaths.html for details of these cases (Mary Frances "Fannie" Zeanah and Alfred "Alf" McDade [or McDay]).

11. According to Singleton family history, the girl was hospitalized at Salter Hospital along with her father, Sam Singleton, for Brill's fever (typhus). It is not known if the child's father was also treated with Elixir Sulfanilamide; regardless, the father survived his illness, which necessitated hospitalization for two or three weeks beyond the time of his daughter's death. Email correspondence with Hugh Singleton, October 2010.

12. FDA records indicate that the child's name was Bettie (or Betty) Joe Story; however, the girl's transcribed death record provides the name of Nettie Joe Story.

13. Associated Press. No more Texas deaths expected. *Galveston Daily.* October 25, 1937 (p 12, col 4).

14. The official notation was, perhaps, an indicator of the general confusion between the two poisonous glycols: ethylene glycol and diethylene glycol.

15. Anonymous. Medicine is fatal to Texas City man. *Galveston Daily.* October 25, 1937 (p 12, col 4).

16. The injections of liver extract in this case were manufactured by Eli Lilly. The product, which was given intramuscularly and intended for the treatment of pernicious anemia, was made with ground livers from "edible animals." See for instance, "Solution liver extract concentrated-Lilly" in Council on Pharmacy and Chemistry. *New and Nonofficial Remedies.* Chicago, IL: American Medical Association; 1939: 311.

17. Part II, Report on Elixir Sulfanilamide manufactured by S. E. Massengill Company, Bristol, Tenn (NARA, Box 935, Central District Sulfanilamide Report). According to Massengill history, Hensley was one of four brothers who worked as notable salesmen for the company in the area of southwestern Louisiana.

18. The local paper reported that 36 "bottles" of Elixir Sulfanilamide had been distributed by Hensley. See Anonymous. S. A. elixir is removed. *San Antonio Light.* October 28, 1937 (p 1, col 3).

19. For further details of this death, see Appendix A and http://bmartinmd.com/elixir-sulfanilamide-deaths.html.

20. See also, Anonymous. Rites for Hatchel baby conducted. *Abilene Reporter News.* October 15, 1937 (p 16, col 3).

21. Part I, Elixir Sulfanilamide Investigation (NARA, Box 935, Central District Sulfanilamide Report).

22. Part III, Report on Elixir Sulfanilamide manufactured by S. E. Massengill Company, Bristol, Tenn (NARA, Box 935, Central District Sulfanilamide Report).

23. Anonymous. Roundup of fatal remedy is too late to save child. *Akron Beacon Journal.* October 26, 1937 (pp 1, 19).

24. Kaempffert W. The week in science: cause of the Tulsa deaths. *New York Times.* October 25, 1937 (p 6, cols 1, 2).

25. Anonymous. Warn surgeons to be cautious with new drug. *Chicago Daily Tribune.* October 26, 1937 (p 11); Anonymous. Drug has life saving quality. *Edwardsville Intelligencer.* October 26, 1937 (p 2, col 2).

26. Associated Press. Deaths from elixir pass half-hundred; little girl dies. *Laurel Leader-Call.* October 27, 1937.

27. For descriptions of Pitts, see FDA Oral History Transcripts. Interview with Samuel Alfend, June 8, 1978, and interview with Malcolm R. Stephens, December 4, 1984.
28. Bulletin from A. E. Lowe to Chief, Central District. October 20, 1937; Special Report from A. E. Lowe to Chief, Central District. October 26, 1937; General Report from A. E. Lowe to Chief, Central District. October 27, 1937 (all in FDA historical records). A brief account of the investigation of Ruth Jeanell Long is also given in Young JH. Sulfanilamide and diethylene glycol. In: Parascandola J, Whorton JC, eds. *Chemistry and Modern Society: Historical Essays in Honor of Aaron J. Ihde.* Washington, DC: American Chemical Society; 1983: 105-125.
29. The FDA records conflict on the sex of this so-called itinerant negro. One report indicates that the patient was a man; another, that the patient was a woman.
30. It is unclear what immediately happened to this "colored" woman who consumed Massengill's elixir, but she apparently survived. Her name is neither listed among the official fatalities, nor is it found in Arkansas death records for 1937. Significantly her name appears in the 1940 census record for Arkansas.
31. Anonymous. M'caskill child is first reported victim in state. *Hope Star.* October 27, 1937 (p 1, col 8). The paper also reported that Dr. Gentry exhumed the girl's body the day after her burial and conducted an autopsy. Her organs were sent to a pathologist in Little Rock.
32. Associated Press. Deaths from elixir pass half-hundred. *Laurel Leader-Call.* October 27, 1937.
33. Letter from Cesar A. Toro to The S. E. Massengill Co (New York City). October 23, 1937 (NARA, Box 934, Eastern District sulfanilamide correspondence).
34. Letter from S. E. Massengill Company to Mr. Toro. October 26, 1937 (NARA, Box 934, Eastern District sulfanilamide correspondence).
35. Anonymous. Agents speed up drug hunt as Georgia reports 5 deaths. *Atlanta Constitution.* October 26, 1937 (pp 1, 12).

Chapter 11: Passive Resistance or Deliberate Opposition

1. For background, see McManus JJ. Review and reminiscences—the Act of 1906. *Food Drug Cosmet Law J.* 1956;11:187-196; Young JH. The early food and drug inspector. *J His Med Allied Sci.* 1987;42:30-53; and US Department of Agriculture. *Directory of Organization and Field Activities of the Department of Agriculture.* Washington, DC: US Government Printing Office; February 1938. McManus also provided scattered reminiscences of his years with the FDA in the FDA Oral History Transcripts (Interview of John J. McManus and Clarence D. Schiffman by James Harvey Young, May 10, 1968).
2. Now known as the Martin Luther King, Jr., Federal Building.
3. A detailed and lengthy chronicle of the Atlanta Station's investigation of Elixir Sulfanilamide in Georgia, Florida, South Carolina, and North Carolina is

provided in a report from J. J. McManus to Chief, Eastern District (William J. Wharton). November 11, 1937 (FDA historical records). McManus wrote that members of the Atlanta Station were first alerted to the elixir-related deaths in Oklahoma and Mississippi by means of "brief" press reports on October 15th and 19th, respectively; however, these dates are likely premature, given that the first wire stories of the Tulsa deaths were not printed until October 19th. The first news reports of deaths in Mississippi, specifically in the *Laurel Leader-Call*, were printed on October 22nd.

4. For the FDA's investigation of this death, that of Arnette (or Anett) Lewis, see Appendix A and http://bmartinmd.com/elixir-sulfanilamide-deaths.html.

5. A more detailed description of the investigation of Leonard Dees in McManus's report indicates that the autopsy was actually performed on October 21st. For more information on this death, see Appendix A and http://bmartinmd.com/elixir-sulfanilamide-deaths.html.

6. In addition to McManus's report, information about the distribution and confiscation of Elixir Sulfanilamide in Florida (as well as in Georgia, North Carolina, and South Carolina) is supplemented by Part I, Elixir Sulfanilamide Investigation (NARA, Box 935, Central District Sulfanilamide Report).

7. In addition, one North Carolina doctor had received 24, two-ounce samples.

8. The Charleston deaths were those of 26-month-old Oscar Chisolm, three-year-old Ella Blanche Washington, 37-year-old Pearl Locklair, 10-year-old James Stewart, and 36-year-old Ward St. John O'Brien. See Appendix A and http://bmartinmd.com/elixir-sulfanilamide-deaths.html for further details.

9. For the paper's coverage, see Anonymous. 10 Georgians hunted in race to prevent elixir deaths. *Atlanta Constitution*. October 24, 1937 (pp 1A, 2A); Anonymous. 'Bottles of death' are object of nation-wide search. *Atlanta Constitution*. October 24, 1937 (p 2A); Anonymous. Federal agents meet difficulty in tracing drug. *Atlanta Constitution*. October 25, 1937 (p 1); Anonymous. Agents speed up drug hunt as Georgia reports 5 deaths. *Atlanta Constitution*. October 26, 1937 (pp 1, 3, col 4); and Anonymous. Drug toll climbs to 6 in Georgia. *Atlanta Constitution*. October 27, 1937 (pp 1, 9, col 2).

10. According to McManus's report, the one remaining elixir consignee in Florida (Capitol Pharmacy in Tallahassee) was not visited by inspectors until October 28th. It is presumed, but not recorded in the report, that the consignee was first contacted by phone, and investigators were informed that the pharmacy's supply of Elixir Sulfanilamide (one pint) had been returned intact to the manufacturer on October 19th (the amount received and return date were documented by McManus). In his interview for the FDA's Oral History project in 1979, Allan Rayfield recalled his role in the confiscation of Elixir Sulfanilamide: "I got a telegram [on October 20th] from Mr. McManus to phone the office. He told me what it was, who made it, and that there were several consignments in Jacksonville that he wanted me to investigate, and collect samples, and to report. He wanted me to do it that day, this was around noon time, and report back the end of the day, even at home." FDA Oral History Transcripts. Interview between Allan E. Rayfield and Robert G. Porter, May 1, 1979.

11. McManus wrote that Florida officials were involved in more than 75% of the state's elixir investigations, all of which were located in the far northern part of the state.

12. According to McManus's report, Rayfield began surveying vendors in southeast Georgia on October 21st. On that date, he visited by himself (without state support) two drug stores in Jesup (approximately 100 miles north of Jacksonville), two drug stores in Metter (about 70 miles north of Jesup), and a drug store in Swainsboro (about 25 miles northwest of Metter). An FDA agent, possibly Grey, returned to Jacksonville to collect the remaining three ounces of Cauley's prescription on October 29th. For details of the deaths in Florida, as determined later by the FDA, see Appendix A and http://bmartinmd.com/elixir-sulfanilamide-deaths.html.

13. McManus's report identified the name of the county health officer as "R. L. Smith." Alternative primary and secondary sources suggest that this physician may have been DeSaussure Dugas "Dessie" Smith.

14. Anonymous. Drug toll climbs to 6 in Georgia. *Atlanta Constitution.* October 27, 1937 (pp 1, 9, col 2). In the newspaper's October 26th edition ("Agents speed up drug hunt as Georgia reports 5 deaths"), Portwood was mistakenly identified as a "negro of Swainsboro."

15. Identified in FDA records as C. R. Williams, who was probably Charles Roy Williams, a white physician living in Wadley, according to the 1940 US census.

16. Anonymous. 10 Georgians hunted in race to prevent elixir deaths. *Atlanta Constitution.* October 24, 1937 (pp 1A, 2A).

17. These included a visit to a drug store in Murphy, North Carolina, just across the Georgia border.

18. To complete the investigation of Dr. West and his third elixir-consuming patient, Cochran, the FDA sent Inspector Simms to the doctor's office in mid-November. At that time, West claimed that Cochran said the elixir "was the best medicine he had ever taken." Through unexplained circumstances, Simms finally located Cochran, who was working as a stone crusher "10 miles back in the mountains." From Cochran, Simms learned a contradictory story: "Cochran did not praise the medicine, stating that each dose he had taken almost killed him, causing dizziness, weakness and a terrible backache, but that it had not effected [sic] his kidneys. When he had consumed the 4 ounces he had gone to another physician, and he stated that that was his reason for misleading Dr. West as to the effect of the medicine." See letter from J. J. McManus to Chief, Eastern District. November 16, 1937 (NARA, Box 934, Eastern District sulfanilamide correspondence).

19. The prescribing doctor, whose practice had "all the appearance of quackery" despite the fact that he was an AMA member, reported the FDA, was probably Ernest Monroe Perry. The FDA apparently did not complete its investigation of Dr. Perry's patients until April 1938, when the agency finally reported that three of the four elixir-consuming patients were "in good health"; however, the fourth patient, an adult schoolteacher, could not be found. Part I, Elixir Sulfanilamide Investigation (NARA, Box 935, Central District Sulfanilamide Report; letter from J. J. McManus to Chief, Eastern

District. November 16, 1937 (NARA, Box 934, Eastern District sulfanilamide correspondence).

20. Associated Press. Elixir round-up is accomplished. *News and Observer (Raleigh)*. October 28, 1937 (NARA, Box 933, sulfanilamide clippings).

21. John (not James) Thomas Tanner died at the age of 59 years at the Parkview Hospital on October 31, 1937. He became the last known American to have died of Elixir Sulfanilamide poisoning. For further details on this case, see Appendix A and http://bmartinmd.com/elixir-sulfanilamide-deaths.html. Repeated visits by Inspector Grey to Dr. Martin (and even interviews with the doctor's wife and son) failed to uncover the names of other possible elixir-treated patients.

22. The white patients were Susie Mae DeLoach and Harry M. Terry. For further details of their cases, see Appendix A and http://bmartinmd.com/elixir-sulfanilamide-deaths.html.

23. In actuality, McDaniel's South Carolina death certificate was not signed by any doctor. Written in faint ink under the cause-of-death section is, "Cause unknown no doctor."

24. A search of the death indexes for South Carolina and Georgia failed to return a death certificate for this Willie Badger.

25. As of December 6, 1937, an analysis of the bottle's contents had not been made by the FDA. See letter from W. G. Campbell to George Warren. December 6, 1937 (NARA, Box 931, Folder 501-.20S).

26. According to McDaniel's South Carolina death certificate, he was buried in Bush Cemetery in Hampton County. If McDaniel's grave was recognizable in the 1950s, it may have been moved along with the entire town of Ellenton, South Carolina, as a result of the construction of the Savannah River nuclear reservation.

27. Anonymous. Drug toll climbs to six in Georgia. *Atlanta Constitution.* October 27, 1937 (pp 1, 9, col 2).

28. Dr. Foster was out of town at the time of Henry's initial investigation of this prescription, on October 22nd. Sources for the investigation of Mrs. Weeks are McManus's official FDA report, along with two letters from J. J. McManus to Food and Drug Administration (Attention: Mr. [George] Larrick), dated November 6, 1937, and November 9, 1937, respectively (NARA, Box 931, Folder 501-.20S). McManus also recalled the investigation of Mrs. Weeks in Review and reminiscences—the Act of 1906. *Food Drug Cosmet Law J.* 1956;11:187-196. Although he misidentified the subject as "Lula Rakes."

29. The nurse was investigating the prescription for Mrs. Weeks at the instigation of Georgia's State Board of Health, which had been prompted to investigate Dr. Foster's prescription by Chief McManus about a week earlier.

30. The 1930 census for Cherry Log (in Gilmer County, Georgia) provides an entry for Kelley Weeks and his wife "Lola."

31. For details of the possible elixir-related death of this boy, J. C. Donalson, see Appendix A and http://bmartinmd.com/elixir-sulfanilamide-deaths.html.

32. This sale resulted in the death of a taxi driver from Millen. For further details of Inspector Rayfield's persistent and thorough investigation of this death, see

Appendix A and http://bmartinmd.com/elixir-sulfanilamide-deaths.html.
33. Anonymous. Drug recovered, fears subsiding, US toll put at 55. *Atlanta Constitution.* October 28, 1937 (p 4).

Chapter 12: Pursuing a Tiger With a Flyswatter

1. Anonymous. Makers of fatal elixir face $100 fine as penalty. *Chicago Daily News.* October 31, 1937 (p 15). The number of reported deaths was actually 59; however, the newspaper graphic omitted the lone death in Ohio (that of six-year-old Jo Anne Cramer) from its map.
2. Letter from W. G. Campbell to Chief, Central District. November 12, 1937 (NARA, Box 931, Folder 501-.20S).
3. Associated Press. Claims damages from medicine co. *Ada Evening News.* November 2, 1937 (p 2, col 5).
4. Anonymous. Two new moves in elixir suits. *Tulsa Daily World.* November 4, 1937.
5. United Press. Autopsy is ordered after elixir deaths. *Delta Star.* November 4, 1937 (p 1, col 1).
6. United Press. Victims of elixir set at sixty-one in medical report. *Atlanta Constitution.* November 3, 1937 (p 11).
7. AMA Chemical Laboratory. Elixir Sulfanilamide-Massengill: Part I—introduction. *J Am Med Assoc.* 1937;109:1531; Schoeffel EW, Kreider HR, Peterson JB. Part II: chemical examination of Elixir of Sulfanilamide-Massengill. *J Am Med Assoc.* 1937;109:1532; Geiling EMK, Coon JM, Schoeffel EW. Part III: preliminary report of toxicity studies on rats, rabbits, and dogs. *J Am Med Assoc.* 1937;109:1532-1536; Cannon PR. Part IV: pathologic effects following the ingestion of diethylene glycol, Elixir of Sulfanilamide-Massengill, "synthetic" elixir of sulfanilamide and sulfanilamide alone. *J Am Med Assoc.* 1937;109:1536-1537; Ruprecht HA, Nelson IA. Part V: clinical and pathologic observations. *J Am Med Assoc.* 1937;109:1537; Hagebusch OE. Part VI: necropsies of four patients following administration of Elixir of Sulfanilamide-Massengill. *J Am Med Assoc.* 1937;109:1537-1538; AMA Chemical Laboratory. Part VII: survey of deaths. *J Am Med Assoc.* 1937;109:1539; AMA Chemical Laboratory. Part VIII: conclusions. *J Am Med Assoc.* 1937;109:1539. Complementary articles in the same *JAMA* issue confirmed the relative toxicity of diethylene glycol in rats (the toxicity was somewhere between that of ethylene glycol and propylene glycol) and sulfanilamide's putative mechanism of antibacterial action. See respectively, Holck HGO. Glycerin, ethylene glycol, propylene glycol and diethylene glycol. *J Am Med Assoc.* 1937;109:1517-1520; and Bliss EA, Long PH. Observations on the mode of action of sulfanilamide. *J Am Med Assoc.* 1937;109:1524-1528.
8. In laboratory rats, a dosage of one cubic centimeter (cc) per kilogram (kg) three times daily (3 cc/kg/day) began to reliably produce toxic effects. This weight-based, experimental dosage of Elixir Sulfanilamide was considerably proportionally higher than the recommended dosages taken by human victims. Massengill's directions were to take two to three teaspoons (about 10-

15 cc) of elixir in water every four hours for the first 24-48 hours and then to decrease the dose to one to two teaspoons (about 5-10 cc) every four hours. Therefore, for a 70-kg man, the recommended divided dosage of Elixir Sulfanilamide ranged from about 0.07 to 0.21 cc/kg six times daily (or 0.42-1.26 cc/kg/day). This weight-based dosage, of course, would be higher in children.

9. Anonymous. Deaths following Elixir of Sulfanilamide-Massengill: III. *J Am Med Assoc*. 1937;109:1544-1545.

10. Anonymous. Food and drugs legislation. *J Am Med Assoc*. 1937;109:1546.

11. The *JAMA* editorial referred to the bill as the "Tugwell-Copeland bill of the [73rd] Congress and passing through various phases in the [74th] and [75th] Congress." The congressional bill championed by Senator Copeland in 1937 was actually known eponymically as the Copeland-Chapman bill, or S. 5 no. 2. This bill was a highly moderated version of the original Tugwell-Copeland bill (S. 1944), which had been introduced by Copeland in the spring of 1933 at a session of the 73rd Congress. For further discussion, see Chapter 14.

12. Anonymous. Sulfanilamide elixir deaths bring demand for US curb. *St. Louis Post-Dispatch*. November 2, 1937 (p 1A).

13. Letter from W. G. Campbell to Dr. George A. Denison. November 6, 1937 (NARA, Box 931, Folder 501-.20S).

14. Dutcher R. Behind the scenes in Washington. *Ames Daily Tribune*. November 8, 1937 (p 4, cols 6, 7).

15. Herzog SA. The first authentic digest of new state laws affecting pharmacy: January 1935 to October 1936. *American Druggist*. 1936;94:46,47,136,138, 140,142,144,146,148.

16. Anonymous. '36 law is barrier to fatal elixir. *New Orleans Tribune*. October 20, 1937 (NARA, Box 931, sulfanilamide clippings). In the news article, an analyst for the Louisiana health board, Cassius L. Clay, claimed that diethylene glycol had been banned in the state as a substitute for glycerin in food products, because it was feared to be poisonous. On November 3, 1937, Clay wrote to FDA Chief Campbell, stating that Elixir Sulfanilamide had been shipped illegally into the state. There was no record of the product's submission for registration (NARA, Box 934, miscellaneous correspondence on sulfanilamide).

17. Anonymous. State health law praised by Campbell. *Ruston Daily Leader*. November 20, 1937 (p 1, col 2). The New York City *Herald Tribune* also claimed, "Untried remedies are under rigid control in New York City to guard against deaths such as those attributed lately to a sulfanilamide preparation in the West." Specifically a patent medicine could not be sold in the city until it had been registered with the local health department. See Anonymous. City has its own restrictions on sale of medical remedies. *Herald Tribune*. October 31, 1937 (NARA, Box 933, sulfanilamide clippings). However, it did not appear that Massengill ever complied with the municipal law, or that there was any reliable way to enforce the regulation generally.

18. Anonymous. The deadly "elixir." *Drug Cosmet Ind*. 1937;41:611; Anonymous. The "elixir" and the industry. *Drug Cosmet Ind*.

1937;41:614,615,619. In a separate source, an unnamed Kansas City pharmacologist said that an "elixir of sulfanilamide has been sought almost since sulfanilamide first was placed on the market in the United States two years ago." Anonymous. Details of deadliness of sulfanilamide revealed in comprehensive news story. *Amarillo Globe.* November 17, 1937 (p 7, cols 2-5).

19. Anonymous. Pharmaceutical tragedy. *St. Louis Post-Dispatch.* November 9, 1397 (p 2C). (Editorial reprinted from the *Oil, Paint and Drug Reporter.*)

20. Anonymous. Fatal remedy. *Time.* November 1, 1937;30(18):61.

21. Associated Press. $50,000 is asked in 'elixir' death. *Atlanta Constitution.* November 13, 1937 (p 9); United Press. First suit for elixir death filed. *Delta Star.* November 13, 1937 (p 1, col 4); and Associated Press. Sues firm that sold sulfanilamide elixir. *Bristol Herald Courier.* November 13, 1937 (p 3, col 2). The wire report in Massengill's hometown newspaper, the *Bristol Herald Courier,* merely identified the plaintiffs in the suit as a Memphis drug store and "the manufacturer."

22. Anonymous. Life on the American newsfront: bad medicine leaves trail of dead patients. *Life.* November 8, 1937 (p 33). All but one photograph in the pictorial was credited to Mississippi author Eudora Welty (p 112). See also, McHaney PA, ed. *Eudora Welty as Photographer.* Jackson, MS: University Press of Mississippi; 2009: 16.

23. Parsons LO. Elixir deaths used as basis of new films. *Chicago Herald and Examiner.* October 30, 1937 (p 14) (NARA, Box 933, sulfanilamide clippings). The *New York Times* later reported that the Warner Brothers film was retitled *One Hundred Million Suckers.* Larry Kimble and Ring Lardner, Jr., were writing the screenplay (Anonymous. Screen news here and in Hollywood. *New York Times.* March 18, 1938 [p 23]). No film, however, appears to have made it to production.

24. Letter from F. C. Sinton to D. M. Walsh forwarded to Chief, Eastern District. October 29, 1937 (NARA, Box 934, Eastern District sulfanilamide correspondence).

25. Associated Press. All sulfanilamide removed from reach. *Ada Evening News.* November 15, 1937 (p 4, cols 2, 3).

26. Letter from Frank W. DeFriece to Dr. Morris Fishbein. November 13, 1937; letter from Paul Nicholas Leech to Frank W. DeFriece. November 17, 1937; letter from Paul Nicholas Leech to Mr. Campbell. November 17, 1937 (all in NARA, Box 934, miscellaneous correspondence on sulfanilamide).

27. Anonymous. Details of deadliness of sulfanilamide revealed in comprehensive news story. *Amarillo Globe.* November 17, 1937 (p 7, cols 2-5).

28. The use of diethylene glycol as a humectant in cigarettes was promoted by a number of manufacturers, including Philip Morris, in the 1930s and later. For a discussion of the use of scientific studies, including those with diethylene glycol, to support health claims in the marketing of cigarettes, see Garner MN, Brandt AM. "The Doctor's Choice Is America's Choice": the physicians in US cigarette advertisements, 1930-1953. *Am J Public Health.* 2006;96:222-232.

29. Old Timer. "Time" article is unfair to Massengill Company, one of leading drug manufacturers. *Bristol Herald Courier.* November 21, 1937 (p 1, col 1). The Bristol Chamber of Commerce wrote a rebuttal letter to the editors of *Time*, parroting much the same objections. See Pully, DeFriece (p 168).
30. Leech PN, AMA Chemical Laboratory. Elixir of Sulfanilamide-Massengill: II. *J Am Med Assoc.* 1937;109:1724-1725.

Chapter 13: The Baby I Grieve for Day and Night

1. Wallace report. The report was produced in response to Senate resolution 194 of November 16, 1937 (submitted by Senator Copeland), and House resolution 352 of November 18, 1937.
2. Specifically Charles "Charley" Crawford, Principal Chemist in charge of the FDA's Interstate Division, according to then-Assistant Chief and later FDA Commissioner Paul Dunbar. At the time, Crawford was becoming a recognized go-to source within the agency for legislative drafting. Dunbar PB. Memories of early days of federal food and drug law enforcement. *Food Drug Cosmetic Law J.* 1959;14:87-138.
3. From October 20th to November 17th, 25 libels were filed in 15 district courts by US attorneys "praying seizure and condemnation of 47 gallon bottles, 603 pint bottles, 12 eight-ounce bottles and 103 sample bottles of elixir sulfanilamide in various lots" at New York, NY; San Francisco, CA; San Juan, Puerto Rico; Jackson, MS; Church Road and Richmond, VA; Salisbury, MD; Detroit, Highland Park, and Dearborn, MI; Alton, Cisne, and East St. Louis, IL; Fort Worth, TX; Williston and Hampton, SC; Wainsboro, Swainsboro, Wrens, and McDonough, GA; Bristol, TN; and Kansas City, MO. See *US v 5 Gallons and 3 Pints of Elixir Sulfanilamide (and 24 other seizure actions against the same product).* Adulteration and misbranding of elixir sulfanilamide (28324). FDA Notices of Judgment collection.
4. Wallace perhaps undermined his case for new legislation by then overreaching: "It is worthy of note that, shocking as these instances have been, the actual toll in deaths and permanent injury from potent drugs is probably far less than that resulting from harmless nostrums offered for serious disease conditions. In these cases the harmful effect is an indirect one. Sick people rely on false curative claims made for worthless concoctions, and thus permit their disease to progress unchecked. It may be too late when they lose confidence in the nostrum and seek rational treatment," he offered.
5. Anonymous. 'Death drug' hunt covered 15 states. *New York Times.* November 26, 1937 (p 42, col 1).
6. Anonymous. 'Elixir' report urges control of new drugs. *Washington Post.* November 26, 1937 (p 3).
7. Associated Press. Stronger drug law requested. *Beckley Post-Herald.* November 26, 1937 (p 5, col 1); United Press. Drug safety laws sought. *El Paso Herald-Post.* November 26, 1937 (p 9, col 3); International News

Service. More 'teeth' in federal food, drug laws asked. *Charleston Gazette (West Virginia)*. November 26, 1937 (p 1, cols 2, 3; p 6, cols 2, 3).

8. United Press. Food law to be strengthened. *Bakersfield Californian*. November 26, 1937 (p 2, col 5).

9. Associated Press. Copeland asks drug ban. *Niagara Falls Gazette*. December 1, 1937 (p 26, col 6).

10. Anonymous. Reform the drug law! *St. Louis Post-Dispatch*. November 27, 1937 (p 4A, col 2).

11. Associated Press. Legislation favored control new drugs. *Kingsport Times*. November 26, 1937 (p 3, col 5).

12. Anonymous. Massengill avers false statements made about elixir. *Bristol Herald Courier*. November 27, 1937 (p 1). Massengill's rebuttal, with a less strident headline, was also published in the *Bristol News Bulletin* (Anonymous. Dr. Massengill in defense of sulfanilamide. *Bristol News Bulletin*. November 27, 1937 [p 7, col 1]).

13. American Medical Association. *New and Nonofficial Remedies, 1937*. Chicago, IL: American Medical Association; 1937: 115-116.

14. Winthrop Chemical. Advertisement for Luminal Sodium. *Can Med Assoc J*. 1937;36(6);xi.

15. American Medical Association. *New and Nonofficial Remedies, 1935*. Chicago, IL: American Medical Association; 1935: 132-133.

16. E. R. Squibb and Sons. Advertisement for Neoarsphenamine Squibb. *Bull N Y Acad Med*. 1939;15(11):viii.

17. See for instance, Hanzlik PJ, Barnett CW, Richardson AP. Modified composition of iodobismitol. *Arch Derm Syphilol*. 1935;32:284-287.

18. American Medical Association. *New and Nonofficial Remedies, 1939*. Chicago, IL: American Medical Association; 1939: 126-127.

19. Letter from W. G. Campbell to Mrs. Maise Nidiffer. November 30, 1937 (NARA, Box 931, Folder 501-.20S).

20. Anonymous. Massengill and firm endorsed by doctors. *Bristol Herald Courier*. December 2, 1937 (pp 1, 2).

Chapter 14: Drafting a Sane, Sensible, Workable Bill

1. Chief support for the antecedent history and ultimate enactment of the Federal Food, Drug, and Cosmetic Act of 1938 (FDCA) is derived from Charles O. Jackson's definitive *Food and Drug Legislation in the New Deal* (Princeton, NJ: Princeton University Press; 1970)), and readers are urged to refer to his work for authoritative details and primary sources on the subject. Reference here is also made to Dunn CW. *Federal Food, Drug, and Cosmetic Act: A Statement of Its Legislative History*. New York, NY: G. E. Stechert and Company; 1938; and Cavers DF. The Food, Drug, and Cosmetic Act of 1938: its legislative history and its substantive provisions. *Law Contemp Prob*. 1939;6:1-42. A more recent, albeit abbreviated, source for the enactment of the FDCA may be found in Carpenter D. *Reputation and Power: Organizational Image and Pharmaceutical Regulation at the FDA*. Princeton, NJ: Princeton University Press; 2010: 73-117.

2. Associated Press. Copeland asks drug ban. *Niagara Falls Gazette.* December 1, 1937 (p 26, col 6).

3. Copeland obtained a medical doctorate from the University of Michigan in 1889 and served as a professor at the university's Homeopathic Medical College from 1895 to 1908. In fact, Harold Cole Watkins was a pharmacy student at the University of Michigan while Copeland served on the faculty; however, there is no indication that the paths of the two men ever crossed at the Ann Arbor campus.

4. *Senate Hearings on Food and Drugs Act* (1930), 1892-93. Cited in Jackson (p 15).

5. FDA correspondence from Ruth Lamb to James Rorty. April 11, 1934. Cited in Jackson (p 27).

6. Anonymous. Copeland revising Tugwell drug bill. *New York Times.* December 16, 1933 (p 4).

7. Anonymous. New foods and drugs legislation. *J Am Med Assoc.* 1933;101:1882-1883.

8. See Jackson (p 59) and Robins N. *Copeland's Cure: Homeopathy and the War Between Conventional and Alternative Medicine.* New York, NY: Alfred A. Knopf; 2005: 189-190, 200.

9. Anonymous. Conclude hearings on Pure Food Bill. *Zanesville Signal.* December 9, 1933 (p 1, col 1).

10. Anonymous. Tugwell bill opposition. *Billings Gazette.* January 1, 1934 (p 4, cols 1, 2).

11. Copeland's first rewrite of S. 1944 was S. 2000, the content of which was guided by the senator's discussions with trade interests. S. 2000 was introduced in the Senate on January 4, 1934, and became the hot target of organized criticism from the drug industry, despite concessions to it. The bill was thereafter altered in committee and renamed S. 2800 by Copeland to emphasize its distinction from S. 2000. See Jackson (pp 49-51).

12. Durno G. The national whirligig. *Sandusky Register.* February 9, 1934 (p 4, col 2).

13. Anonymous. The week. *The Nation.* 1934;77:264-265. Cited in Jackson (p 61).

14. Anonymous. The Tugwell-Copeland Pure Food, Drugs and Cosmetics Bill. *J Am Med Assoc.* 1934;102:696.

15. Anonymous. Copeland plans pure food bill. *New York Times.* January 15, 1935 (p 17).

16. Bureau of Legal Medicine and Legislation, American Medical Association. Food, drug, therapeutic device, and cosmetic legislation pending in Congress. *J Am Med Assoc.* 1935;105:2055-2062. To support the AMA's disapproval of S. 5, Jackson (pp 85-87) also cited the Senate testimony of Dr. William Woodward, director of the AMA's Bureau of Legal Medicine and Legislation, from March of 1935.

17. Anonymous. Roosevelt urges new pure food act. *New York Times.* March 23, 1935 (p 2).

18. Anonymous. Drug advertisers see threat in bill. *New York Times.* April 7, 1935 (p F12).

19. Chicago Tribune Press Service. Democrat leads fight in Senate on drug bill. *Chicago Daily Tribune.* April 4, 1935 (p 6).
20. Anonymous. Copeland balked again on drug bill. *New York Times.* April 6, 1935 (p 8).
21. Chicago Tribune Press Service. Congress may not act on new food and drug bill. *Chicago Daily Tribune.* April 9, 1935 (p 2).
22. Associated Press. Hope for drug bill rises. *New York Times.* May 5, 1935 (p 39).
23. Anonymous. Modified food and drug bill passes Senate. *Chicago Daily Tribune.* May 29, 1935 (p 5). According to Cavers (citing the Congressional Record), the bill was passed without a recorded vote. A notice in the *New York Times* indicated that the bill was passed by the Senate "without a record or dissenting vote" (Anonymous. May act this week on Copeland bill. *New York Times.* July 7, 1935 [p F9]).
24. Anonymous. 6 major bills left as Congress quits. *New York Times.* August 28, 1935 (p 10).
25. Anonymous. Early action seen on drug measure. *New York Times.* April 12, 1936 (p F9).
26. The FDA no longer lent out its Chamber of Horrors exhibit (owing to the risk of violating the 1919 Deficiency Appropriation Act), but it did provide various photographs and slides to requesting professional groups to demonstrate weaknesses of the 1906 law. Moreover the agency allowed the 1936 publication of the *American Chamber of Horrors* by Ruth Lamb, the FDA Information Officer; although the book was not an official publication of the FDA.
27. Particularly those stipulated by the Bailey amendment. See for instance, Anonymous. Food, drug, and cosmetic legislation. *J Home Econ.* 1936;28(3):176.
28. Anonymous. Food and drug bill adopted by House. *New York Times.* June 20, 1936 (p 7).
29. Woodward WC. Comments on the Copeland food, drugs, therapeutic device, and cosmetic bill. *J Am Med Assoc.* 1936;106:1896-1898.
30. Pease O. *Responsibilities of American Advertising.* New Haven, CT: Yale University Press; 1958: 123; Lamb to Mary Ross. June 12, 1936; and Consumers Union *Reports.* June 19, 1936. All cited in Jackson (p 121).
31. Correspondence from Campbell to Wallace. May 25, 1936. Cited in Jackson (p 122).
32. In 1935.
33. Anonymous. Congress closes shop with filibuster fatal for Guffey coal bill. *San Antonio Light.* June 21, 1936 (p 1, col 2; p 5, col 2).
34. Correspondence from Crawford to Cavers. June 25, 1936. Cited in Jackson (p 125).
35. Anonymous. New food and drug bill. *New York Times.* July 1, 1936 (p 46).
36. A companion bill in the House (H.R. 300) was concurrently launched by Representative Chapman. While both measures gave the FDA regulatory power over drug advertising, there were important differences—which were sources of confusion for interested spectators, including industry

representatives (See Anonymous. Copeland fosters altered drug bill. *New York Times.* Jan 7, 1937 [p 3]). Chief among these differences were clauses defining the penalties for misleading advertising. The Copeland bill merely stated that violators were subject to injunction, while Chapman's bill stipulated civil and criminal prosecution.

37. Anonymous. Drug bill weak, President fears. *New York Times.* February 24, 1937 (p 4).
38. Anonymous. Bolt on Roosevelt long threatened. *New York Times.* June 22, 1936 (p 3).
39. Anonymous. Food, drug bill voted by Senate. *New York Times.* March 10, 1937 (p 16); Associated Press. Senate passes Copeland food and drug bill. *Washington Post.* March 10, 1937 (p 3).
40. From January 1935 to October 1936, 92 drug-related laws had been passed in 39 states. Herzog SA. The first authentic digest of new state laws affecting pharmacy, January 1935 to October 1936. *American Druggist.* 1936;94:46,47,136,138,140,142,144,146,148.
41. Even the original Tugwell bill had been stripped of its drug-licensing provisions before it was introduced in the Senate by Copeland in 1933.
42. Anonymous. Bristol calls ads safety insurance. *New York Times.* December 8, 1937 (p 38). Bristol's primary point, however, was that public advertising of over-the-counter remedies represented an important form of consumer protection.
43. Anonymous. Drug producers told US licensing looms. *New York Times.* December 7, 1937 (p 46).
44. Anonymous. Congress and potent drug regulation. *Drug Cosmet Ind.* 1938;42(3):316.
45. United Press. Death elixir found in use by food firms. *Ogden Standard-Examiner.* December 9, 1937 (p A-8, col 6).
46. Anonymous. Poison flavorings are seized by US. *Washington Post.* December 11, 1937 (p 10); Associated Press. Fatal elixir's drug seized in Baltimore. *Evening Sun.* December 10, 1937 (latter in NARA, Box 931, sulfanilamide clippings). In the Associated Press report, FDA Assistant Chief Paul Dunbar revealed that the agency had known "for some time" of the use of diethylene glycol in flavoring extracts "but had no authority to prohibit it until the extent of its toxic qualities on humans was revealed through use of the sulfanilamide elixir." There were no known deaths in the United States from the contaminated extracts, but the agency reported "two or three" related fatalities in Canada. Editors of *Drug and Cosmetic Industry* lamented the aggressive tactics of the FDA in its seizure of the contaminated flavorings, writing in January of 1938: "There is as yet no definite evidence that these products have any cumulative toxic effect" (Anonymous. Glycols inspire FDA activity. *Drug Cosmet Ind.* 1938;42[1]:32-33).
47. By January 7, 1938, the FDA had obtained records of nine additional persons who had died after consuming Elixir Sulfanilamide (in addition to the 93 confirmed or probable elixir-related deaths described in Secretary Wallace's report of November 1937). At the time, the FDA concluded that at least four of these deaths were caused by Elixir Sulfanilamide. Letter from

W. G. Campbell to Dr. I. M. Rubinowitch. January 7, 1938 (NARA, Box 47).

48. Letter from J. J. McManus to Chief, Central District. December 13, 1937 (FDA historical files). For further details of this death, see Appendix A and http://bmartinmd.com/elixir-sulfanilamide-deaths.html.

49. Letter from R. D. Sherman to Chief, Central District (Death of Jerry Strickland). December 9, 1937; letter from R. D. Sherman to Chief, New Orleans Station (Death of Sallie Louise Brown). December 14, 1937; letter from R. D. Sherman to Chief, New Orleans Station (Death of Walter Bell). December 14, 1937; letter from R. D. Sherman to Chief, New Orleans Station (Death of Joe Hewitt). December 14, 1937; and letter from Roland D. Sherman to Chief, Central District (Death of William Corneel Howell). December 9, 1937 (all in FDA historical files). Inspector Sherman also recounted his investigations of these deaths for the FDA Oral History project in 1978; however, some details of his recollections do not agree with accounts in the official, contemporaneous reports. FDA Oral History Transcripts. Interview between Roland D. Sherman and Robert G. Porter, July 4, 1978. For further details of these deaths in Mississippi and Texas, see Appendix A and http://bmartinmd.com/elixir-sulfanilamide-deaths.html.

50. Associated Press. Sulfanilamide case before US board. *New York World Telegram.* December 16, 1937; Associated Press. US agents push new drug inquiry. *Tulsa Daily World.* December 16, 1937; and Anonymous. Dr. S. E. Massengill cited by US in elixir shipments. *Kansas City Journal-Post.* December 15, 1937 (all in NARA, Box 931, sulfanilamide clippings).

51. Anonymous. Drug firm paying on sulfanilamide elixir claims. *St. Louis Post-Dispatch.* December 10, 1937; Anonymous. Pays on elixir deaths. *Kansas City Star.* December 10, 1937; and Anonymous. $2000 claim paid for elixir death of St. Louis man. *St. Louis Star-Times.* December 10, 1937 (all in NARA, Box 931, sulfanilamide clippings).

52. Pully, DeFriece (p 168).

53. Associated Press. Sulfanilamide maker pays. *Kansas City Times.* December 22, 1937; Anonymous. Five elixir death claims settled here. *St. Louis Post-Dispatch.* December 28, 1937 (both in NARA, Box 931, sulfanilamide clippings).

Chapter 15: Simple Persecution

1. Associated Press. Denial is issued on adulteration. *Kingsport Times.* January 12, 1938 (p 1, col 6); Associated Press. Deny adulteration of fatal elixir of sulfanilamide. *Times Recorder (Ohio).* January 13, 1938 (p 1, col 8).

2. Letter from W. G. Campbell to the Solicitor. February 17, 1938 (NARA, Box 47).

3. In composite, elixir shipments from San Francisco (which resulted in one death) and those from New York City were considered a continuation of the violations originating from the company's Bristol headquarters. Therefore, the FDA did not advise prosecutions against Massengill in these jurisdictions.

P. B. Dunbar to Chief, Eastern District. February 11, 1938; W. G. Campbell to Chief, Western District. February 19, 1938 (both in NARA, Box 47).

4. It appeared that the FDA was wrestling with the basis of its charges against Massengill under the existing Food and Drugs Act. In a separate, contemporaneous letter, the FDA's Chief Medical Officer, Theodore Klumpp, wrote, "A manufacturer could market cyanide in instantly lethal doses and this Administration would have no power under the law to stop him unless in some way the drug was adulterated or misbranded." Theodore G. Klumpp to Dr. James K. Gray. January 28, 1938 (NARA, Box 47). Klumpp's statement undermined Campbell's argument to the Solicitor that a poisonous drug was adulterated on the mere basis that it was poisonous and not therapeutic.

5. Letter from W. G. Campbell to Chief, Central District. February 4, 1938 (NARA, Box 47).

6. Letter from W. G. Campbell to Chief, Central District (with enclosure of letter from C. Falstrom to FDA). January 31, 1938; letter from W. G. Campbell to Mr. C. Falstrom. January 31, 1938 (both in NARA, Box 47).

7. See for example, P. B. Dunbar to Lindsay, Young and Atkins. January 10, 1938; S. A. Postle to Mr. S. W. Polk. January 27, 1938; P. B. Dunbar to Lindsay, Young and Atkins. January 28, 1938; P. B. Dunbar to Lindsay, Young and Atkins. February 10, 1938; G. P Larrick to Mr. R. S. Young. March 4, 1938; P. B. Dunbar to Hill, Hill, Whiting, and Rives. May 2, 1938; and G. P. Larrick to Hon. B. W. Gearhart. September 21, 1938 (all in NARA, Box 47). When agent testimony was requested, the FDA's policy was to require a subpoena, and the agency would "consent to the taking of depositions of our employees when the information sought is not available through other sources, and when revelation of the information contained in the Department's file is not contrary to the public interest." (W. G. Campbell to Embry, Johnson, Crowe and Tolbert. March 9, 1938 [NARA, Box 47].) In December of 1937, a Bristol civic leader, writing to Senator Kenneth McKellar of Tennessee, urged the consolidation of damage suits against Massengill and that they be "called in the court at Greeneville, Tennessee." Harry L. Brown to Hon. Kenneth McKellar. January 3, 1938 (NARA, Box 47).

8. Anonymous. Massengill will face damage suit. *Kingsport Times.* March 11, 1938 (p 3, col 2).

9. Jackson (p 172).

10. Chicago Tribune Press Service. Roosevelt gets bill on control of advertising. *Chicago Daily Tribune.* March 15, 1938 (p 21); Anonymous. Wheeler-Lea bill passed by Senate. *New York Times.* March 15, 1938 (p 37).

11. Press release: "Remarks of Senator Royal Copeland Relative to the Conference on S. 1077." Cited in Jackson (p 173).

12. Regulation of prescription-drug advertising was finally transferred to the FDA with the passage of the Kefauver-Harris Drug Amendments in 1962.

13. Jackson (p 168).

14. Correspondence from Copeland to Lea. April 11, 1938. Cited in Jackson (p 176).

15. For instance, see Hoge JD. Effects of conflicting food and drug legislation. *Printer's Ink.* 1938;183:57,60. Cited in Jackson (p 177).
16. Anonymous. Drug control. *Washington Post.* April 4, 1938 (p X6).
17. Browning B. Women debate change in US Constitution. *Chicago Daily Tribune.* April 29, 1938 (p 5).
18. Anonymous. Drug bill opposed. *New York Times.* April 22, 1938 (p 34).
19. Associated Press. Death takes New York's Senator Royal Copeland. *Nebraska State Journal.* June 18, 1938 (p 1, col 1; p 4, col 3).
20. Cavers DF. The Food, Drug, and Cosmetic Act of 1938: its legislative history and its substantive provision. *Law Contemp Prob.* 1939;6:10.
21. Anonymous. Copeland's rise typifies America. *New York Times.* June 18, 1938 (p 3).
22. International News Service. US accuses maker of sulfanilamide. *El Paso Herald-Post.* June 3, 1938 (p 1, col 4). See also, *US v Samuel Evans Massengill (S. E. Massengill Co).* Adulteration and misbranding of Elixir of Sulfanilamide (29752). FDA Notices of Judgment collection. According to the government record, the Kansas City charges were based on 30 shipments, with multiple charges alleging adulteration and misbranding per shipment. Massengill's general counsel, Frank DeFriece, wrote that a capias was issued for Massengill in Kansas City on information "charging 95 shipments [...] with 3 counts on each shipment." DeFriece also claimed that, because Massengill was a resident of Tennessee, the Kansas City court could not serve process on the defendant. See Pully, DeFriece (pp 169-173 [Appendix 7]).
23. Associated Press. Manufacturer accused. *New York Times.* June 12, 1938 (p 14); Associated Press. Bristol druggist to face prosecution elixir cases. *Kingsport Times.* June 12, 1938 (p 1, cols 6, 7; p 8, col 1); and Associated Press. Federal charged lodged against Massengill Co. *Greeneville Sun.* June 13, 1938 (p 1, cols 3, 4). For reasons currently unknown to this writer, the Justice Department apparently did not agree with Campbell that chemist Watkins should also be prosecuted.
24. *United States of America v Samuel Evans Massengill, trading as The S. E. Massengill Company.* March term, 1938. National Archives, Atlanta Regional Archives Branch, RG21. US District Court, Eastern District of Tennessee, Greeneville Division. Criminal no. 4058. Box 105 at B/87/07/16. See also, *US v Samuel Evans Massengill (S. E. Massengill Co).* Adulteration and misbranding of Elixir of Sulfanilamide (29751). In FDA Notices of Judgment collection.
25. Theodore G. Klumpp to Mr. A. Singleton. May 10, 1938 (NARA, Box 47). See also an abstract for the proceedings at the 30th Annual Meeting of the American Society for Clinical Investigation, held in Atlantic City, New Jersey, on May 2, 1938. Klumpp TG, Calvery HO. The toxicity for human beings of diethylene glycol with sulphanilamide. *J Clin Invest.* 1938;17(4):520-521.
26. Anonymous. Massengill enters plea of not guilty. *Greeneville Sun.* June 14, 1938 (p 1, col 5); Associated Press. Massengill posts appearance bond. *Bristol Herald Courier.* June 14, 1938 (p 2, col 4).
27. DeFriece evidently used a penalty of $1,000, not $100, and one year of imprisonment per shipment to calculate Massengill's possible fine and

sentence from the federal government. DeFriece also calculated the total number of federal counts against Massengill at 261 (not 259), by adding 95 (not 93) and 166 counts out of Kansas City and Tennessee, respectively. See Pully, DeFriece (pp 169-173 [Appendix 7]). Text in the appendix indicates that DeFriece's rebuttal to the federal indictments was written in July of 1938: "About a month ago the Department of Justice in Washington proceeded in the Federal District Court in Kansas City to issue a capias for Massengill..."

28. DeFriece claimed that the government had counteroffered a settlement sum of $50,000 and then later $87,000.

29. P. B. Dunbar to Drug Division. July 23, 1938 (NARA, Box 47).

Chapter 16: To Secure Justice for the Public

1. Walter G. Campbell to Mr. Appleby. July 23, 1938 (NARA, Box 47). Campbell learned of DeFriece's allegation against FDA inspectors by way of a letter sent from Virginia Congressman John W. Flannagan, Jr., of Bristol, to the Executive Secretary of the Department of Agriculture. Despite Campbell's denial, it is reasonable to speculate that the FDA may have been looking for other, recent violations of the 1906 Food and Drugs Act by Massengill, to bolster the federal indictments and to exact greater penalties against the company because of a second violation of the federal law.

2. Ibid.

3. P. B. Dunbar to the Solicitor. August 31, 1938; memo re Dr. Kenneth M. Lynch. September 2, 1938 (both in NARA, Box 47).

4. Geiling EMK, Cannon PR. Pathologic effects of Elixir of Sulfanilamide (diethylene glycol) poisoning: a clinical and experimental correlation—final report. *J Am Med Assoc.* 1938;111:919-926.

5. Lynch KM. Diethylene glycol poisoning in the human. *South Med J.* 1938;31:134-137.

6. It should be noted that three of Dr. Lynch's cases were also considered in the human autopsy series of Geiling and Cannon.

7. *United States of America v Samuel Evans Massengill, trading as The S. E. Massengill Company.* March term, 1938. National Archives, Atlanta Regional Archives Branch, RG21. US District Court, Eastern District of Tennessee, Greeneville Division. Criminal no. 4058. Box 105 at B/87/07/16.

8. FDA. Federal Food and Drugs Act of 1906. Available at http://www.fda.gov/regulatoryinformation/legislation/ucm148690.htm. Last accessed August 13, 2013.

9. Nevertheless the government could possibly argue that diethylene glycol was an alcohol derivative; although this interpretation would directly contradict the FDA's basis for seizing Elixir Sulfanilamide in the first place.

10. *US v Samuel Evans Massengill (S. E. Massengill Co).* Adulteration and misbranding of Elixir of Sulfanilamide (29751). FDA Notices of Judgment collection. See also, *United States of America v Samuel Evans Massengill, trading as The S. E. Massengill Company.* March term, 1938. National Archives, Atlanta Regional Archives Branch, RG21. US District Court,

Eastern District of Tennessee, Greeneville Division. Criminal no. 4058. Box 105 at B/87/07/16.

11. Notably Judge Taylor cited the 1911 Supreme Court case of *US v Johnson*, a case that hinged on the failure of the 1906 law to address false or misleading advertising, as opposed to the accuracy of a drug label's ingredients.

12. Telegram (text) from P. B. Dunbar to Hartigan. September 14, 1938 (NARA, Box 47).

13. Associated Press. Druggist pleads guilty to charge. *Kingston Times.* October 3, 1938 (p 1, col 5); Anonymous. Massengill pleads guilty, is fined $16,800. *Greeneville Sun.* October 3, 1938 (p 1, col 8; p 6, cols 5, 6).

14. See endnote 10.

15. Anonymous. Deaths following Elixir of Sulfanilamide-Massengill: VIII. *J Am Med Assoc.* 1938;111:1567-1568.

16. W. G. Campbell to FDA, San Francisco [regarding October 19th telegram], October 20, 1937; letter from John L. Harvey to Western District Stations, October 20, 1937 (both in NARA, Box 934, miscellaneous correspondence on sulfanilamide).

17. Council on Pharmacy and Chemistry. Sulfanilamide solutions. *J Am Med Assoc.* 1937;109:1567.

18. A. G. Murray to Chief, Central District. December 14, 1937 (NARA, Box 931, Folder 501-.20S).

19. In 1939, Clarence A. Vogenthaler, working for Donley-Evans, filed a patent with the US government (US patent 2,252,822 [Serial No. 267,619]) for a "stable solution" of sulfanilamide at a concentration of approximately 5%. The proposed solvent was glucose "cut with glycerin," and the antibiotic was kept in solution through a "proper application of heat" followed by natural cooling. The patent application was a "continuation in part of an application for US patent filed [...] on October 1, 1937, Serial No. 166, 831." In 1942, the company announced that it was changing the name of its product (presumably along with its composition) from "Sulfanilamide with Citra-Lactate" to "Gluco-Sulfanilamide" (see Donley-Evans advertisement in *Am Prof Pharm.* 1942;8:194).

20. Christiansen WG, inventor; E. R. Squibb and Sons, assignee. Stable solutions of sulphanilamide. US patent 2,161,407. August 26, 1937.

21. Anonymous. Dr. S. E. Massengill president of Bristol's Chamber of Commerce: membership campaign opens. *Bristol News Bulletin.* January 10, 1939 (p 1, cols 5-7; p 10, cols 5-8).

22. Anonymous. H. C. Watkins victim wound. *Bristol News Bulletin.* January 17, 1939 (p 1, col 6); Anonymous. Harold Cole Watkins victim of gunshot. *Bristol Herald Courier.* January 18, 1939 (p 2, col 2); and Anonymous. Maker sulfanilamide formula is suicide. *Greeneville Sun.* January 19, 1939 (p 1, col 6). See also Tennessee death certificate no. 1921.

23. Watkins's widow claimed that the self-inflicted gunshot was an accident, not a suicide.

24. Correspondence from W. T. Ford to Chief, Cincinnati Station. July 21, 1938. Cited in Young JH. Sulfanilamide and diethylene glycol. In: Parascandola J, Whorton JC, eds. *Chemistry and Modern Society: Historical*

Essays in Honor of Aaron J. Ihde. Washington, DC: American Chemical Society; 1983: 105-125.

25. Pully, DeFriece (pp 162-164 [Appendix 5]).
26. To the widow, two children, and mother of Robert Montgomery Goode. Anonymous. Texas Citians given damages in poison case. *Galveston Daily News*. May 29, 1938 (p 21, col 8).
27. Anonymous. $2000 claim paid for elixir death of St. Louis man. *St. Louis Star-Times*. December 10, 1937 (NARA, Box 931, sulfanilamide clippings).
28. Court records for *Gibbons v Massengill* (1939); *Williams v Massengill* (1939); *Beard v Massengill* (1939); *Cauley v Massengill* (1940); *Voorhees v Massengill* (1940); and *Wilson v Massengill* (1942) are all housed at the National Archives Southeast Region. Atlanta, GA. See also, *Cauley v S. E. Massengill*, 35 F Supp 371 (ED Tenn 1940); *Wilson v Massengill*, 124 F2d 666 (6th Cir 1942); and *Massengill v Wilson*, 316 US 686; 62 S Ct 1274; 86 L Ed (US SC 1942).
29. A jury trial was waived by the plaintiff and defendant.
30. In 1967, DeFriece incorrectly stated that the last claim stemming from Elixir Sulfanilamide was settled by the company in 1939. See Pully, DeFriece (p 141).
31. Notably significant amounts of protein were not detected in urine samples taken at the time of the boy's illness.
32. Specifically there were no reports of BUN or creatinine levels in the blood. The assessment of liver function was performed after the child's convalescence by means of a galactose tolerance test and the assessment of bile in the stool. The results of both tests were normal or negative.
33. Dr. Helwig and another expert witness for the defendant, Dr. Robert M. Isenberger, both from the University of Kansas (Missouri) School of Medicine, reportedly performed numerous experiments on dogs with sulfanilamide, relatively high doses of diethylene glycol, and a mixture of the two compounds. In sworn depositions, they both testified that, among dogs surviving the ingestion of diethylene glycol, the livers and kidneys of the animals showed no abnormalities weeks or months later. A search of the medical literature failed to return any publications of these doctors' animal experiments with diethylene glycol.
34. Massengill's attorneys also attempted to imply during discovery that, whatever physical limitations the boy (whose estimated life expectancy was less than 49 years) may have suffered, they were due to an intervening case of laboratory-confirmed malaria.
35. Pully, DeFriece (pp 163-164).
36. Ibid (p 175).
37. Ibid (p 160).
38. Determined by searching the FDA Notices of Judgment collection.
39. *US v The S. E. Massengill Company*. Adulteration Bethiamin, Livitamin, and calcium gluconate (2204). FDA Notices of Judgment collection.
40. *US v 1,365 Jars*. Misbranding of Massengill powder (3475). FDA Notices of Judgment collection.

41. Hammer AR. Beecham, Ltd., plans acquisition offer for Massengill Co. *New York Times*. February 23, 1971 (p 49).
42. Dougherty P. Advertising: life salesmen get a pep talk—Massengill picks an agency. *New York Times*. April 30, 1970 (p 65).
43. Freudenheim M. SmithKline and Beecham in talks. *New York Times*. April 3, 1989 (pp D1, D5); Reuters. SmithKline, Beecham to merge. *Chicago Tribune*. April 13, 1989 (p A3).
44. See entries for King Pharmaceuticals in *Standard & Poor's Guide to Health Care, Pharmaceutical, and Biotech Stocks*. New York, NY: McGraw-Hill; 2003; and *International Directory of Company Histories*, Vol. 54. Detroit, MI: St. James Press; 2003. The purchase was actually made from RSR Pharmaceutical, which was housed at Bristol in the former site of Beecham Laboratories. Beecham had moved its headquarters to Philadelphia, after the merger with SmithKline.
45. In 2010, Pfizer purchased King Pharmaceuticals for $3.6 billion in cash and then announced a year later that it would cease manufacturing at the Bristol plant by 2014. De La Merced. Pfizer bids to buy King, a painkiller producer. *New York Times*. October 13, 2010 (p B3); Brown R. Pfizer ending manufacturing work at Bristol plant. *Bristol Herald Courier* [e-edition]. August 10, 2011. Available at http://www.tricities.com/news/article_dbb87c92-c5ba-551a-909d-f9518616fd66.html. Last accessed August 13, 2013. In May 2013, Maryland-based UPM Pharmaceuticals purchased the Bristol plant from Pfizer. Notably UPM CEO John Gregory was an original founder of King Pharmaceuticals. Palmer E. Pfizer sells King Pharma plant to UPM Pharmaceuticals. *Fierce Pharma Marketing*. Available at http://www.fiercepharmamanufacturing.com/story/pfizer-sells-king-pharma-plant-upm-pharmaceuticals/2013-05-30. Last accessed August 13, 2013.
46. Sorkin AR. Merger talks by SmithKline and Glaxo. *New York Times*. January 15, 2000 (p C1).
47. In January of 1969, the National Association of Broadcasters softened its Code Authority, by permitting the television advertising of feminine-hygiene products, including douches. See for instance Anonymous. Revised code flirts with rich new market. *Broadcasting*. 1969;76(3):25.
48. MMR/IRI H&BA Report. April 13, 2009.
49. Pully, DeFriece (p 164).
50. Ibid (p 129).
51. See deposition of Dr. Archie Calhoun in records for *Gibbons v Massengill*. National Archives Southeast Region. Atlanta, GA.
52. Anonymous. Thousands attend rites for Dr. H. H. Weathers, national known surgeon. *St. Louis American*. August 10, 1950 (pp 1, 16); Vaughn AN. St. Mary's Infirmary as a hospital for colored people. *J Natl Med Assoc*. 1938;30:16-17; and Kennedy JA. The Homer G. Phillips Hospital of St. Louis, Mo. *J Natl Med Assoc*. 1938;30:17-18.
53. Anonymous. Sews up heart, rare feat saves man's life. *Chicago Defender*. July 17, 1943 (p 1); Anonymous. Performs feat. *Chicago Defender*. July 24, 1943 (p 3).

54. Anonymous. Appoint 3 to faculty of St. Louis University. *Chicago Defender.* December 25, 1948 (p 1); Anonymous. University names three Negroes to medical faculty. *North Country Catholic Edition of Our Sunday Visitor.* January 2, 1949 (p 2A, cols 4, 5)
55. Anonymous. Doctors Hospital cofounder dies. *Tulsa World.* June 7, 1996.
56. W. G. Campbell to Distributors of Sulfanilamide and Related Drugs. August 26, 1938 (NARA, Box 47).
57. See Lesch JE. *The First Miracle Drugs: How the Sulfa Drugs Transformed Medicine.* New York, NY: Oxford University Press; 2007: 175, 180. According to Lesch, six US companies, including Merck, submitted their applications for sulfapyridine to the FDA. Sulfapyridine is also credited for saving the life of Winston Churchill in 1942, when the Prime Minister was suffering from pneumonia on a trip to North Africa.
58. Although toward the end of the war, the utility of sulfanilamide in these kits was questioned. The issue may have had something to do with the fact that GIs, in the heat of battle, didn't so much judiciously sprinkle the antibiotic on wounds as dump it on in a big clump.
59. The liberal, prophylactic use of sulfanilamide during World War II probably contributed to the development of antibiotic resistance.
60. For instance, with recognized inhibitors of folic acid, like methotrexate.

Chapter 17: Nothing to Prevent Incidents Like This Occurring in the Future

1. Calvery HO, Klumpp TG. The toxicity for human beings of diethylene glycol with sulfanilamide. *S Med J.* 1939;32:1105-1109. The authors also presented their preliminary report of 104 elixir-related deaths at the 30th Annual Meeting of the American Society for Clinical Investigation at Atlantic City, New Jersey, on May 2, 1938. See Klumpp TG, Calvery HO. The toxicity for human beings of diethylene glycol with sulphanilamide. *J Clin Invest.* 1938;17(4):520-521.
2. Klumpp and Calvery apparently did not perform analyses to determine the statistical difference, if any, between the mean cumulative doses consumed by the deceased victims and those taken by survivors.
3. Although it should be remembered that, in several cases, Elixir Sulfanilamide was compounded with other liquid medications at the direction of the prescribing physician. Therefore the mean volume of consumed diethylene glycol is probably overestimated.
4. In a contemporaneous report on the toxicity of glycols, published in May of 1939, FDA pharmacologists estimated that the LD50 of diethylene glycol in humans—meaning the dose at which 50% of a population is killed—was 1 mL per kilogram (mL/kg) of body weight (or about 0.015 fluid ounces per pound of body weight). For a person weighing 70 kg (approximately 154 pounds), the LD50 is therefore about 70 mL, or 2.4 ounces. By comparison, the lethal dose of ethylene glycol in humans was estimated to be, on the basis of case reports, about 100 mL. In animals, the LD50 for diethylene glycol was consistently lower than that for ethylene glycol, and ethylene glycol was more acutely toxic (Laug EP, Calvery HO, Morris HJ, Woodard G. The toxicology

of some glycols and derivatives. *J Ind Hyg Toxicol.* 1939;21:173-201). In the pharmacologists' calculation of the LD50 for diethylene glycol in humans, it is unclear if they accounted for the fact that Elixir Sulfanilamide was 72% diethylene glycol and thereby underestimated the LD50 of the solvent.

5. Linton FB. Leaders in food and drug law: part five. *Food Drug Law J.* 1995;50:49-58 (originally published in *Food Drug Cosmet Law J.* 1950;5:771.) Linton based his projected death tally on the total volume consumed, estimated at about six gallons, by 107 deceased.

6. Geiling EMK, Cannon PR. Pathologic effects of Elixir of Sulfanilamide (diethylene glycol) poisoning: a clinical and experimental correlation—final report. *J Am Med Assoc.* 1938;111:919-926.

7. According to the August 28, 2006, issue of *Chemical Market Reporter* (http://www.icis.com/chemicals/channel-info-chemicals-a-z/), the price of pharmaceutical grade glycerin was approximately three times higher than that of diethylene glycol ($0.84-$1.25 versus $0.39 per pound, respectively).

8. Bowie MD, McKenzie D. Diethylene glycol poisoning in children. *S Afr Med J.* 1972;46:931-934.

9. Cantarell MC, Fort J, Camps J, Sans M, Piera L. Acute intoxication due to topical application of diethylene glycol. *Ann Intern Med.* 1987;106:478-479.

10. Both diethylene glycol and diethylene glycol stearate (essentially diethylene glycol linked up with a fatty acid) were present in the ointment.

11. Blau R. US warns about deadly chemical in Austrian wine. *Chicago Tribune.* July 24, 1985 (p A2); Prial FJ. Wine talk: Austrian wine contaminated with antifreeze is discovered in Washington and Chicago. *New York Times.* July 24, 1985 (p C10); Siegart A. Poison scandal contaminates market for wine. *Chicago Tribune.* July 29, 1985 (p 20); Tagliabue J. Scandal over poisoned wine embitters village in Austria. *New York Times.* August 2, 1985 (p A1); Molotsky I. US finds poison in 12 brands of wine imported from Austria. *New York Times.* August 2, 1985 (p A6); Molotsky I. Testing Austrian wine taxes staff of US lab. *New York Times.* August 3, 1985 (p 5); Reuters. Austrian scandal grows. *New York Times.* August 6, 1985 (p B11); Curry K. Doctored wine: Rx mostly harmless, within limits. *Chicago Tribune.* August 15, 1985 (p G30); Curry KN. Toxic chemical scandal in European wines expands. *Chicago Tribune.* August 22, 1985 (p F13E); Anonymous. List of tainted imported wines grows. *New York Times.* August 28, 1985 (p C12); Reuter. Austria's wine laws tighten in scandal. *New York Times.* August 30, 1985 (p A3); Anonymous. Those contaminated wines. *New York Times.* August 30, 1985 (p B6); Goldberg HG. US tests for tainted wines continue. *New York Times.* October 16, 1985 (p C12); Reuters. Austrian wine dealer guilty. *Chicago Tribune.* October 18, 1985 (p 26); Reuters. Austrian wine controls. *New York Times.* October 30, 1985 (p C16); Molotsky I. Popular wines found to hold toxic chemical. *New York Times.* November 1, 1985 (p A16); Anonymous. US tests for 3 chemicals. *New York Times.* November 6, 1985 (p C16); Associated Press. Chemical found in more wines. *New York Times.* November 9, 1985 (p 32); Reuters. German tests conclude on adulterated wines. *New York Times.* March 19, 1986 (p C15); Molotsky I. Study faults US response to 1985 wine threat. *New York Times.* April 12,

1986 (p 9); Molotsky I. Antifreeze poison found in 10 wines. *New York Times*. April 16, 1986 (p C10); Steyer RW. Drama behind a wine crisis. *New York Times*. May 18, 1986 (p LI12); Anonymous. Alcohol agency warns of highly tainted brand of Austrian wine. *New York Times*. June 17, 1986 (p A19); Goldberg HG. Testing confirms safety. *New York Times*. August 6, 1986 (p C8); and Anonymous. Austria battles to recover from wine scandal. *Los Angeles Times*. September 28, 1986 (p 8).

12. Most of the implicated imported wines were Austrian labels. German wines were likely contaminated in the process of making blends with the intentionally laced Austrian wines, and wines with only trace amounts of the solvent (for instance, implicated Italian wines) were suspected to have been inadvertently contaminated through tainted equipment.

13. A brief news item in *The Lancet*, published August 3, 1985, indicated that the highest yet-detected concentration of diethylene glycol in Austrian wine was three grams per liter (g/L), and that a single lethal dose of the toxin in humans was about one gram per kilogram (g/kg) (Anonymous. Some wine to break the ice. *Lancet*. 1985;326:254).

14. A preliminary Dutch report, published in September of 1985, suggested that the contaminated wine had not caused any major kidney abnormalities in identified consumers (van der Linden-Cremers PMA, Sangster B. Medical sequelae of the contamination of wines with diethylene glycol [Dutch]. *Ned Tijdschr Geneeskd*. 1985;129:1890-1891). However, a later report suggested that at least one case of significant nephrotoxicity, in a 54-year-old man, was due to the consumption of diethylene glycol–tainted wine (Van Leusen R, Uges DRA. A patient with acute necrosis of the renal tubules due to consumption of wine containing diethylene glycol [Dutch]. *Ned Tijdschr Geneeskd*. 1987;131:768-771). In 1995, Hanif et al indicated that 21 cases of renal impairment in The Netherlands were due to the tainted Austrian wine. They cited *The Lancet* news item and two Dutch articles as support (Hanif M, Mobarak MR, Ronan A, Rahman D, Donovan JJ, Jr, Bennish ML. Fatal renal failure caused by diethylene glycol in paracetamol elixir: the Bangladesh epidemic. *BMJ*. 1995;311:88-91).

15. Pandya SK. An unmitigated tragedy. *BMJ*. 1988:297:117-119. The glycerin, a hyperosmolar agent, was presumably administered to reduce intracranial pressure. See for instance, Frank MS, Nahata MC, Hilty MD. Glycerol: a review of its pharmacology, pharmacokinetics, adverse reactions, and clinical use. *Pharmacotherapy*. 1981;1:147-160.

16. Anonymous. Acute renal failure secondary to ingestion of adulterated paracetamol syrup, Plateau and Oyo States, June-September 1990. *Nigeria Bull Epidemiol*. 1991;1:5-7. See also, Okuonghae HO, Ighogboja IS, Lawson JO, Nwana EJC. Diethylene glycol poisoning in Nigerian children. *Ann Trop Pediatr*. 1992;12:235-238.

17. Hanif M, Mobarak MR, Ronan A, Rahman D, Donovan JJ, Jr, Bennish ML. Fatal renal failure caused by diethylene glycol in paracetamol elixir: the Bangladesh epidemic. *BMJ*. 1995;311:88-91.

18. According to a 2007 *New York Times* report, pediatrician Michael L. Bennish (the anchor author of the 1995 *BMJ* article) had to smuggle samples

of the contaminated syrup out of Bangladesh in a suitcase for testing in the United States. See Bogdanich W, Hooker J. From China to Panama, a trail of poisoned medicine. *New York Times*. May 6, 2007 (p 1).

19. On October 19, 2011, the Bangladeshi *Daily Star* reported that "all documents" relating to the adulteration of the acetaminophen syrup in early 1990s had "vanished from the Directorate General of Drug Administration (DGDA), the public institution responsible for checking drug adulteration and prosecuting those committing the crime." The outcomes of "three relevant cases" against drug manufacturers (two of which were under "High Court stay orders" and the hearings for which had been pending for 17 years) hinged on the availability of the records, which were "deliberately destroyed" by the DGDA, the paper alleged. The write-up further revealed that the tainted syrup had been created by five companies in 1992. Some interviewed doctors who were involved in the 1992 investigation claimed that adulteration of the drug had begun as early as 1972 and had killed more than 2,000 children over the course of 20 years.

20. Ferrari LA, Giannuzzi L. Clinical parameters, postmortem analysis and estimation of lethal dose in victims of a massive intoxication with diethylene glycol. *Forensic Sci Int*. 2005;153:45-51. See also, Anonymous. Natural tonic poisoning death toll reaches 20. *Houston Chronicle*. August 21, 1992 (p 12); Anonymous. 20 die, 17 injured in natural tonic poisoning. *New Mexican*. August 21, 1992 (p A2, col 1). The pathologic findings of seven victims were reported by Drut R, Quijano G, Jones MC, Scanferla. Hallazgos patologicos en la intoxicacion por dietilenglicol. *Medicina (Buenos Aires)*. 1994;54:1-5.

21. By weight per volume. In their toxicologic study of 15 adult victims, Ferrari and Giannuzzi estimated that the lethal dose of diethylene glycol in humans was very small, from 0.014 to 0.170 mg/kg of body weight, especially when compared with the LD50 calculated by FDA pharmacologists after the Elixir Sulfanilamide disaster (1.12 g/kg). However, a subsequent letter to the editor by Schep and Slaughter indicated that Ferrari and Giannuzzi had underestimated the lethal dose of diethylene glycol by a factor of 1,000 (meaning, the estimated LD50 was actually 0.014-0.170 g/kg). The letter writers argued that the corrected range (although still relatively low) better approximated the LD50 reported in 1939. See Schep LJ, Slaughter RJ. Comments on diethylene glycol concentrations. *Forensic Sci Int*. 2005;155:233.

22. Bogdanich W. A toxic pipeline: hunting an elusive killer—as FDA tracked poisoned drugs, a winding trail went cold in China. *New York Times*. June 17, 2007 (p 1).

23. Baffi P, Elneser S, Baffi M, De Melin M. Quantitative determination of diethylene glycol contamination in pharmaceutical products. *J AOAC Int*. 2000;83:793-801.

24. Centers for Disease Control and Prevention. Fatalities associated with ingestion of diethylene glycol-contaminated glycerin used to manufacture acetaminophen syrup—Haiti, November 1995-June 1996. *MMWR Morb Mortal Wkly Rep*. 1996;45:649-650; O'Brien KL, Selanikio JD, Hecdivert C, et al. Epidemic of pediatric deaths from acute renal failure caused by

diethylene glycol poisoning. *JAMA*. 1998;279:1175-1180; and Junod SW. Diethylene glycol deaths in Haiti. *Public Health Rep*. 2000;115:78-86. For an investigative, journalistic report of the Haiti investigation, see Bogdanich W. A toxic pipeline: hunting an elusive killer—as FDA tracked poisoned drugs, a winding trail went cold in China. *New York Times*. June 17, 2007 (p 1).

25. The median consumed dose of the toxic solvent among 32 affected children was calculated at 1.34 mL/kg (range, 0.22-4.42 mL/kg); however, toxic doses were often less than 1 mL/kg, the investigators noted.

26. The implication being, the records had been destroyed. In 2007, the *New York Times* reported that the Tianhong Fine Chemicals Factory had also shipped about 50 tons of tainted glycerin to the United States in 1995. Recipients included a Chicago-based supplier of bulk pharmaceuticals and nonmedicinal products. The supplier reportedly detected the diethylene glycol before passing it on to an unsuspecting buyer. The FDA denied knowledge of the incident (Bogdanich W, Hooker J. From China to Panama, a trail of poisoned medicine. *New York Times*. May 6, 2007 [p 1]). In October of 2007, the *New York Times* provided a brief update of the Haitian episode, stating that "Chinese authorities took no action" against the Tianhong Fine Chemicals Factory or the "giant state-owned trader, Sinochem International Chemicals," which had exported the diethylene glycol–tainted glycerin (Bogdanich W. Chinese chemicals flow unchecked to market. *New York Times*. October 31, 2007 [p A1]).

27. Singh J, Dutta AK, Khare S, et al. Diethylene glycol poisoning in Gurgaon, India, 1998. *Bull World Health Organ*. 2001;79:88-95.

28. Hari P, Jain Y, Kabra SK. Fatal encephalopathy and renal failure caused by diethylene glycol poisoning. *J Trop Pediatr*. 2006;52:442-444.

29. Haramburu F. Plantes: suspension d:AMM du Pilosuryl. *Bulletin d'information du Département de Pharmacologie du CHU de Bordeaux*. 2003;57(July-August); Haramburu F. Pilosuryl: un nouveau cas d'insuffisance rénale. *Bulletin d'information du Département de Pharmacologie du CHU de Bordeaux*. 2003;58(September). In January 2004, the sale of an herbal diuretic, Urosiphon, was also suspended because it contained diethylene glycol monoethyl ether (Haramburu F. Urosiphon: suspension d'AMM. *Bulletin d'information du Département de Pharmacologie du CHU de Bordeaux*. 2004;63[February]).

30. Vial T, Harry P, Eftekhart P, et al. Severe toxicity due to a drug containing diethylene glycol ethyl-ether as an excipient: report of six cases. *Fundam Clin Pharmacol*. 2004;18:218. Abstract O-24. In 2006, the Scientific Committee on Consumer Products of the European Commission determined that "the use of diethylene glycol monoethyl ether (DEGEE) in all cosmetic products, except products for oral hygiene and eye products at a concentrations [sic] up to 1.5% does not pose a risk to the health of the consumer, provided that the level of ethylene glycol in DEGEE used is <0.2%. The opinion relates to the dermal application. It does not include any other cosmetic exposure, such as exposure from possible aerosol/spray products." Scientific Committee on Consumer Products (SCCP). Opinion on diethylene glycol monoethyl ether (DEGEE). December 19, 2006.

31. Lin B-L, Zhao Z-X, Chong Y-T, et al. Venous diethylene glycol poisoning in patients with preexisting severe liver disease in China. *World J Gastroenterol.* 2008;14:3236-3241; Peng XM, Huang MX, Gu L, Lin BL, Chen GH. Characteristics of patients with liver disease intravenously exposed to diethylene glycol in China 2006. *Clin Toxicol.* 2009;47:124-131; and Luo M-Y, Lin B-L, Gao Z-L. Clinical features, laboratory findings and imaging appearances of venous diethylene glycol poisoning in patients with liver disease. *Chinese Med J.* 2009;122:2315-2320.

32. In 2008, the *New York Times* reported "at least 18" deaths due to the tainted drug. Hooker J, Bogdanich W. Tainted drugs linked to maker of abortion pill. *New York Times.* 31 January 31, 2008 (p A1).

33. The tainted version of armillarisin-A was recently introduced by the company as a result of price bidding, which was sponsored by the local Chinese government (Peng XM, Huang MX, Gu L, Lin BL, Chen GH. Characteristics of patients with liver disease intravenously exposed to diethylene glycol in China 2006. *Clin Toxicol.* 2009;47:124-131). In 2007, the *New York Times* reported that Qiqihar had also used the toxic solvent in four other drug products: "a special enema fluid for children; an injection for blood vessel diseases; an intravenous pain reliever; and an arthritis treatment." It was not reported (and it is possibly unknown) if any of these contaminated therapies caused illness or death in China (Bogdanich W, Hooker J. From China to Panama, a trail of poisoned medicine. *New York Times.* May 6, 2007 [p 1]).

34. Anonymous. Five jailed over lethal fake medicine scandal. Xinhua News Agency. April 30, 2008. Available at http://www.china.org.cn/2008-04/30/content_15038787.htm. Last accessed August 13, 2013; Anonymous. Key figure in fake drug scandal gets life sentence. *Shanghai Daily.* June 4, 2008. Available at http://www.china.org.cn/china/local/2008-06/04/content_15623981.htm. Last accessed August 13, 2013; and Reuters, Beijing Newsroom. China ingredient supplier gets life for killer drug. June 4, 2008. Available at http://www.med24.ee/eng/services/contact/article_id-3538. Last accessed August 13, 2013.

35. See Bogdanich W, Hooker J. From China to Panama, a trail of poisoned medicine. *New York Times.* May 6, 2007 (p 1).

36. Rentz ED, Lewis L, Mujica OJ, et al. Outbreak of acute renal failure in Panama in 2006: a case-control study. *Bull World Health Organ.* 2008;86:749-756. The growing outbreak was also reported by the *New York Times* in October of 2006 (Lacey M, Grady D. A killer in a medicine bottle shakes faith in government. *New York Times.* October 16, 2006 [p A4]).

37. In March of 2008, the *New York Times*, citing Panamanian officials, reported that 174 people were poisoned and 115 people died as a result of consuming the diethylene glycol–tainted cough syrup (Story L, Fabrikant G. 4 executives are charged over tainted toothpaste. *New York Times.* March 7, 2008 [p C3]). The internal, retrospective investigation of deaths reportedly included a limited number of exhumations by Panamanian officials (Bogdanich W, Hooker J. From China to Panama, a trail of poisoned medicine. *New York Times.* May 6, 2007 [p 1]).

38. Bogdanich W, Hooker J. From China to Panama, a trail of poisoned medicine. *New York Times*. May 6, 2007 (p 1); Hooker J. Chinese company linked to deaths wasn't licensed. *New York Times*. May 9, 2007 (p A13).

39. The *Times* reporters indicated that the contamination of the glycerin "was hiding in plain sight." All of the barrels were shipped from the Taixing Glyerine Factory with the name "TD glycerin." The interim brokers preserved the "TD" modifier but remained clueless about its meaning. Only the *Times* reporters learned, after interviewing a former salesman of the Taixing Glyerine Factory, that TD was short for the Mandarin phrase "tì dài" (the English-letter phonetics for 替代), which means "substitute."

40. Bogdanich W. The everyman who exposed tainted toothpaste. *New York Times*. October 1, 2007 (p A1). See also, Bogdanich W, McLean R. Poisoned toothpaste in Panama is believed to be from China. *New York Times*. May 19, 2007 (p A3); Barboza D, Bogdanich W. China questions 2 companies in contaminated toothpaste exports. *New York Times*. May 22, 2007 (p C1); Reuters. Dominican Republic bans 2 toothpastes. *New York Times*. May 23, 2007 (p C4); Bogdanich W. FDA to test toothpaste sent to US from China. *New York Times*. May 24, 2007 (p C3); Anonymous. Costa Rica seizes contaminated toothpaste imported from China. *New York Times*. May 26, 2007 (p A4); Anonymous. Nicaragua seizes Chinese toothpaste. *New York Times*. May 28, 2007 (p A6); Bogdanich W. Toxic toothpaste made in China is found in US. *New York Times*. June 2, 2007 (p A1); Mulier T, Wolf C. Fake Colgate toothpaste is found in four US states. *Bloomberg*. June 14, 2007. Available at http://www.bloomberg.com/apps/news?pid=newsarchive&sid=aaMIgss9jleM. Last accessed August 13, 2013; Bogdanich W. Wider sale seen for toothpaste tainted in China. *New York Times*. June 28, 2007 (p A1); and Bogdanich W. China prohibits poisonous industrial solvent in toothpaste. *New York Times*. July 12, 2007 (p C4).

41. According to a *New York Times* report, most of the contaminated toothpaste in the United States was brought in through Long Beach, California, by two Los Angeles–based importers. In March of 2008, a Los Angeles city attorney filed criminal charges against executives from the importers. Story L, Fabrikant G. 4 executives are charged over tainted toothpaste. *New York Times*. March 7, 2008 (p C3).

42. Hooker J, Bogdanich W. China says 2 of its companies played a role in poisonings. *New York Times*. June 1, 2007 (p A6); Bogdanich W. Toxic toothpaste made in China is found in US. *New York Times*. June 2, 2007 (p A1). See also, Bogdanich W. Chinese chemicals flow unchecked to market. *New York Times*. October 31, 2007 (p A1).

43. Barboza D, Bogdanich W. China shuts 3 companies over safety of products. *New York Times*. July 21, 2007 (p C1).

44. Kahn J. China quick to execute drug official. *New York Times*. July 11, 2007 (p C1).

45. Hooker J, Bogdanich W. Agreement with China to regulate some drugs. *New York Times*. December 12, 2007 (p C3).

46. CDC. Fatal poisoning among young children from diethylene glycol-contaminated acetaminophen—Nigeria, 2008-2009. *MMWR Morb Mortal Wkly Rep.* 2009;58:1345-1347. See also, Akuse RM, Eke FU, Ademola AD, et al. Diagnosing renal failure due to diethylene glycol in children in a resource-constrained setting. *Pediatr Nephrol.* 2012;27:1021-1028.

47. In January of 2012, Akuse et al reported 59 related deaths. In February of 2009, the *New York Times* reported 84 deaths. Polgreen L. 84 children are killed by medicine in Nigeria. *New York Times.* February 7, 2009 (p A7); Associated Press. Nigeria: 12 held over tainted syrup. *New York Times.* February 12, 2009 (p A10).

48. Barewa had reportedly purchased the fake propylene glycol in spouted jerrycans instead of the original (barrel) containers.

49. Alam S. Babies die slowly after Bangladesh drug scam. Agence France-Presse. July 29, 2009; Anonymous. Probe body may submit report today. *Daily Star.* July 29, 2009. Available at http://archive.thedailystar.net/newDesign/news-details.php?nid=99071. Last accessed August 13, 2013; Anonymous. Tests confirm toxic substance in paracetamol syrup. bdnews24.com. July 29, 2009. Available at http://dev-bd.bdnews24.com/details.php?id=139034. Last accessed April 13, 2013; Hossain MR. Medication safety for children. *Daily Star.* August 15, 2009. Available at http://archive.thedailystar.net/newDesign/news-details.php?nid=101369. Last accessed August 13, 2013; Our Correspondent, Brahmanbaria. Rid Pharma case hearing today. *Daily Star.* August 17, 2009. Available at http://archive.thedailystar.net/newDesign/news-details.php?nid=101743. Last accessed August 13, 2013; Our correspondent, Brahmanbaria. Rid Pharma officials defy court order: warrant issued for third time as they do not show up in court. *Daily Star.* September 4, 2009. Available at www.thedailystar.net/newDesign/print_news.php?nid=104307. Last accessed August 13, 2013; Our correspondent, B'baria. 28 children's death, toxic paracetamol: Rid owner gets bail; 4 in hiding. *Daily Star.* October 1, 2009. Available at http://archive.thedailystar.net/newDesign/news-details.php?nid=107766. Last accessed August 13, 2013; Anonymous. Rid Pharma case deposition finally starts. bdnews24.com. February 12, 2012. Available at http://ns.bdnews24.com/details.php?id=218285. Last accessed August 13, 2013; Court correspondent. 'Toxic' Rid syrup, 28 deaths: case hearing deferred again. *Daily Star.* March 1, 2011. Available at http://archive.thedailystar.net/newDesign/news-details.php?nid=175971. Last accessed August 13, 2013; Halder CC. No charge framed. *Daily Star.* January 11, 2011. Available at http://archive.thedailystar.net/newDesign/news-details.php?nid=170545. Last accessed August 13, 2013; Halder CC. Trial of Rid Pharma finally starts. *Daily Star.* February 15, 2012. Available at www.thedailystar.net/newDesign/print_news.php?nid=222513. Last accessed August 13, 2013.

50. Follow-up reports of the trial proceedings, after February 15, 2012, were not found in a search of the *Daily Star* archives.

51. For a review of diethylene-glycol metabolism, see Schep LJ, Slaughter RJ, Temple WA, Beasley DMG. Diethylene glycol poisoning. *Clin Toxicol.* 2009;47:525-535.

52. For those who care, 2-hydroxyethoxyacetic acid and diglycolic acid, respectively.

53. Landry GM, Martin S, McMartin KE. Diglycolic acid is the nephrotoxic metabolite in diethylene glycol poisoning inducing necrosis in human proximal tubule cells in vitro. *Toxicol Sci.* 2011;124:35-44.

54. Besenhofer LM, Adegboyega PA, Bartels M, et al. Inhibition of metabolism of diethylene glycol prevents target organ toxicity in rats. *Toxicol Sci.* 2010;117:25-35. For related animal data, see Besenhofer LM, McLaren M, Latimer B, et al. Role of tissue metabolite accumulation in the renal toxicity of diethylene glycol. *Toxicol Sci.* 2011;123:374-383. Fomepizole is a well-established antidote for methanol and ethylene-glycol poisoning. See for instance, Brent J. Fomepizole for the treatment of pediatric ethylene and diethylene glycol, butoxyethanol, and methanol poisonings. *Clin Toxicol (Phila).* 2010;48:401-406.

55. Ming Xing Huang, Xiao Mou Peng, Lin Gu, Gui Hua Chen. Pre-existing liver cirrhosis reduced the toxic effect of diethylene glycol in a rat model due to the impaired hepatic alcohol dehydrogenase. *Toxicol Ind Health.* 2011;27:742-753.

56. CDC. Fatal poisoning among young children from diethylene glycol-contaminated acetaminophen—Nigeria, 2008-2009. *MMWR Morb Mortal Wkly Rep.* 2009;58:1345-1347.

57. Brophy PD, Tenenbein M, Gardner J, Bunchman TE, Smoyer WE. Childhood diethylene glycol poisoning treated with alcohol dehydrogenase inhibitor fomepizole and hemodialysis. *Am J Kidney Dis.* 2000;35:958-962.

58. Peng XM, Huang MX, Gu L, Lin BL, Chen GH. Characteristics of patients with liver disease intravenously exposed to diethylene glycol in China 2006. *Clin Toxicol.* 2009;47:124-131. There was also no apparent difference in the extent of liver damage between the two groups; however, the symptomatic patients were more likely to have baseline renal dysfunction. Therefore, while liver disease may have been protective in these Chinese cases of diethylene-glycol poisoning (by reducing the breakdown of the toxin), there were probably other patient-specific factors that influenced the clinical manifestations of toxicity.

59. Reported as 20% of 140 controls. Rentz ED, Lewis L, Mujica OJ, et al. Outbreak of acute renal failure in Panama in 2006: a case-control study. *Bull World Health Organ.* 2008;86:749-756.

60. A reader-friendly explanation of the metabolism of alcohol by ADH and ALDH can be found at the website of the National Institute on Alcohol Abuse and Alcoholism. Available at http://pubs.niaaa.nih.gov/publications/AA72/AA72.htm. Last accessed August 13, 2013.

61. Peng XM, Huang MX, Gu L, Lin BL, Chen GH. Characteristics of patients with liver disease intravenously exposed to diethylene glycol in China 2006. *Clin Toxicol (Phila).* 2009;47:124-131. It is also probable, if not certain, that

the quantity of diethylene glycol that is metabolized by the liver after oral consumption is significantly different from that after intravenous administration (eg, like in the Chinese inpatients with liver disease). With oral consumption of diethylene glycol, the intestinally absorbed toxin would be immediately transported to the liver, where it would undergo metabolism to the putative toxic metabolites. (This phenomenon is known as first-pass metabolism.) In the case of intravenous administration, the percentage of diethylene glycol initially metabolized by the liver would theoretically be less than that after oral consumption.

62. Heilmair R, Lenk W, Lohr D. Toxicokinetics of diethylene glycol (DEG) in the rat. *Arch Toxicol.* 1993; 67:655-666. Cited in Schep LJ, Slaughter RJ, Temple WA, Beasley DMG. Diethylene glycol poisoning. *Clin Toxicol.* 2009;47:525-535.

63. Rollins YD, Filley CM, McNutt JT, Chahal S, Kleinschmidt-DeMasters BK. Fulminant ascending paralysis as a delayed sequela of diethylene glycol (Sterno) ingestion. *Neurology.* 2002;59:1460-1463.

64. In this case, the alcohol presumably competed with the diethylene glycol for the metabolic enzymes ADH and ALDH, thereby deterring the breakdown of diethylene glycol to its toxic metabolite(s).

65. Hasbani MJ, Sansing LH, Perrone J, Asbury AK, Bird SJ. Encephalopathy and peripheral neuropathy following diethylene glycol ingestion. *Neurology.* 2005;64:1273-1275.

66. Marraffa JM, Holland MG, Stork CM, Hoy CD, Hodgman MJ. Diethylene glycol: widely used solvent presents serious poisoning potential. *J Emerg Med.* 2008;35:401-406. The wallpaper stripper was 26% diethylene glycol.

67. Alfred S, Coleman P, Harris D, Wigmore T, Stachowski E, Graudins A. Delayed neurologic sequelae resulting from epidemic diethylene glycol poisoning. *Clin Toxicol (Phila).* 2005;43:155-159.

68. Approximately 83% of exposed victims versus 51% of control patients. Self-reported neurologic symptoms included dysarthria, numbness, paralysis, weakness, loss of sensation, loss of consciousness, convulsion, dysphagia, and facial paralysis. Rentz ED, Lewis L, Mujica OJ, et al. Outbreak of acute renal failure in Panama in 2006: a case-control study. *Bull World Health Organ.* 2008;86:749-756.

69. Although ethylene glycol is more commonly used.

70. Schep LJ, Slaughter RJ, Temple WA, Beasley DMG. Diethylene glycol poisoning. *Clin Toxicol (Phila).* 2009;47:525-535.

71. Marraffa JM, Holland MG, Stork CM, Hoy CD, Hodgman MJ. Diethylene glycol: widely used solvent presents serious poisoning potential. *J Emerg Med.* 2008;35:401-406.

72. FDA. FDA advises manufacturers to test glycerin for possible contamination. Available at http://www.fda.gov/NewsEvents/Newsroom/PressAnnouncements/2007/ucm 108909.htm. Last accessed August 13, 2013.

73. US Department of Health and Human Services, FDA. *Guidance for Industry: Testing of Glycerin for Diethylene Glycol.* Washington, DC: US DHHS; 2007. Available at

http://www.fda.gov/downloads/Drugs/GuidanceComplianceRegulatoryInform
ation/Guidances/UCM070347.pdf. Last accessed August 13, 2013.

74. Maurer JE, Kessler C. Identification and quantification of ethylene glycol and diethylene glycol in plasma using gas chromatography-mass spectrometry. *Arch Toxicol.* 1988;62:66-69. Cited in Baffi P, Elneser S, Baffi M, De Melin M. Quantitative determination of diethylene glycol contamination in pharmaceutical products. *J AOAC Int.* 2000;83:793-801.

75. O'Brien KL, Selanikio JD, Hecdivert C, et al. Epidemic of pediatric deaths from acute renal failure caused by diethylene glycol poisoning. *JAMA.* 1998;279:1175-1180.

76. Singh J, Dutta AK, Khare S, et al. Diethylene glycol poisoning in Gurgaon, India, 1998. *Bull World Health Organ.* 2001;79:88-95.

77. Kenyon AS, Shi X, Wang Y, Ng WH, Prestridge R, Sharp K. Simple, at-site detection of diethylene glycol/ethylene glycol contamination of glycerin and glycerin-based raw materials by the thin-layer chromatography. *J AOAC Int.* 1998;81:44-50. In 2007, the FDA advised that this field test could also be used on site to identify diethylene glycol in propylene glycol.

78. For a brief history of how the cheaper field test was created and adapted, see Junod SW. Diethylene glycol deaths in Haiti. *Public Health Rep.* 2000;115:78-86.

Appendix B: Elixir Distribution by State

1. The total amount of Elixir Sulfanilamide distributed in commercial packages was calculated by adding values provided in primary FDA and NARA sources. The calculated number of direct recipients of commercial packages, 620, is lower than the shipment tally (633) provided by Secretary Wallace in his November 1937 report to Congress. The difference is probably because Wallace's tally accounted for indirect shipments (eg, shipments to drug stores from other, direct-recipient drug stores.)

2. Wallace report (p 1).

3. See Pully, DeFriece (p 162).

4. This amount presumably included the volume of Elixir Sulfanilamide that remained at Massengill's warehouses. The large majority of elixir was found during the last two weeks of October. However, stray bottles and sample vials were collected by the agency in early November and later. A notice in a 1949 issue of *Food and Drug Review* reported the government's collection of "what may have been the last unrecalled bottle of Elixir Sulfanilamide." The bottle was handed over to an FDA inspector on March 10, 1949, by Dr. Claire F. Miller of Waco, Texas. Miller found the bottle "among some old physician's samples taken over from another clinic." See Anonymous. They still turn up! *Food Drug Rev.* 1949;33:117.

Appendix C: Racial Breakdown of Elixir Sulfanilamide Victims

1. Carpenter D. *Reputation and Power: Organizational Image and Pharmaceutical Regulation at the FDA*. Princeton, NJ: Princeton University Press; 2010: 89.
2. Ibid (p 92, footnote).
3. Ibid (pp 92-93). It should be noted that there was never any link between Elixir Sulfanilamide and syphilis, per se, because the drug was used to treat gonorrhea—an entirely different venereal disease.

INDEX

ABOUT THE AUTHOR

A native East Tennessean, Barbara J. Martin is a formerly practicing neurologist who received her undergraduate and medical doctorate from Duke University before completing her postgraduate training in general neurology and neuromuscular diseases at the Hospital of the University of Pennsylvania in Philadelphia. She has worked in academia, private practice, medical publishing, drug market research, and continuing medical education. She is the owner of and sole contributor to Pathophilia (www.bmartinmd.com), a blog covering the drug and health care industries (as well as providing the occasional movie recommendation). She currently lives in Evanston, Illinois. *Elixir: The American Tragedy of a Deadly Drug* is her first book.

This book is set in Baskerville Old Face and is edited by using a modified version of the *AMA Manual of Style* (10th edition).

Made in the USA
San Bernardino, CA
04 March 2014